Na

Please return or renew this
item by the last date shown.
You may renew books by phone
0345 60 80 195 or the internet

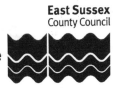
East Sussex
County Council

Library and Information Service
eastsussex.gov.uk/libraries

D1337547

Nature's

Medicines

Published by
The Reader's Digest Association Limited
London • New York • Sydney • Montreal

Contents

About this book

Nature's Medicines is an introduction and practical guide to the properties of many plants used to treat illness and its symptoms in the Western world. In the first part the book outlines the history of herbalism and modern plant research, then explains how to find a qualified medical herbalist and the regulations governing the sale of herbal products. It also tells you how to cultivate and make use of your own herbs.

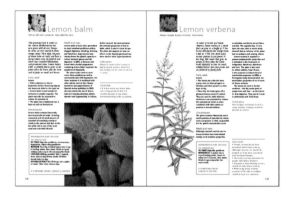

A to Z of Plants

The Plant pages feature 184 species, listed A to Z by common name, with the Latin and other names below. We tell you how they are grown and harvested, which parts are used and each plant's chemical properties as demonstrated in scientific research. 'Preparation and dosage' boxes suggest ways in which the plants can be used medicinally; more uses are suggested in the Ailment pages. Take note of the 'Cautions'; these state clearly when the plant should not be used and possible side effects.

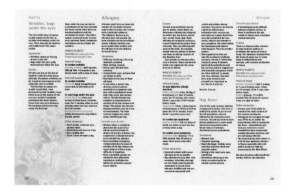

A to Z of Ailments

In the Ailment pages more than 150 common illnesses are described, together with herbs that can be used to treat them. In each case, readers are advised not to use more than one herbal preparation at any given time without consulting a medical herbalist. It is also imperative not to exceed the dosages suggested here and on the plant pages. If you are due to have an operation, tell your doctor which herbs you take: some, such as garlic, cause bleeding and should be stopped before surgery.

Dosages For capsules and tablets, specific strengths in milligrams have often been suggested. If you cannot find products of the same strength, buy the nearest equivalent (if in doubt choose a lower strength) and do not exceed the recommended daily dose. Tincture strengths are usually stated. If not, our consultants have selected a dose for the most common tincture strength – 1:4 in 25% alcohol. If you cannot find the tincture strength suggested, consult a medical herbalist before attempting self-medication.

Over-the-counter products More than 200 Licensed Herbal Medicines are listed on pages 310-317. These preparations have been licensed for use by the Medicines and Healthcare products Regulatory Agency – making them the safest herbal preparations available. They can be identified on the label either by the product licence (PL) number or MHRA Marketing Authorisation.

Important

While the creators of this work have made every effort to be as accurate and up to date as possible, medical and pharmacological knowledge is constantly changing. Readers are recommended to consult a qualified medical specialist for individual advice. The writers, researchers, editors and the publishers of this work cannot be held liable for any errors and omissions, or actions that may be taken as a consequence of information contained in this book.

Nature's medicine chest

The plant world is an immense store of active chemical compounds. Nearly half the medicines we use today are herbal in origin, and a quarter contain plant extracts or active chemicals taken directly from plants. Many more have yet to be discovered, recorded and researched; only a few thousand have been studied. Across the globe, the hunt is on to find species that could form the bases of new medicines.

From the dawn of time

Humans have always used plants to ease their pains. They imbued them with magical powers and then gradually learnt to identify their properties. We can now enjoy the benefits of herbal medicines because, over thousands of years, our ancestors discovered which plants were medicinally beneficial and which were highly toxic.

Modern paleobotanists, studying ancient burial sites, are confirming much of the herbal folklore handed down over the centuries. Remains of seeds preserved in these sites have substantiated what early doctors and herbalists wrote about the medicinal plants they used. In recent years, this folklore has been supported by scientific studies that confirm both the safety and efficacy of many herbal treatments.

Thousands of years ago, the ancient Egyptians discovered simple ways to extract and use the active ingredients within plants. Egyptian papyrus manuscripts from 2000 BC record the use of perfumes and fine oils, and aromatic oils and gums were an essential part of the embalming process.

In ancient Greece in the 5th and 4th centuries BC, Hippocrates, known as the father of medicine, was already recommending asparagus and garlic for their diuretic qualities, poppy as a way of inducing sleep and willow leaves to relieve pain and fever. In the 1st century AD, another Greek doctor, Dioscorides, established the first collection of medicinal plants. His treatise on the subject was translated into Arabic and Persian. Centuries later, his work was also used by the Muslim scholars who influenced great universities of the period, particularly at Montpellier, Europe's most famous centre for the study of botany.

As a result of trade with Africa and Asia, the Western world's store of herbal medicines was enriched by the inclusion of camphor, cinnamon, ginger, ginseng, nutmeg, sandalwood, turmeric and senna.

For a long time, however, the use of both local plants and those with more distant origins was based on more or less fanciful

At Abidjan in the Ivory Coast, women pound plants that will be used to make medicines.

beliefs. Throughout the Middle Ages herbal medicine consisted of a mixture of magic, superstition and empirical observation.

From the Renaissance onwards, scientists came to the fore, rejecting alchemists' elixirs and other magical remedies. Local plants were carefully collected and widely used to make infusions, decoctions and ointments. These plants make up the major part of the traditional cures that we have inherited.

The active principles

In the late 1700s, Carl Wilhelm Scheele, a gifted Swedish chemist, obtained tartaric acid from grapes, citric acid from lemons and malic acid from apples. The techniques that he and his contemporaries used led to the isolation of the first purified compounds from plants that could be used as drugs.

First came the isolation of morphine from the opium poppy in 1803, then caffeine from coffee beans in 1819, quinine from cinchona bark and colchicine from meadow saffron both in 1820 and atropine from deadly nightshade in 1835.

Similarly, Dr William Withering, an 18th-century English doctor and botanist, began to take an interest in the common foxglove, which was widely used in popular medicine as a treatment for water retention. In 1785 he published a paper on the plant, describing the foxglove's diuretic property and its beneficial effect on 'cardiac weaknesses'.

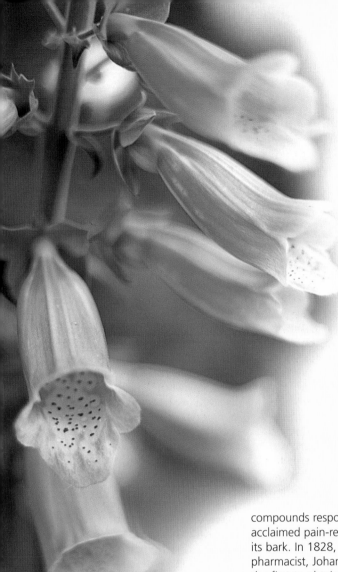

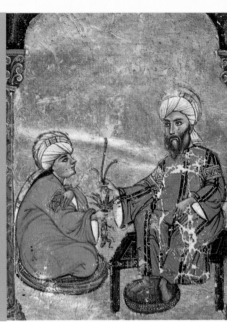

A miniature painting illustrating a 12th-century manuscript copy of *De Materia Medica* which shows Dioscorides and a student. Of the 500 plants included in the treatise written by this Greek doctor, who lived in the 1st century AD, 54 are still on the list of essential medicinal plants compiled by the World Health Organization in 1978.

Clinical trials using extracts from the leaf began in 1809 but it was not until around 1835 that French chemist, Claude Adolphe Nativel, succeeded in isolating the plant's active principle, digitalin. Today, the related species, woolly foxglove, is the basis of numerous medicines and drugs that treat heart problems.

Aspirin from willow

One tree that generated great interest among scientists was the willow. In the early 1800s, chemists from Germany, Italy and France began the search for the compounds responsible for the acclaimed pain-relieving effects of its bark. In 1828, the German pharmacist, Johann Buchner, was the first to obtain salicin, the major compound in a pure form. In 1838, the Italian chemist Raffaele Piria also obtained salicylic acid from the bark by various chemical processes. But these early compounds caused blisters in the mouth, and stomach upsets when ingested.

In 1853, a French chemist, Charles Frederic Gerhardt, synthesised a modified form of salicylic acid – acetylsalicylic acid. But still it wasn't further developed for more than 40 years until a German chemist, Felix Hoffman, working for Bayer, rediscovered Gerhardt's compound. Hoffman gave it to his father who suffered from arthritis and reported the beneficial effects.

Bayer decided to market the acetylsalicylic acid as a new drug for pain relief and patented the compound acetylsalicylic acid in 1899. At last from the willow, the first modern drug was born and, with 12,000 tonnes of aspirins sold every year throughout the world, it has kept its number one position.

A new era

From the 1930s onwards, advances in chemistry have made it much easier to reproduce the active ingredients in plants. But plants will continue to have a medicinal importance in their own right.

Their active constituents may be slightly modified to improve their efficiency or to reduce undesirable side effects, but they are still the bases of drugs that are vital for the treatment of disorders such as cancers and heart diseases or as a means of combating malaria. And they remain the essence of herbal medicine – an area that has still not been fully understood and explored.

From plant to potent drug

There is a huge amount of collecting to be done if we are to benefit from the great diversity and therapeutic potential of plants. Many species have yet to be discovered, especially those in the forests of equatorial Africa, South America and South-east Asia or on the Pacific islands. Local people also have a lot to reveal about their traditional uses of healing herbs.

Across the world, a wide range of experts is engaged in the search for new plant species. There are teams of ethnobotanists, phytochemists, pharmacognosists, ethnopharmacologists (scientists who study people and their plants) and herbalists. Hundreds of thousands of plants are collected, then analysed in high-tech research laboratories, where up to 50,000 a day are examined.

Some scientists will target the species of a particular family of plants known to contain specific active substances. Attempts will be made to collect plants from these families in order to find and compare their active constituents.

Others – the so-called ethnobotanists – begin their search by talking to traditional healers among native populations, who understand the powers of plants. They select plants that seem promising, note their names in the local dialect, the parts used and what they are used for. This approach is proving particularly successful in uncovering evidence that may lead to new drugs, as such plants are already used medicinally and are therefore much more likely to contain active chemical constituents.

Scientists have also begun to observe what plants animals eat when they are ill. Swans with injured necks often eat willow leaves and twigs. Scientists know that this plant contains the pain-relieving compounds that are the basis of aspirin. When they are infested with hair lice, badgers dig holes under elder, whose roots contain insecticidal compounds.

Known as zoopharmacognosy, this research area is also providing a means of discovering compounds and new herbal medicines.

A lengthy process

When samples have been identified and gathered in sufficient numbers, chemists take extracts from the raw materials to isolate a plant's pure chemical constituents. These extracts are tested, first to discover any possible toxicity, then to define their biological effects. The selection process is rigorous. It is estimated that, at this stage, only one out of every 10,000 analysed is kept.

Thorough clinical studies are then carried out, first with animals and then with human volunteers. If the results are positive, the real work of preparing medicines can begin. The active constituent is developed into a suitable form for ingestion, such as capsules, tablets or liquid solutions.

For the pharmaceutical laboratory, the final step is to get permission to market the medicine from the appropriate government authority. In the UK, this is usually the Medicines and Healthcare products Regulatory Agency (MHRA), although with many herbal products classified as food supplements (see pages 16-17) it could also involve the Food Standards Agency.

In total, 12-15 years, or even more, can elapse between finding the plant in the forest and marketing the end product.

The wealth in plants

It is no accident that plants play an important role in contemporary pharmacological research: the substances that interest us are those the plant itself uses to survive.

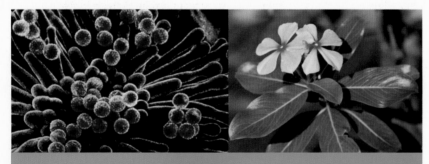

Once used to bring down fevers in traditional Chinese medicine, artemisen, taken from *Artemesia annua*, is now the fastest and most effective antimalarial drug, and it has no adverse side effects.

The Madagascar periwinkle is nowadays cultivated on a large scale in Europe. Constituents have been extracted from it that have helped to create some of the most effective anticancer drugs.

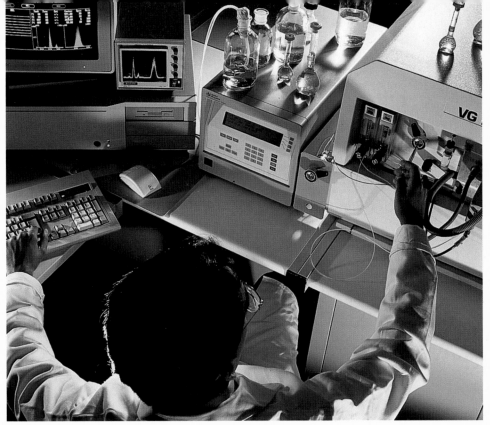

In the past few decades increasingly sophisticated machines for analysing chemical substances have led to a significant advance in medical knowledge.

More than 100,000 of these special substances have been found in the plant world and, because of their complex and diverse chemical structures, they are the basis of many medicines.

The struggle against malaria

Quinine, the active principle in the bark of the cinchona tree first isolated in 1820, still has a role to play in the treatment of severe cases of malaria. But most strains of the parasites responsible for this illness have developed a resistance to the synthetic antimalarial drugs, modelled on quinine. The search for new chemicals is, therefore, a major medical priority, as some 300 million people catch malaria every year and 2 million die from it.

The qing-hao or *Artemesia annua*, a plant used in traditional Chinese medicine, has recently given rise to a new class of anti-malarial drug that is now used worldwide and especially in Africa and South-east Asia.

Fighting cancer

The Madagascar periwinkle was reputed to be a cure for diabetes in its native country, but the scientists who studied it noticed a reduction of white corpuscles in the blood of the animals involved and used the plant to treat leukaemia, in which white cells multiply abnormally. Two alkaloids with powerful effects, vinblastine and vincristine, were subsequently isolated in the periwinkle's leaf. A French team then created highly active derivatives from other constituents present in greater amounts in the plant. These drugs increased the life expectancy of patients suffering from Hodgkin's disease and acute leukaemia.

The anticancer property of an extract of bark from the Pacific yew tree was detected completely by accident in the mid Sixties. The active substance, taxol, was isolated a few years later. The clinical trials came to an abrupt halt, however, when it became clear that to get enough taxol to treat each patient, six 100-year-old trees would have to

be felled. Fortunately, a solution was found; in the needles of the European yew, a French team isolated a compound that could be chemically converted into products similar to and even more effective than taxol. They are successfully used nowadays to treat certain breast and ovarian cancers.

In the rhizome of the American mandrake, there are anticancer substances similar to those in the alkaloids found in the Madagascar periwinkle. A substance extracted from *Camptotheca acuminata,* a tree found in southern China, was the source of two synthetic drugs, irinotecan, developed in Japan, and topotecan, developed in the United States. Both are used to treat certain forms of cancer.

Over the past few years, plants have enabled some amazing advances to be made in all areas of medicine. Such progress requires time, persistance and investment, but across the world it is now generally recognised that plants hold out great hopes for the future health of mankind.

Herbal medicine in the West

Over thousands of years traditional ways of using plants medicinally have developed in different societies. Today the study of herbs has become a medical science and new ways of using plants therapeutically have been found such as the advent of 'nutraceuticals' or aromatherapy and its essential oils.

What is herbal medicine?

Herbal medicine, also known as phytotherapy, is the treatment of illnesses using measured doses of specific plants. A qualified medical herbalist can prescribe plants to be taken internally or used externally in various forms and concentrations, depending on the ailment.

The herbalist may suggest the addition of certain edible plants to the diet – such as celery, radish or cabbage – or may prescribe a medicinal preparation, such as a suspension, powder, infusion, tincture or extract. The herbalist may also recommend an essential oil, distilled from the plant.

A holistic approach

Conventional drug research tends to be focused on identifying a single active constituent in a plant and this approach has yielded a significant number of blockbusting drugs. Herbalists take a holistic approach believing that the whole of the plant should be used, because all the constituents are important, not just the compounds that have been shown to be active.

A herbal medicine consists of hundreds of phytochemicals – plant-based compounds that herbalists believe interact in a 'synergistic' way. Together they achieve a greater effect than the sum of all their individual effects. An analogy can be made to music – we can appreciate that when single notes are played together in a certain way they make up the pleasing sound of a chord. The pharmaceutical industry is still focused on producing 'single notes', while herbalists argue that the 'chords' found in herbal medicines are more effective.

Recent studies have demonstrated this effect. For example, research at Middlesex University, London in 1999 showed that an extract of common sage was more potent as an inhibitor of acetylcholinesterase (so helping to maintain memory function) than any of the pure compounds found in the plant.

Using mixtures of compounds is an approach that is now also beginning to be used in orthodox medicine. HIV/AIDS patients, for instance, are often given a cocktail of drugs because the combination appears to work more effectively than using one single drug.

New herbal trends

A recent development in herbal medicine is the creation of extracts with higher concentrations of certain active constituents. For example, St John's wort (Hypericum perforatum) has been shown clinically to be beneficial in the treatment of mild to moderate depression, an effect due, in part, to a compound called hypericin. As a result, herbal manufacturers now produce extracts 'standardised' to contain at least 0.3 per cent of hypericin.

Whether in fact these standardised extracts are more effective than traditional preparations is not currently known. This is partly because clinical data is often available only from the standardised version of the herb – because a manufacturer has funded the study. Herbalists do not have the means to test traditional herbal medicine tinctures in the same way.

Several pharmaceutical companies have also started to research and develop pharmaceutical versions of herbal medicines. Like conventional synthetic drugs these will have to undergo rigorous controls that may take years and could cost millions of pounds.

Examples in the UK include the development of cannabis as a prescription drug for pain relief for people with multiple sclerosis and of a Chinese herbal medicine to treat premenstrual syndrome.

Dr Bach's flowers

In the 1930s the English physician Edward Bach developed a holistic system of healing based on plants. He believed that certain flowers give off 'vibrations' that directly influence the human spirit. Through trial and error, he established 38 remedies to be used to correct various states of emotional distress, which he believed were at the root of all illnesses.

The remedies are taken in the form of drops that contain a floral elixir. Bach flower remedies have no adverse side effects and many people find that they help them to regain inner harmony and balance. However, scientific research has yet to substantiate the effectiveness of the remedies.

Creating 'nutraceuticals'

Herbal medicines are now also being incorporated into food. Plant extracts are being formulated to create food products that will help to cure ailments, prevent disease and maintain health. These so-called functional foods or 'nutraceuticals' will enable people to take herbal medicines in a different way: rather than swallowing a capsule, tablet or tincture, they will be able to consume the herbs in soft drinks, bread or chocolate bars.

Aromatherapy

For many people, one of the most pleasurable ways of enjoying the benefits of herbs is through aromatherapy. This involves the use of aromatic essential oils obtained from plants. The oils are usually produced by means of steam distillation. In the UK, the practice of aromatherapy, has gained widespread acceptance and some hospitals have even introduced it for their patients.

There are about 40 plant oils currently in common use. Some, such as basil, cinnamon and rosemary, have a stimulating effect and others, like anise, neroli and chamomile, a sedative one. Some oils, however, have a double effect, stimulating certain areas of the brain and calming others.

How to use the oils

The essential oils are almost always diluted but there are different ways of using them. A familiar method is massage, whereby a few drops are added to a carrier oil, such as almond or grapeseed, which is applied to the skin. If preparing this at home, use the proportions suggested on the Plant or Ailment pages and do not keep the mixture for more than a few days.

Essential oils can also be dispersed into the atmosphere; water and a little essential oil are put into a vaporiser and then heated. When the water evaporates, the oil is dispersed creating a powerful aroma. The oil can also be added to near-boiling water and inhaled.

You can add oil to bath water; a few drops will usually suffice. They will form a film on the surface which will be partially absorbed as skin pores open in the heat.

However, not all essential oils can be used this way. If in doubt, consult a professional. Some oils can also provoke an allergic reaction and some should not be used during pregnancy. Never take essential oils by mouth unless under the supervision of a qualified herbalist.

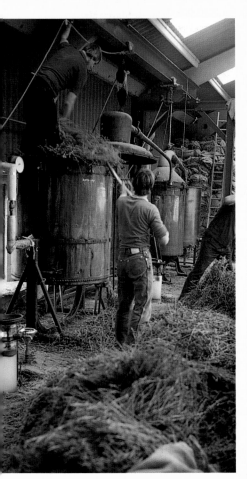

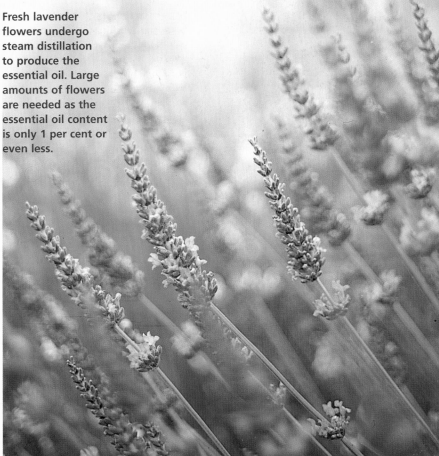

Fresh lavender flowers undergo steam distillation to produce the essential oil. Large amounts of flowers are needed as the essential oil content is only 1 per cent or even less.

Herbs in Eastern medicine

In most Asian countries, traditional forms of medicine are still widely practised.
Plants play a crucial role, but they are used according to ways of thinking that
are often very different from ours in the West. These medicinal plants are now
being intensively studied by scientists, which should help to clarify their role
in the various treatments, and perhaps to discover new applications for them.

India is the birthplace of Ayurvedic medicine, the oldest medical system known to man. It is still in use today and takes a holistic approach, in which health is seen in terms of the whole being. Herbal remedies play a central role in it.

An enduring inheritance

Born on the banks of the river Indus, Ayurvedic medicine has been practised for over 5,000 years, and was greatly influenced by Hindu philosophy. At first, the knowledge was passed on orally by spiritual teachers. But from around the 8th century BC, it was gradually set out in a number of medical treatises. Its use spread throughout Asia at the same time as Buddhism in the 1st and 2nd centuries AD, and has influenced other medical traditions, particularly in Tibet and China.

A holistic approach

In Ayurvedic medicine, it is thought that good health depends on a harmonious relationship between the three fundamental forces of energy, or *doshas*, which govern all living processes. They are the *vata* – the principle of air and movement, the *pitta* – the principle of fire and transformation, and the *kapha* – the principle of water, which ensures cohesion and support.

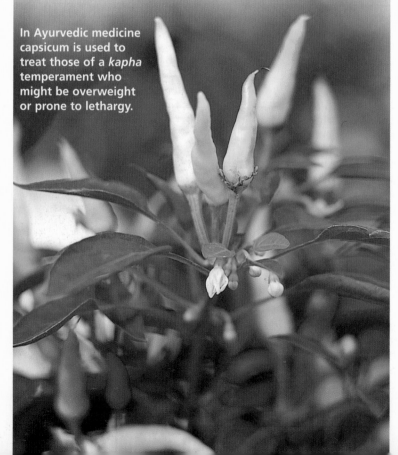

In Ayurvedic medicine capsicum is used to treat those of a *kapha* temperament who might be overweight or prone to lethargy.

At birth all people receive a personal combination of *doshas*, which determines their basic physical constitution and susceptibility to illness. Ayurvedic medicine takes into account the temperament conferred by the doshas as well as an individual's current emotional state and way of life.

Plants that cure

Ayurvedic remedies are based essentially on plants; about 1,250 are used. Patients are given their own personal plant mixture, to be used, as appropriate, in the form of infusions, lotions, poultices or pills.

For example, someone with a *kapha* temperament – which is thought to lead to excess weight and lethargy – will be treated with ginger and capsicum. The *pitta* temperament requires chiretta or dandelion root, plants that must not be given to the *vata* type, who will benefit from rosemary, which is too hot a plant for the *pitta* individual.

Recently in the UK, however, heavy metals have been detected in a number of Ayurvedic medicines. Certain plants have also been misidentified and the safety of some Indian herbal products has been questioned. The safety of Indian plants is now being reviewed by the government as part of its work on a new directive. (See page 16.)

In China and Japan

Traditional forms of medicine, many based on the use of medicinal plants, have been practised for thousands of years in China and Japan. They now live side-by-side

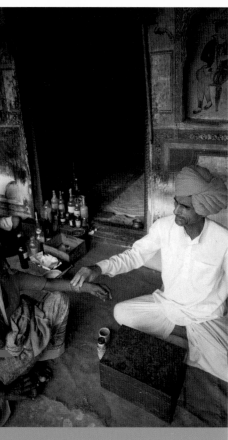

For Ayurvedic doctors, taking the patient's pulse is essential before making a diagnosis.

earth, metal, water and wood. Each of these elements is associated with specific emotions, tastes, bodily organs and plants.

'Hot' and 'cold' plants

In the 1st century AD, the herbal treatise *Shen Nong* recorded over 250 medicinal plants and also listed their 'temperature' and 'taste'. The combination of these two factors determines the healing potential of each plant. A plant that is 'hot' (*yang*), pungent, sweet and invigorating, like ginseng, is used to treat 'cold' conditions (*yin*). In order to reduce an excess of *yang*, 'cold', bitter and salty plants such as Chinese skullcap are needed.

The therapeutic qualities of plants also depend on where they grow. A low-altitude plant will have different healing powers to one that grows high up a mountain. The way they are prepared, whether with heat or water or a combination of the two, also has a bearing on their effects. The same is true of substances like honey, rice water and vinegar that are added to target the action on a particular organ.

A tradition that lives on

Traditional herbal medicines are still in widespread use in China and are now the subject of scientific study in many universities: more than 8,000 plants have been investigated.

The research institute at the Academy of Beijing, the largest in China, has the task of establishing connections between the theories of traditional and modern medicine. Around 3,000 scientists, doctors and technicians are working there on hundreds of projects.

Traditional Chinese medicine is now the most popular form of practitioner-based herbal treatment in the UK. However, due to recent reports of the illegal adulteration of herbal preparations produced in China, their quality control and

safety is currently being monitored by the UK government. There have been, for example, reports of two traditional Chinese medicines, *Qian Er* and *Mazin dol*, containing the prescription-only drug fenfluramine. The Medicines and Healthcare products Regulatory Agency is now working to ensure that all traditional Chinese medicines that are sold in the UK are safe.

Kampoh medicine

Chinese medicine was introduced to Japan in the 6th or 7th century AD and developed there under the name of kampoh, which means 'Chinese method'.

At the end of the 19th century, the Japanese government adopted Western medicine but there has now been a significant change of policy. A research institute in traditional medicine has been set up in Tokyo, many universities have courses in herbalism and kampoh is again part of the medical-school curriculum. Japan's state health insurance scheme will pay for plant-based preparations, and doctors often prescribe kampoh remedies.

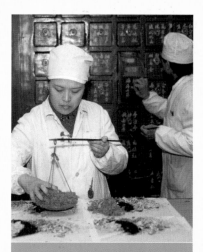

China has the richest store of herbal medicines in the world and a vast legacy of experience, recorded over the centuries by its herbalist doctors.

with Western medicine. Official plant research programmes have been set up; cooperation between practitioners of the old and the new is beginning to yield results.

Man within the universe

According to Taoist philosophy, everything in the universe rests upon the interplay of two opposing principles, *yin* and *yang*. Their interaction generates the lifeforce or *qi*, which circulates in the body through 12 key points. Illness is thought to be the result of a blockage or imbalance in this flow, and any treatment involves restoring the correct *yin-yang* balance.

Traditional Chinese medicine has also been influenced by another system of thought, based upon the theory of the five elements – fire,

Harnessing the healing power

When you drink a cup of coffee, or sip mint tea, you are also taking a form of herbal medicine. The coffee gives you a lift, while the mint tea settles your stomach. Although these two beverages are often consumed simply for pleasure, they illustrate the principle on which herbal medicine is based – that plants can have a potent physiological effect on the body.

A plant's effect on the body will vary considerably according to its active constituents. Coffee beans, for example, contain caffeine, which stimulates the cardiovascular and nervous systems, making you more alert. Mint leaves contain menthol, which is calming and antispasmodic; it relaxes the stomach and aids digestion.

Coffee and mint are just two of the hundreds of plants that medical herbalists have at their disposal – each with its own individual properties. As a result of both training and experience, a good herbalist knows which herb or combination of herbs is best for treating a particular disorder.

Generations of herbalists have handed down that knowledge over the centuries. In recent years scientific research has verified the biochemical actions of many plant extracts, which now form the basis of thousands of modern drugs.

But herbalists do not simply look up an ailment and prescribe the corresponding herb – they take a holistic approach, looking at other less obvious factors that may be contributing to a problem. Their use of herbs is also holistic; herbalists believe that the whole plant is more effective medicinally than any of its constituents in isolation.

A warning

Like many common herbs, coffee and mint tea are relatively harmless, but some herbs can have a more potent effect. Certain combinations of herbs can also have adverse side effects, and the action of some plants can interfere with that of conventional drugs. For example, St John's wort can reduce the effect of some of the drugs used to treat cardiac and circulatory disorders and has also been known to interfere with the contraceptive pill.

The 'Cautions' included in the Plant section of this book list possible interactions and also which herbs should be avoided if you have a particular medical problem. If you are already taking prescribed medicines it is imperative that you consult your doctor before trying any herbal remedy.

In the case of essential oils, you are advised never to ingest them unless under the supervision of a medical herbalist who has sufficient knowledge of their effects and possible toxicity.

Consulting a herbalist

It is always advisable, therefore, to consult a qualified medical herbalist (see Box) before treating anything but the mildest of illnesses. In addition, there is a danger of misdiagnosis. What seems to be bronchitis, for example, might be tuberculosis or even bronchial cancer; or you might treat yourself with a herbal preparation for haemorrhoids when the problem is far more serious.

Expect your first visit to a herbalist to be at least an hour long. As well as discussing your complaint, the herbalist will use the time to get to know you as an individual and take a full medical history, including lifestyle factors, such as whether you smoke and how much alcohol you drink – in confidence, of course, as in the case of a medical doctor.

The prescription you are given can then be tailored to your specific needs. Herbalists use herbs in three ways: to cleanse and detoxify; to restore to normal function; and to maintain health. They often prepare

How to find a medical herbalist

It is best to choose a herbalist, who is a member of one of the professional bodies listed below. These organisations have their own ethical codes and require members to take out full professional insurance. They should be able to give you details of herbalists in your area:

National Institute of Medical Herbalists. Members have the initials MNIMH or FNIMH after their names.

Association of Master Herbalists. Members have MAMH after their names.

International Register of Consultant Herbalists and Homeopaths (IRCH). Registered members, who have completed their course can use the initials MIRCH.

The **College of Phytotherapy** runs a distance learning course (BSc) in herbal medicine and will soon have a postgraduate diploma in phytotherapy aimed at health professionals such as GPs.

For addresses see page 324.

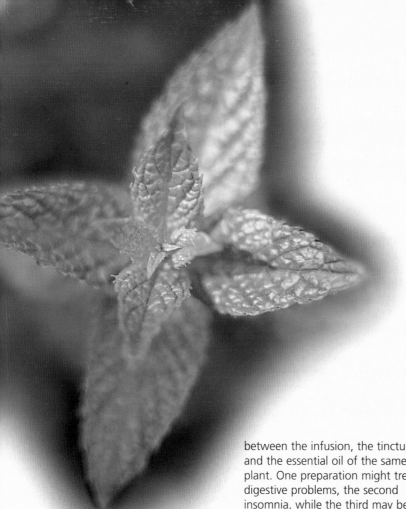

Training to become a herbalist

Entry requirements for the many courses available vary but will soon be standardised by the European Herbal Practitioners Association. Some are based on distance learning and are made up of modules, which allows for study on a part-time basis.

The professional bodies listed opposite can supply details of accredited training establishments. For instance, those recommended by the National Institute of Medical Herbalists (NIMH) include: The Scottish School of Herbal Medicine, Middlesex University, the University of Westminster and the University of Central Lancashire, all of which offer a BSc in medical herbalism.

The IRCH (see box, page 14) offers a two-tier system of training to suit both aspiring professionals and those who simply want to gain an under-standing of herbal medicine but do not wish to practise.

their own formulations, in the form of creams, ointments, tinctures or in a dry form (which will normally need to be boiled in water).

Fresh preparations made up by a herbalist are closer to their natural state and are often more effective than over-the-counter remedies. The herbalist will tell you how and when a remedy should be taken.

As with other holistic therapies, the effect of the herbs may not be immediately apparent and it may be a few months before you see any improvement. Chronic ailments that have been present for a long time generally take longer to treat.

Different strengths

The active principles contained in plants differ according to the medicinal form that is used. There is, for example, a big difference between the infusion, the tincture and the essential oil of the same plant. One preparation might treat digestive problems, the second insomnia, while the third may be used to relieve insect bites.

Qualified herbalists know, through training and experience, how a plant should be taken and the most effective dose. They should also be able to modify a treatment for a baby or young child or suggest an alternative treatment.

Using a combination

Groups of plants can also be combined to treat the same illness, either because they have similar and complementary effects or because they have properties that are different but that work together to achieve the desired result.

For example, artichoke and turmeric both act upon the liver and the gall bladder in a similar way. Boldo, fumitory and peppermint, when combined in a treatment, have various beneficial effects – anti-inflammatory, antispasmodic, stimulating the secretion of gastric juices in the stomach – which all benefit the upper digestive tract. Finally, liquorice, sweet fennel and hyssop have different properties but when combined can effectively treat bronchial congestion.

A qualified herbalist will know which plants to combine to achieve the optimum effect and which might have conflicting effects. Generally no more than two or three extracts would be mixed together so that the properties of each plant are preserved.

It is then essential to keep to the herbalist's prescribed dosage, as in conventional medicine. Failure to do so can lead to adverse side effects or cause the treatment to fail.

Using herbal medicines safely

Many people who use herbal medicines assume that they must be completely safe because they are natural. In fact, they contain powerful, active organic compounds and great care should be taken with their use.

Although some herbal preparations can be made safely at home, it is often best to visit a medical herbalist or buy quality herbal products from pharmacies or health-food stores.

Plants are potent. The alkaloid galanthamine, from daffodils, for instance, may one day provide a breakthrough drug for Alzheimer's disease but other alkaloids in the plant are highly toxic. Echinacea and dandelion are considered 'safe', but as members of the family Asteraceae (Compositae), which includes many allergenic plants, they must also be used with care, especially by those who have a history of allergic reactions such as skin rashes or asthmatic attacks.

Current concerns

The UK government has recently begun to investigate the safety of commonly used herbal medicines because some plants, which have been in common use, are now causing concern. Comfrey, for instance, a popular herb traditionally used to heal wounds, has come under close scrutiny in recent years because it contains pyrrolizidine alkaloids, which are known to cause liver cancer. Its use internally has been banned in Britain and medical herbalists now prescribe it only for external application. More recently kava kava, a popular natural sedative found in the Polynesian Islands, was banned from use for similar reasons.

One of the problems of assessing the safety of particular herbs is that they contain a complex mixture of compounds, only some of which may be toxic. However, isolating the toxic compounds and conducting extensive toxicity studies can be an expensive procedure, which is often

beyond the budget of many herbal manufacturers. The EU Traditional Herbal Medicines Directive means that the government will consider the historical use of plants as a guide to their possible safety and will also investigate the type of constituents in the plant, and whether these or similar compounds have been shown to be toxic in other separate studies. A new directive has been developed and was introduced in October 2005. This legislation should eventually ensure that only safe herbal medicines will be on offer and necessary quality controls will be in place to ensure their efficacy.

UK rules and regulations

Herbal medicines are available in a variety of forms and outlets in the UK. You can buy fresh or dried herbs, tinctures, capsules, tablets, ointments and creams. They are sold in supermarkets, pharmacies, by mail order and via the internet. The biggest selection is usually found in health-food shops.

Their sale is regulated in various ways. Most herbal products are sold as food supplements. In this case the manufacturer is not allowed to make claims on the label for the use of the products, since legally they are considered to be foods. In fact, many food supplements are available as capsules and tablets and most consumers buy them for self-medication, having read about their use in books on herbal medicine or in the press.

Aware of this anomaly, the government is currently reviewing the status of food supplements. A body called the Novel Foods Committee (NFC), part of the Food Standards Agency and originally set

up to review genetically modified foods, is now also looking at herbal ingredients and products that may be new to Europe. It is now likely that many of the food supplements currently on sale will eventually need NFC approval, if they have not been sold in the EU prior to 1997.

In addition, the introduction of the new EU Food Supplement Directive, though mainly concerned with vitamins and minerals, will lead to a review of herbal products that contain vitamins or minerals.

Licensed herbal products

In certain cases, manufacturers want their product approved as a medicine and submit it for approval to the Medicines and Healthcare products Regulatory Agency (MHRA). This usually involves sending bibliographic evidence for the efficacy of the product along with expert reports on its safety and appropriate quality controls.

Newly licensed products get a Marketing Authorisation; products that have been on the market for a while have a product licence; both are identified by a product licence (PL) number on the label. Unlike food supplements, the label also includes a statement about the intended use of the product. Thus if echinacea, which is used for the treatment of colds and flu, is in a licensed product, it will state: 'A traditional herbal remedy for the symptomatic relief of colds and flu'.

Because of the high standards required, licensed herbal medicines are probably the safest and most effective forms of herbal medicines that consumers can buy. Many of them are listed at the back of this book (*see* Licensed Herbal Medicines on pages 310-317).

The government has also set controls on which herbs are allowed to be sold with or without medical supervision. In certain cases, licensed herbal medicines and other herbal products may also be marked with a 'P' to indicate 'pharmacy-only' – that is, that they should not be sold in an outlet that does not have a pharmacy. Such medicines include hawthorn (*Cratageous oxyacantha*), which is used for heart problems. Others, such as deadly nightshade (*Atropa belladonna*) can only be administered by a medical herbalist.

Unlicensed herbal medicines

Under current legislation, herbal medicines may not necessarily require a licence. Under Section 12 of the Medicines Act, herbs can be sold to the public in dried, crushed or powdered form without any claims on the label, but stating the botanical name of the product. For example, you can purchase dried sage, but the label would contain only its botanical name *Salvia officinalis* and no recommendations about how it should be used.

Under the same act, practitioners of herbal medicine are permitted to make their own remedies to treat patients, for example, in the form of tinctures or capsules, without the need to obtain a Marketing Authorisation. In certain cases, a manufacturer can make a product on behalf of a herbalist, under a Special Manufacturing Licence.

A new directive

The European Commission has developed a new directive for herbal medicines that takes into account their traditional uses, while at the same time tightening up their safety and quality control. It defines 'traditional' generally as at least 30 years of continuous use in the European Union. However, for medicines used continually outside the EU for at least 15 years, only a further 15 years of use within the EU is required. This directive became law in 2005.

A registration scheme, introduced in autumn 2005, and known as the Traditional Herbal Medicines Registration Scheme (THMRS) applies only to manufactured over-the-counter (OTC) traditional herbal remedies. It may take some time for the first registered products to appear on the market, while a seven-year transitional period means that products do not have to be registered until 30 April 2011.

Meanwhile, manufactured traditional herbal medicines will need, progressively, to be registered. Such products will be given a registration number, which shows that they comply with the required safety and quality standards, and are accompanied by appropriate information for patients to help ensure safe use of the medicine.

For the most up-to-date information, visit the MHRA web site at http://www.mhra.gov.uk

In *Nature's Medicines*

When using this book, the Plant section highlights which plants should only ever be used under the supervision of a medical herbalist. For other products as well as fresh or dried herbs, shop around. It is always worth buying the best quality you can afford.

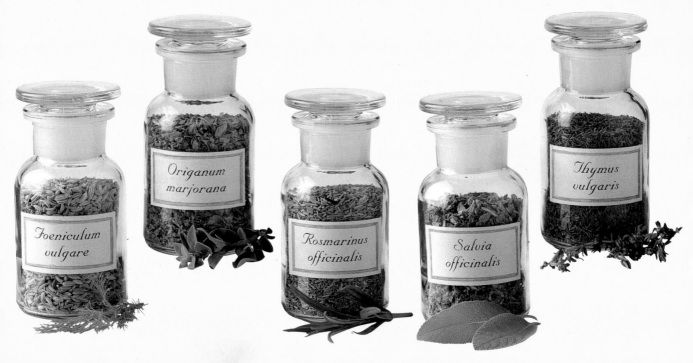

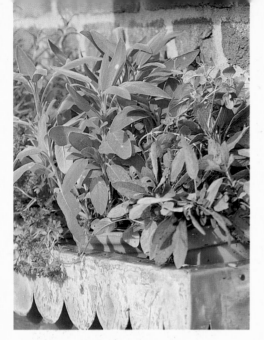

Cultivating your own herbs

There are many advantages to growing your own herbs: they look pretty; several can be used in cooking; and if you wish to use herbs medicinally, you can be confident about their freshness and purity. Furthermore, many medicinal plants are becoming increasingly rare in the wild – some are even threatened with extinction – so growing your own herbs rather than gathering them will help to preserve those that remain.

Space no object

You do not need a lot of space to grow herbs. A successful and varied herb garden can be grown in a container, hanging basket, window box, or in a row of pots on a windowsill.

You may like to dedicate a specific plot to your herb garden, or you may prefer to grow herbs among the flowers in a border: herbs like coriander and basil – particularly the purple-leaved varieties – have lovely foliage and taste delicious.

It is important to plant herbs well away from busy roads, as they are prone to contamination by exhaust fumes. Do not use pesticides, again because of the risk of contamination. However, because they exude such strong aromas, herbs are targeted by very few insects – although aphids seem drawn to the sweet aniseed-like scent of caraway and dill. Make a note of what you have planted where – a simple diagram of the area and plant labels will help.

Soil and situation

Drainage is probably the most important single factor in successful herb growing. Few herbs will grow well in waterlogged soils, though marshmallow and peppermint do not mind wetter ground.

The soil does not have to be rich. In fact highly fertile soils tend to produce plants with masses of foliage but a poor flavour. Instead of adding fertilisers, dig in homemade compost or buy organic compost. Most herbs do best in a sunny sheltered position.

Growing from seed

Many herbs can be grown from seed. Be sure to buy seeds or seedlings from a reputable supplier, so you can be confident of what you are planting and using. Seeds must be dry and free from mould. Sow seeds in trays in late winter, and transplant the seedlings outdoors in spring after the last frost.

Use fine seed compost and do not cover the seeds too deeply with soil. The smaller the seed, the shallower it should be sown.

Some seeds should be sown outdoors where they are to grow – coriander and dill, for example, do not like to be moved. If you can work your soil into a fine tilth, your seeds will be happy. But if your garden is very stony or on heavy clay, it may be worth importing a layer of sandy topsoil.

Sow seeds in very shallow drills and firm the soil over them. Mixing fine seeds such as oregano or thyme with sand will enable you to spread them more evenly. The soil needs to be kept moist in order for the seeds to germinate: stop it from drying out by soaking some sacking or newspapers in water and spreading them over the seedbed.

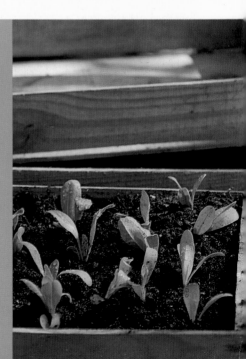

Other forms of propagation

Some herbs spread so fast that division is an easy way to increase them. Dig up the plant and ease it into separate smaller plants, making sure that each section has plenty of root attached. Lemon balm, lady's mantle and stinging nettle are good candidates for division.

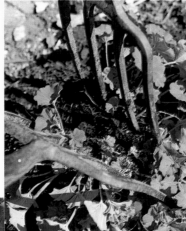

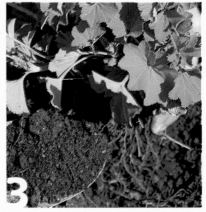

2 If old, drive two garden forks, back to back, into the clump. Push the handles together, then pull them apart. Separate the roots into four pieces.

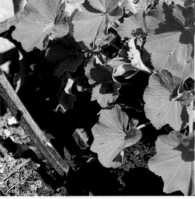

1 Dig up the plant, with all its roots, in spring or autumn. If it is young, divide the roots by hand.

3 Cut away each woody centre. Split the remainder into pieces of six buds or shoots. Remove any excess soil and unhealthy growth. Plant and water.

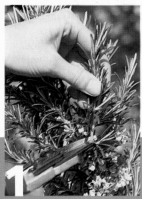

1 Cut off 15-20cm of non-flowering, leafy sideshoots. Remove the lower leaves.

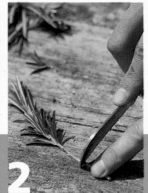

2 Cut the shoot just below a leaf joint and remove the soft tip to leave cuttings 5-10cm long.

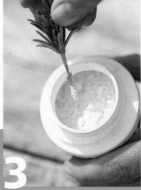

3 Dip the base in hormone rooting agent. Fill a pot with cutting compost (8cm wide for 5 cuttings, 13cm for 10).

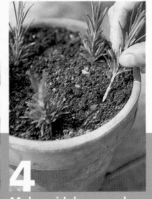

4 Make widely spaced holes around the pot edge and insert the cuttings to a third of their length. Firm the soil. Water.

Growing from cuttings

Plants such as lavender and rosemary take a long time to grow from seed and are best propagated from cuttings. Pick a healthy young plant and choose shoots of the current year's growth – this will ensure that the tips of the shoots are soft and the lower stem is firm. Using a rooting hormone powder will help the cutting to root more quickly.

Protect from frost

Perennial and biennial herbs are more likely to overwinter successfully if you protect them. This involves covering them with good thick mulch. Straw, oak leaves or the prunings from evergreens make a good blanket, which should be left in place until the herbs begin to show signs of growth in early spring.

Harvesting and preserving herbs

All herbs have a peak harvesting time, when leaves, flowers, seeds or roots have their highest concentration of active constituents. Dry the herbs as soon as possible after cutting. Once dry, store them in sterilised, airtight, dark glass jars (Marmite jars are ideal) away from sunlight. Herbs will keep for about a year in a cool dark place. Some remedies are made from bark or resins: it is best to buy these from a herbalist as incorrect methods of collection can kill a shrub or tree.

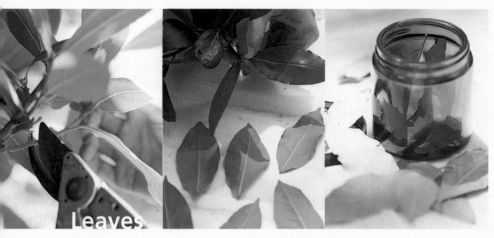

Leaves

Pick leaves when the plant has enough foliage to keep growing. Collect them on a dry day when the dew has gone but before the sun gets too hot; herbs like sage give off their fragrance, and thus lose their volatile oils, in heat. Choose young shoots of healthy plants, and take care not to crush or bruise them. Brush away any soil – do not wash the leaves. Spread them on kitchen paper in a warm, dark, dry place. Alternatively, tie them in small bunches and hang them away from direct sunlight in a sheltered but well-aired place. Most leaves will dry in 24-48 hours.

Fruits and berries

Gather fruits and berries just as they ripen. Line a baking sheet with kitchen paper and spread berries in a thin layer. Put them in a warmed oven, switched off, with the door slightly open, for 3 hours. Afterwards, move the fruits or berries to somewhere dry, warm and dark – such as an airing cupboard – to finish drying.

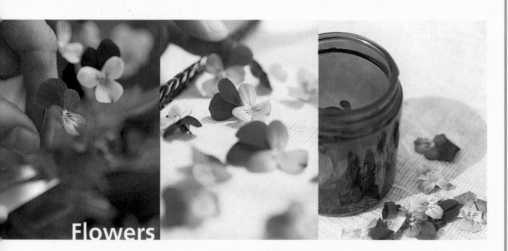

Flowers

Pick flowers as they start to bloom. Small flowerheads can be dried whole: spread them on a rack covered with kitchen paper or muslin in a warm dry place, or hang them upside down over a sheet of muslin or a paper bag; strip the petals from larger flowerheads, such as marigolds, and dry them in a thin layer on a sheet of muslin or kitchen paper.

Seeds

Collect fragile seedheads in late summer. Leave on plenty of stalk so you can tie them in small, loose bunches. Hang stems upside down in clean paper bags – which will catch the seeds as they fall. Once the seeds are dry, shake the bunch to loosen any still attached.

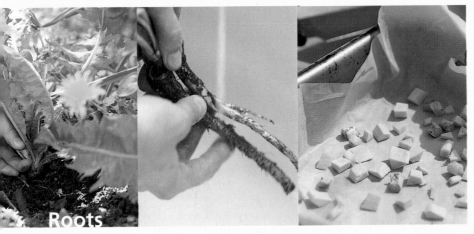

Roots

Collect roots and rhizomes in autumn once the plant has died down, but before the first frosts. Take what you need and replant the remaining underground plant. Wash the root and remove any soft parts or side roots. Slice thinly or chop into small chunks with a sharp knife and spread in a thin layer on kitchen paper on a baking sheet. Dry for 2 hours in a warmed oven, switched off, with the door slightly open, and then keep in a warm place until completely dry.

Microwave drying

Herbs dry quickly in a microwave. Spread them on a layer of kitchen paper, and dry at a low setting for 2-3 minutes, checking and rearranging them every 30 seconds to ensure even drying.

Using fresh aloe vera

Aloe vera contains a thick, colourless gel at the centre of each leaf, which is useful for treating burns, wounds and dry skin conditions. Do not use any of the gel that is tinged green.

Cut off a healthy large leaf near its base.

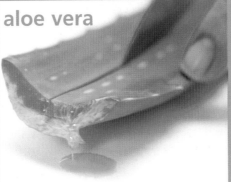

Slice carefully along the leaf centre.

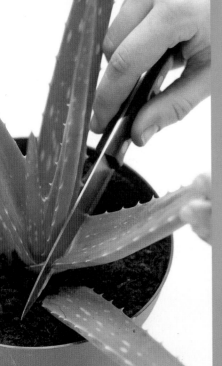

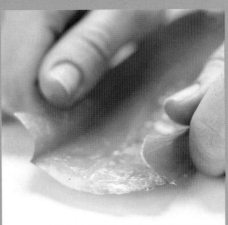

Peel back the edges. Using a blunt edged knife, scrape the clear gel from the centre of the leaf. It should be used fresh as the gel is unstable and quickly loses its consistency.

Harvesting wild herbs

Do
- Collect only where you have the landowner's permission to do so.
- Take a detailed plant guide for reference.
- Gather herbs in dry weather.
- Wear protective gloves when collecting plants that have bristles or caustic sap.
- Take only as much of the plant as you need.
- Make sure you take the correct medicinal part of the plant.

Do not
- Collect rare or endangered species.
- Pick anything you are not sure about – some plants are poisonous.
- Pick plants damaged by disease or insects.
- Harvest from roadsides – exhaust fumes contaminate herbs.
- Mix cut plant materials – you may not be able to identify them when you get home.

Make your own herbal remedies

Herbs can be used in a wide range of medicinal preparations. Some, such as syrups and tinctures, are made for internal use. Others, like creams and poultices, are for external application. Infusions and decoctions can often be taken internally or used externally – in gargles or on compresses, for example. It is not difficult to make your own remedies but it can be time consuming. The following step-by-step guides show you how to make simple herbal preparations at home.

Infusion

An infusion is a tea, and is made in the same way. Infusions are gentle remedies made from flowers and leaves and are best made fresh each day. Use the proportions of dried or fresh herb to water specified in the Plant and Ailment sections of the book, multiplying quantities as required. The usual dose is 1 teacup three times a day. Infusions can also be used cold for gargles and mouthwashes, and hot or cold for a compress.

Compress

A compress is a pad of soft fabric soaked in a herbal infusion or decoction and applied to the painful area. A compress may be hot or cold. Hot compresses are useful to relieve cramp or muscle tension. Cold compresses are used when the skin feels hot to the touch. A cold compress can help to ease a headache.

1 Soak a clean cotton pad in a herbal infusion or decoction.

2 Place pad over the affected part and cover with a towel.

3 Keep refreshing the compress to keep the area warm or cool as required.

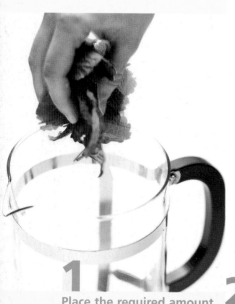

1 Place the required amount of herb in a warmed china or glass (not metal) teapot or in a cafetière.

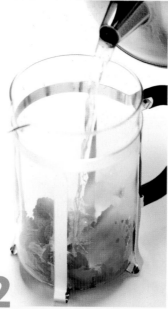

2 Pour on water that has been boiled, then left to stand for 30 seconds.

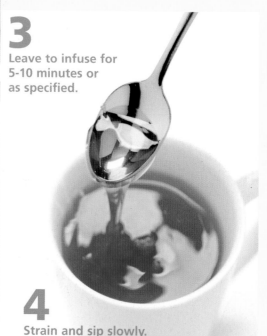

3 Leave to infuse for 5-10 minutes or as specified.

4 Strain and sip slowly. Sweeten with honey if desired.

Decoction

A decoction is a more vigorous way of extracting the active constituents from the tough parts of a herb, such as its bark, roots or seeds. For safety, use only the proportions of plant to liquid specified in the Plants and Ailments sections of the book, multiplying quantities as required.

Decoctions are most effective if prepared fresh each day, but they can be kept for up to three days in a refrigerator.

Syrup

Syrups are a good way of making medicines more palatable. Sugar-based preparations soothe sore throats and other irritated mucous membranes. A standard syrup is made using 500ml infusion or decoction and 500g honey or unrefined sugar. The usual dose is 10ml (5ml for children) three times a day. Syrups keep for up to six months in a cool place.

1 Pour the infusion or decoction into a pan. An infusion should have been steeped for at least 10 minutes; a decoction should have been simmered for an hour.

2 Add the sugar or honey and heat gently until dissolved.

3 Remove from the heat and allow to cool.

4 Pour into sterilised glass bottles (use a funnel).

5 Label and stopper with corks: syrups can ferment and a bottle sealed with a screw-top lid might explode.

1 Crush up seeds or bark in a pestle and mortar.

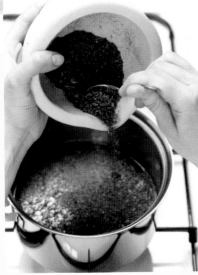

2 Put the required amount of water in a stainless steel or enamel saucepan. Add the broken dried herb or chopped fresh herb.

3 Bring to the boil, reduce heat and simmer for up to an hour, until the volume has reduced by about a third.

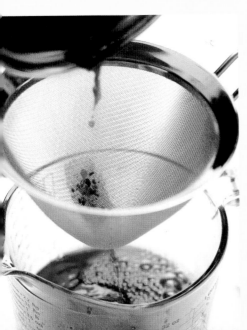

4 Strain and add water to make up to the required amount. Sweeten with honey if desired.

Making a tincture

Tinctures, such as rosehip, are made by steeping dried or fresh herbs in alcohol. For commercial tinctures, specific water-to-alcohol proportions are used for each herb. For homemade tinctures, vodka can be used, but it is safest to check the proportions first with a medical herbalist. Tinctures keep for up to three years if stored in a cool, dark cupboard.

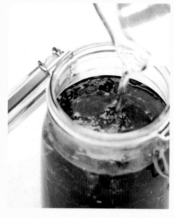

1 Put 225g of rosehips in a large glass jar. Pour in 700ml of vodka and 300ml of water and close the jar tightly.

2 Keep in a warm place for two weeks shaking occasionally.

3 Strain through a muslin cloth, squeezing out the residue.

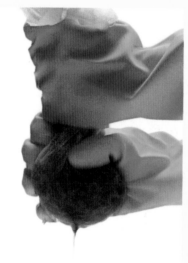

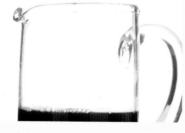

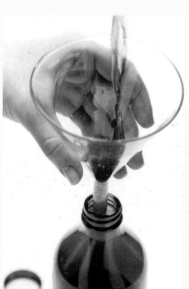

4 Discard the solids and pour tincture into a labelled dark glass bottle.

Poultice

A poultice – usually used hot – is a herb paste applied directly to the skin on strips of gauze. Poultices are mainly used to draw pus from the skin, to reduce inflammation, heal boils and abscesses, and draw splinters. Here the plant is marigold, an effective treatment for cracked skin, insect bites and sunburn.

1 Finely chop 220g of dried marigold.

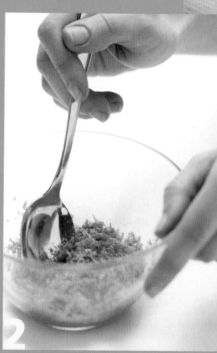

2 Transfer to a bowl and mix with enough boiled water to make a paste.

3 Apply a little olive oil to the skin to stop the poultice from sticking.

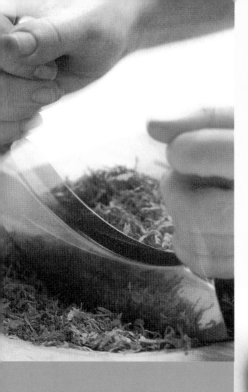

Massage oils

The essential oil of some plants, such as sweet marjoram (see page 192), can be used to make a massage oil to relieve aching bones and joints. Although a few essential oils, such as lavender can be used neat, most should be diluted with a carrier oil, such as a bland odourless vegetable oil, in the proportions specified in the 'Preparation and dosage' boxes on the Plant pages. To prepare a sweet marjoram massage oil, for instance, use 3 drops of the essential oil for every 10ml of the carrier oil.

Fragrant inhalants

Inhalants are used to treat blocked nasal passages, catarrh, asthma and sinus infections. The simplest inhalants are infusions. Suitable herbs include lavender, eucalyptus, pine and peppermint.

1 Put 1-2 tablespoons of dried lavender flowers into a bowl.

2 Pour boiling water over them.

3 Lean over the bowl with a towel covering both your head and the bowl.

4 Inhale the steam until it stops rising. Repeat twice a day or as needed.

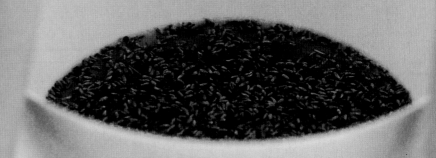

4 Spread the herb paste on gauze or cotton strips and apply to the skin.

5 Keep the poultice in place until cool and replace as often as required.

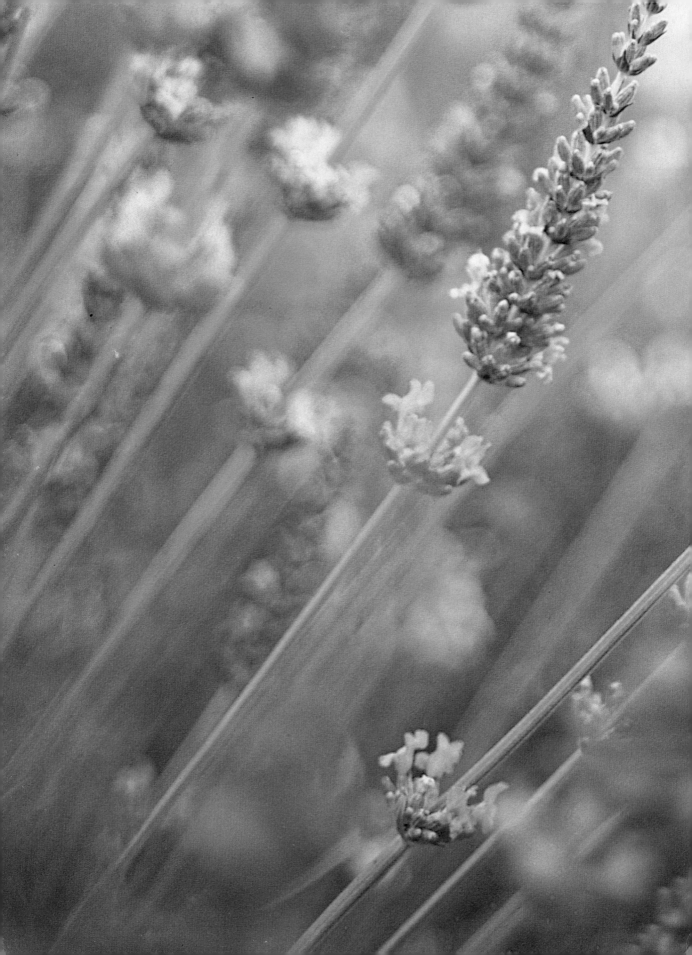

A to Z of Plants

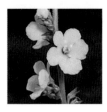

Aaron's rod

Verbascum thapsus Scrophulariaceae **Also called** Great mullein

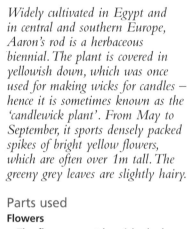

Widely cultivated in Egypt and in central and southern Europe, Aaron's rod is a herbaceous biennial. The plant is covered in yellowish down, which was once used for making wicks for candles – hence it is sometimes known as the 'candlewick plant'. From May to September, it sports densely packed spikes of bright yellow flowers, which are often over 1m tall. The greeny grey leaves are slightly hairy.

Parts used

Flowers

• The flowers must be picked when in full bloom and dried rapidly to preserve their effectiveness.

• They are used in decoctions and infusions, liquid or dry extracts, and also in pharmaceutical products.

Constituents

The Aaron's rod flower contains sugars, mucilage, flavonoids, iridoids, saponins and yellow colorants.

Medicinal uses

The mucilage in Aaron's rod helps to soothe irritation, while its saponins and flavonoids combine to reduce inflammation. The saponins also contribute expectorant properties, which is why a syrup made from Aaron's rod is used to treat throat infections and coughs.

Various preparations made from the plant are used for easing respiratory tract infections, such as asthma, bronchitis, laryngitis and the symptoms of influenza. In addition, the plant's soothing and anti-inflammatory abilities have long been recognised as effective in treating digestive problems, such as diarrhoea, gastritis, enteritis and colitis, and in helping to ease gout.

Applied externally, Aaron's rod will help to heal cuts and leg ulcers and to soothe skin irritations. Olive oil, infused with the dried flowers, is sometimes used to ease the pain of earache and haemorrhoids.

Research has indicated that Aaron's rod has anti-viral properties and it may also help to inhibit the spread of cancer.

Cultivation

Aaron's rod grows easily from seeds, planted in a sunny position in any type of well-drained soil.

CAUTIONS

• No toxicity or undesirable effect has been recorded to date, but medical advice is recommended before using.

• Aaron's rod should not be taken when pregnant or breastfeeding.

PREPARATION AND DOSAGE

For internal use

TO TREAT laryngitis, tracheitis, bronchitis, diarrhoea, gastritis, enteritis, colitis

INFUSION Put 1.5-2g into a cup of boiling water. Leave to infuse for 15 minutes, then strain. Take 3 cups a day.

LIQUID EXTRACT Put 50 drops into a glass of water. Take three to four times a day.

DRY EXTRACT Take 300mg three to six times a day.

SYRUP FOR CHILDREN Take 1 teaspoon three times a day.

For external use

TO TREAT cuts, leg ulcers, skin irritations

COMPRESS Soak 3 teaspoons of dried plant in 300ml of cold water for 30 minutes. Gently bring to the boil. Strain. Soak a cloth in the solution. Apply twice a day.

IF SYMPTOMS PERSIST, CONSULT A DOCTOR

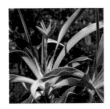

African potato

Hypoxis rooperi (*H. hemerocallidea*) Hypoxidaceae

A native of South Africa, the African potato is a herbaceous perennial that grows from a corm. Like the closely related amaryllis, it is cultivated for its ornamental qualities. Evergreen foliage surrounds its stems which, from June to November, bear luminous yellow, star-shaped flowers.

Parts used

Corm

● Wild plants are harvested after the flowers have bloomed.

● The corms are removed, cleaned, then dried in the open air, before being reduced to a powder.

● The powder is used for infusions and in pharmaceutical preparations.

Constituents

The corm contains sterols and sterolins. Researchers have also identified another constituent – hypoxoside – which has an anti-bacterial and antifungal action.

Medicinal uses

Traditional African medicine uses the African potato for different purposes according to region: for example, in its native South Africa it is used to treat urinary infections, and in Malawi it is given for enlargement of the prostate gland. Its use has even spread to the Caribbean, where it is prescribed for certain cancers. In fact, recent animal studies have shown that rooperol, a derivative of the hypoxoside found in the plant, can inhibit the growth of cancer cells.

Rooperol is also the key to the African potato's ability to act as an antiviral agent and research has demonstrated its benefit in the treatment of certain viral infections. Other properties conferred by the lignins make the African potato highly potent as an antibacterial and antifungal agent.

The African potato is attracting increasing interest from Western medical researchers. Scientists have recently shown that extracts from the plant can help to boost the immune system, and that an aqueous extract is effective in reducing inflammation. The b-sitosterol and its glucoside are thought to be responsible for this anti-inflammatory action. The same research describes the effectiveness of African potato preparations in treating the symptoms of rheumatoid arthritis.

Cultivation

The African potato is a wild plant that grows easily, even in poor stony soils. As it should only be taken as prescribed, cultivation for home use is not recommended.

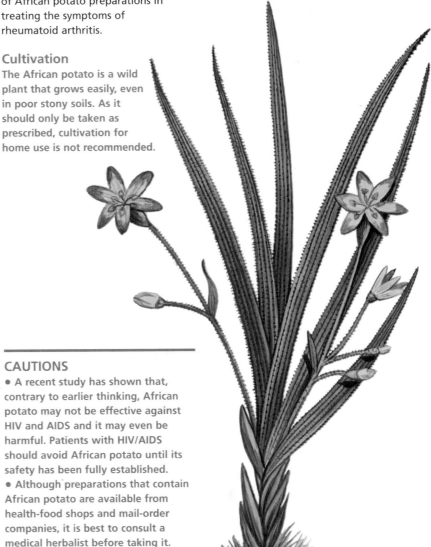

PREPARATION AND DOSAGE

African potato – taken in any form, including commercially available products – should only be used in consultation with a qualified medical herbalist.

IF SYMPTOMS PERSIST, CONSULT A DOCTOR

CAUTIONS

● A recent study has shown that, contrary to earlier thinking, African potato may not be effective against HIV and AIDS and it may even be harmful. Patients with HIV/AIDS should avoid African potato until its safety has been fully established.

● Although preparations that contain African potato are available from health-food shops and mail-order companies, it is best to consult a medical herbalist before taking it.

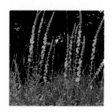

Agrimony

Agrimonia eupatoria Rosaceae **Also called** Cockleburr, Church steeples

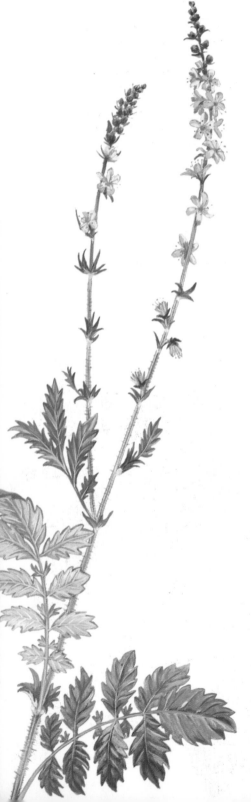

A slender hedgerow plant found throughout Europe, agrimony grows up to a metre in height. It has rough stems and large dark green leaves with a whitish downy underside. The spikes of yellow flowers have a slightly spicy scent and appear from June to early September, followed by burr-like seedpods with hooked spines.

Parts used
Flowerheads
- Gather in full flower in July and August and dry in a warm place.
- For internal use, agrimony is usually made into an infusion, but can be bought as tablets. Externally, it is used in gargles and compresses.

Constituents
The flowers contain three types of active components: tannins – which have antioxidant, antimicrobial and anti-inflammatory properties; flavonoids – antioxidants believed to prevent cardiovascular disease and fight cancer; and terpenes – the plant's volatile oils that give it its pleasing aroma.

Medicinal uses
The anti-inflammatory qualities of agrimony make it useful for treating skin rashes and stomach upsets, as well as sore throats and rheumatism.

Weak infusions can be given to children with diarrhoea and mild tummy upsets. A Swedish study has

CAUTIONS
- Do not use if pregnant or breast-feeding.
- Avoid exposure to bright sunlight when taking agrimony.
- No contraindications have yet been reported, but agrimony is usually combined with other plants, which modifies its effect.

PREPARATION AND DOSAGE

For internal use
TO TREAT mild diarrhoea, sluggish digestion, poor circulation, haemorrhoids
INFUSION Use 2 teaspoons of dried flowers to 250ml of boiling water. Leave to infuse for 5 minutes and then strain. Drink 3-4 cups a day. Haemorrhoid treatments are available over-the-counter.

For external use
For a healthy mouth and throat
GARGLES, RINSES Make an infusion using 1 teaspoon of the dried flowers to 250ml of boiling water. Cool and use as a mouthwash or gargle two or three times a day.

TO TREAT haemorrhoids, circulation problems, skin problems
COMPRESS Use 5 dessertspoons of the dried plant to 250ml of cold water. Bring to the boil and let boil for 5 minutes. Cool and strain. Soak a soft cloth in the liquid and apply four or five times a day.

IF SYMPTOMS PERSIST, CONSULT A DOCTOR

---

confirmed that agrimony infusions can help to ease inflammatory skin conditions. A cooled infusion applied on a cloth soothes skin allergies and improves blood circulation, and a compress may reduce haemorrhoids.

Gargling with an infusion of agrimony can heal sore throats while rinsing is good for mouth ulcers. Drinking infusions of agrimony improves digestion by stimulating the stomach and gall bladder. It can also soothe an irritable bowel.

Historically, agrimony was used to heal gunshot wounds, and research has shown that it helps blood to clot.

Cultivation
Prefers well-drained soil and is suited to sunny positions. Agrimony is harvested when it is in flower.

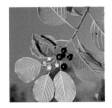

Alder buckthorn

Rhamnus frangula Rhamnaceae **Also called** Black dogwood, Frangula bark

Found throughout Europe, alder buckthorn is a shrub that flourishes in damp woodlands and thickets. It is an upright plant, reaching a height of 3-5m. The brownish grey bark is covered in whitish warty spots. Pale green flowers appear in May and June, followed by small red stone-bearing berries, which turn black when ripe.

Parts used
Bark
• The bark is torn off in strips from the young trunk or branches of shrubs at flowering time.
• It is chopped into small pieces and dried, and is used in a decoction.
• Freshly picked bark is toxic, so it should not be used until it has been dried and stored for at least a year.

CAUTIONS
• Fresh bark is toxic – do not use.
• Avoid alder buckthorn if pregnant or breastfeeding.
• Do not use if suffering from bowel disease such as Crohn's disease, ulcerative colitis or intestinal obstruction.
• Do not give to children under 15.
• Talk to a medical herbalist before using alder buckthorn.
• Overdose can cause convulsions.

PREPARATION AND DOSAGE
As preparations of alder buckthorn may conflict with certain prescribed medicines including certain corticosteroids and anti-arrhythmic heart drugs, it is advisable to seek the advice of a medical herbalist before using the plant.

IF SYMPTOMS PERSIST, CONSULT A DOCTOR

Constituents
The bark of alder buckthorn contains derivatives of anthracene, a well-known and effective laxative.

Medicinal uses
Alder buckthorn has long been used to treat constipation. It works by increasing the absorption of water and electrolytes in the intestine, thereby stimulating intestinal movement. However, studies have also shown that if taken over a long period, alder buckthorn can cause diarrhoea and potassium loss. When produced commercially, the bark is often mixed with other ingredients.

Alder buckthorn is also believed to be a diuretic and to increase bile secretion in the gall bladder. It has been used to treat liver and gall-bladder complaints such as jaundice, hepatitis and cirrhosis.

A decoction rubbed into the gums can cure gingivitis; applied to the scalp, it clears headlice.

Research published in 1976 in the US journal *Llyodia*, showed that an extract from alder buckthorn seeds inhibited the growth of tumours. And in 1991, American researchers demonstrated the antiviral activity of alder buckthorn plant extracts.

Cultivation
Alder buckthorn is best grown from seeds sown in autumn. It likes a sunny or lightly shaded position and a neutral to acid soil. It is a hardy shrub and can withstand freezing temperatures as low as –35°C.

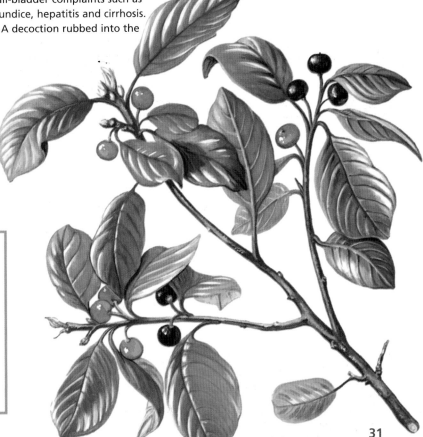

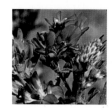

Alfalfa

Medicago sativa Fabaceae **Also called** Lucerne

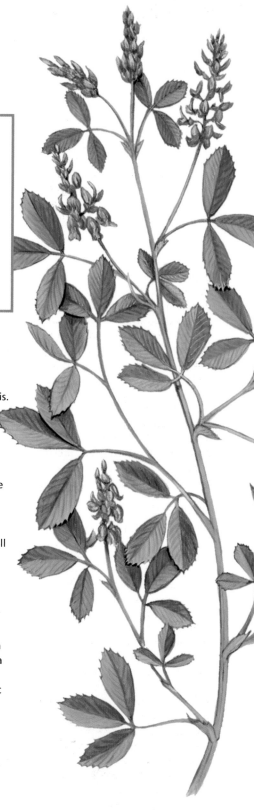

Reaching a height of around 60cm, alfalfa is a perennial herb that grows wild on the edges of fields. It bears purple-blue flowers in summer and its seedpods are coiled spirals. Besides its medicinal use, it is cultivated as livestock feed and its young sprouts are enjoyed in salads.

Parts used

Leaves

• The leaves are harvested up to five times every growing season, just as the plant starts to flower.
• They are used to make tinctures and dry or liquid extracts.

Constituents

Alfalfa is an excellent source of dietary nutrients for the body including protein, calcium and vitamins. It also contains saponins, which dissolve fats, coumarins, phenols, tannins and unsaturated fatty acids. Alfalfa is rich in phyto-estrogens that mimic the action of the female hormone, oestrogen.

Medicinal uses

Due to its oestrogenic effects, alfalfa regulates periods, and stimulates milk-flow in breastfeeding women.

CAUTIONS

• **Alfalfa has shown no signs of toxicity to date.**
• **Do not use to treat lupus (a chronic inflammatory disease).**
• **Not recommended for people with other autoimmune disorders or rheumatic conditions.**
• **If pregnant or breastfeeding, do not consume larger amounts than you would eat in a normal meal.**
• **Alfalfa may induce sensitisation to sunlight, so when using it, it is wise to avoid sunbathing.**
• **Alfalfa can alter blood counts.**
• **Do not exceed prescribed doses.**

Experiments carried out by clinical nutritionists in 1982 showed that eating alfalfa helped to protect monkeys that were on a high cholesterol diet from atherosclerosis. They also proved the effectiveness of alfalfa in decreasing blood cholesterol levels.

In 1990, researchers in Northern Ireland showed that alfalfa affects the metabolism of glucose and, like coriander, eucalyptus and juniper, it also reduces excessive thirst and blood sugar levels.

Alfalfa's fortifying effects are well known and, due to its ability to stimulate the appetite, the plant is often given to induce weight gain and also as a restorative during convalescence. Alfalfa can help to reduce exhaustion and nervous agitation. In India, alfalfa is used in poultices to treat boils; in Colombia it is used to treat coughs. It may have a therapeutic effect on gastric ulcers, and has been used in the treatment of kidney stones.

Cultivation

Plant in a sunny position in a light, well-drained soil. The blue flowers are rich in nectar and attract bees.

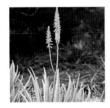

Aloe vera

Aloe vera Liliaceae **Also called** Bitter aloe

A perennial succulent, aloe is native to the dry regions of East and South Africa, and the Mediterranean basin. Its greeny grey, tightly packed, thick, fleshy leaves have jagged, thorny edges. The tissue inside the leaf contains aloe juice – believed to have been used to preserve the body of Jesus.

Parts used
Leaf sap and gel
● Leaves are collected from plants that are two to three years old.
● Sap exudes when the leaf is cut and gel comes from mucilage-rich cells in the heart of the leaf.
● Aloe vera is available in drinks and in skin preparations.

Constituents
The leaf gel contains polysaccharides and lipids, which have healing properties, while the sap contains anthraquinones such as aloin A and B, which provide laxative properties.

Medicinal uses
Aloe's medicinal properties have been known since ancient times. The laxative sap is dried and sold as 'resin'. The gel stimulates the immune system and has antibiotic, anti-inflammatory and antiseptic effects. This makes it useful in the treatment of certain skin problems such as eczema and psoriasis.

In the 1950s, aloe vera became renowned for treating radiation burns. Today the gel is widely used to sooth, moisturise and heal burns (including sunburn), wounds, acne, anal fissures and haemorrhoids.

In 1996, Mexican researchers investigating aloe vera's effectiveness as an anti-inflammatory agent showed that it prevented swelling by inhibiting the migration of inflammatory cells and the chemicals that induce inflammation.

Aloe may also help rheumatic ailments. Research published in 1986 found that a cream containing aloe vera both prevented and treated rheumatoid arthritis in rats.

Because aloe vera is a powerful laxative, herbal practitioners advise that it should be used primarily as

CAUTIONS
● Taken internally, aloe vera causes diarrhoea, which may reduce levels of potassium in the blood.
● It can trigger attacks of colitis.
● It should not be taken by young children, pregnant or breastfeeding women.
● Do not take if suffering from uraemia (excess urea in the blood) or disorders of the kidneys or liver.

an external remedy. However, some commercial preparations can be taken internally. These immune-stimulant drinks have had aloe's laxative principles removed.

Cultivation
This tender plant can be grown as a houseplant if kept above 5°C.

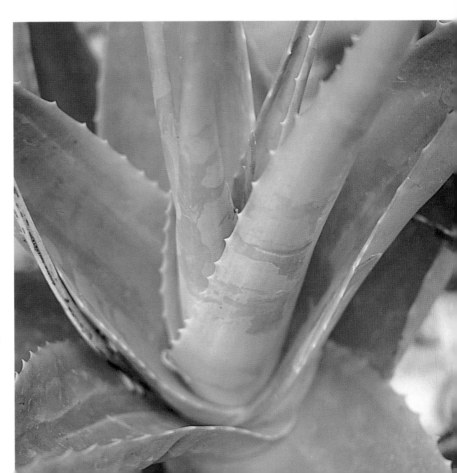

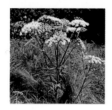

Angelica

Angelica archangelica Apiaceae **Also called** Archangel

Known in the past as the Root of the Holy Spirit, angelica is a striking architectural plant whose thick, hollow stalks can grow to 3m tall. It has finely cut leaves and its oval fruits have wings like those of an angel, hence its name. In the Renaissance, angelica was thought to be able to cure all illnesses.

Parts used
Roots
- The hard roots are collected from one to two-year-old plants.
- Roots are washed, cut up and dried in the open air.
- They are used in decoctions, in capsules or in a drinkable solution.

Constituents
Angelica root is made up of 1 per cent essential oil. This consists mainly of beta-phellandrene, along with the aromatic coumarins angelicin, bergapten and osthole.

Medicinal uses
Angelica root is mainly used to treat common digestive problems such as indigestion and flatulence. It is also recommended for stomach pains and intestinal spasms.

Angelica has long been used as a remedy for coughs, colds and influenza because it acts as an expectorant. It is particularly recommended for bronchitis.

PREPARATION AND DOSAGE
For internal use
TO TREAT digestive problems, colds and coughs, fatigue
INFUSION Put 1-2g dried root in 1 cup of boiling water. Strain and drink three times a day.
DECOCTION Put 1 teaspoon of root into ¾ cup of water, bring to the boil and steep for 5 minutes. Strain. Take as two doses during the day.
LIQUID EXTRACT (1:1 in 25% alcohol) Take 0.5-2ml root extract , three times a day.
TINCTURE (1:5 in 50% alcohol) Take 0.5-2ml three times a day.

IF SYMPTOMS PERSIST, CONSULT A DOCTOR

A root extract may alleviate the painful symptoms of back pain, gout and rheumatism: in 1978, researchers demonstrated angelica's anti-inflammatory and pain-relieving properties. The root oil is also antibacterial and antifungal.

In 1996 researchers found osthole to be an effective anticoagulant, and thus potentially useful for treating thrombosis. And in 1998, researchers described bergapten as a photo-sensitising agent that could benefit psoriasis sufferers.

Angelica can be taken as a bitter tonic. It works by increasing appetite through stimulation of the salivary glands and digestive organs.

Cultivation
Angelica is easily grown from seed. It is a hardy plant suited to moist soils and temperate climates. It is happy in sun or light shade.

CAUTIONS
- There have been no reported adverse effects.
- However, do not use if pregnant or breastfeeding.
- Do not sunbathe when using, as it may cause sensitisation to sunlight in fair-skinned individuals.
- Do not use if you are diabetic.
- Avoid if taking anticoagulants.

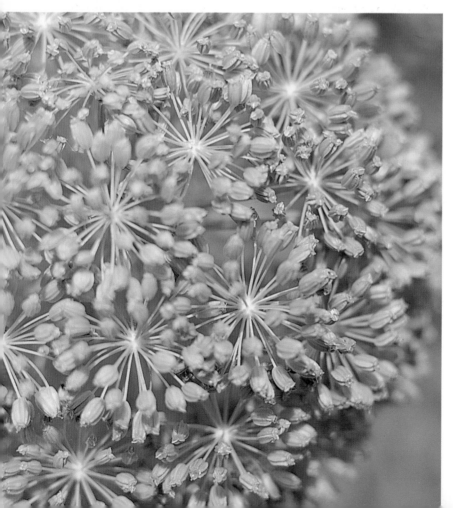

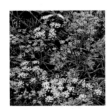

Anise

Pimpinella anisum Apiaceae **Also called** Aniseed, Common anise

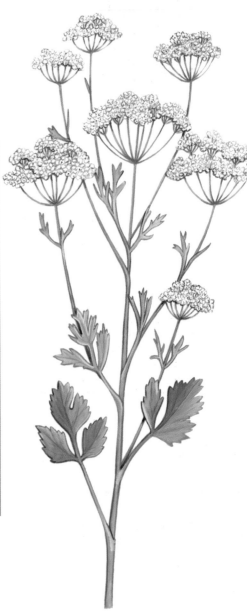

A highly aromatic low-growing plant, anise originated in the Middle East and was cultivated by the ancient Egyptians. Dainty yellow-and-white flowers on upright stems are followed by aromatic greyish fruits (known as seeds) that have a warm, sugary taste.

Parts used

Seeds

● Seeds are gathered in autumn after flowering.
● They are dried, and must then be stored in a dry, dark place.
● The essential oil is extracted and used in cough lozenges and many other pharmaceutical preparations, herbal medicines, foods and drinks.

Constituents

The seeds contain between 1-6 per cent essential oil. Up to 90 per cent of the oil is anethole, which gives anise its distinctive aroma. Other constituents are coumarins – including bergapten, flavonoids and sterols.

Medicinal uses

Anise has long been used in remedies to ease indigestion, infant colic, bloating, belching and flatulence. Its effectiveness is largely due to its antispasmodic action, which is also thought to ease period pains. Anise increases fluid secretion in the intestine, thus helping to stimulate digestion.

Anise has expectorant properties making it useful in the treatment of bronchitis. The expectorant action of both anise and its main active constituent, anethole, have been proven in animal studies cited in the *European Monographs on the Medicinal Uses of Plant Drugs*.

The *European Monographs* also mention studies of the antibacterial, antifungal and insecticidal properties of the essential oil. Externally, the undiluted oil can be applied to get rid of head lice. It is also used in an ointment for treating scabies.

Anise seeds are thought to be mildly oestrogenic and have long been used in traditional medicine to ease childbirth, stimulate milk production and regulate periods. Anise was also reputed to increase libido in both sexes. A study published in the *Journal of Ethnopharmacology* in 1980 showed that certain anethole-based compounds are responsible for many hormone-mimicking effects.

Cultivation

Sow the seeds at the plant's flowering time in late spring. Anise is a hardy plant that likes a rich, well-drained sandy soil. Choose a sunny or lightly shaded spot.

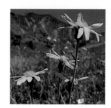

Arnica

Arnica montana Asteraceae **Also called** Mountain tobacco, Leopard's bane

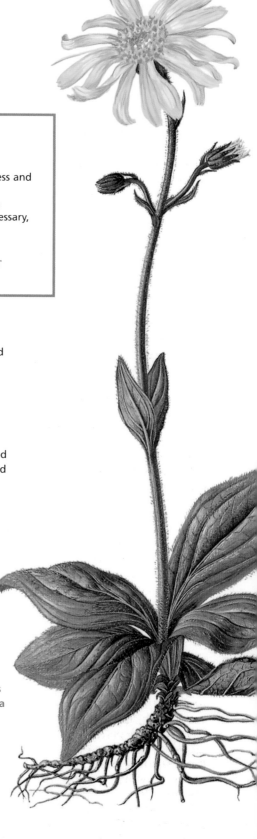

A perennial, native to mountainous regions, arnica is characterised by its bright yellow, daisy-like flowers borne on tall, hairy stems in summer. The name arnica is thought to come from the Greek word 'arnikos', which means lamb's skin and alludes to the downy texture of the plant's leaves. The leaves are pointed and form a rosette around the base.

Parts used

Flowers

• Harvested in June and July and quickly dried, the flowers form the base of numerous preparations – usually tinctures and extracts.

• Mountain arnica is the only species that is used in herbal medicine and should not be confused with its relative *Arnica chamissonis*, a plant grown for ornamental purposes.

Constituents

Arnica contains anti-inflammatory sesquiterpenic lactones – the most important medically is helenalin. Arnica also contains flavonoids which strengthen blood vessels.

CAUTIONS

• Arnica is for external use only; preparations must never be used near the eyes and the mouth, nor on open wounds.

• If there is any contact with an open wound, it must be washed with plenty of distilled water.

• Under no circumstances should arnica be used to treat children under three years old.

• The sesquiterpenoid content may cause skin allergies for some people, and so it is sensible to carry out an initial patch test. Stop the treatment immediately if there is any sign of irritation; the irritation should then gradually disappear.

PREPARATION AND DOSAGE

For external use only

TO TREAT bruising

TINCTURE Use to make a compress and apply to the affected area.

CREAMS, GELS Massage into the affected area, as directed. If necessary, repeat two or three times a day.

IF SYMPTOMS PERSIST, CONSULT A DOCTOR

Medicinal uses

Arnica's primary use is for relieving bruising. The various lactones found in the plant inhibit the leakage of blood under the skin and prevent the inflammation of the tissues surrounding the area.

Arnica is also used to relieve sprains and other minor injuries where there is swelling but no blood loss or broken skin. In studies carried out in 1979 and 1980 using sesquiterpenic lactones, helenalin was found to inhibit swelling and chronic arthritis in rats.

Another use of arnica is for treating bacterial and fungal infections. It should never be taken internally, although there is a homeopathic form that is a remedy for injuries, accidents and shock.

Cultivation

This hardy plant should be planted in well-drained acidic soil. It prefers a sunny location. Picking wild arnica is prohibited because the plant is threatened with extinction in its natural habitats.

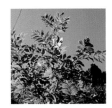

Ash

Fraxinus excelsior Oleaceae **Also called** European ash, Common ash

This large deciduous tree can grow up to 25m tall. Its trunk is upright and is covered in smooth, greyish bark. It was the ability of its bark to reduce fevers that led to ash being called the 'quinine of Europe'. The leaves consist of 9-15 pinnate, serrated leaflets. Clusters of small, brownish flowers are seen among the twigs in April and May, before the leaves. The fruit, called the samara, is a tough, flat wing containing a single seed.

Parts used

Leaves and bark
● The leaves are collected in June and July. The leaflets are then detached from the main stem and spread out in thin layers, out of direct sunlight, to dry.
● The dried leaves can be used in an infusion or are reduced to a powder and put into capsules.
● The bark, which is used for decoctions, is taken from the young branches in spring.

Constituents

The active compounds are iridoids, tannins, flavonoids and coumarins (such as fraxin and fraxinol), which contribute to the anti-inflammatory effects of the plant. The diuretic effect could be due to the presence of manitol and potassium salts.

Medicinal uses

Ash leaves have a recognised anti-inflammatory effect, particularly useful for treating rheumatism. The plant's ability to inhibit several inflammatory processes, was documented in 1995 in German laboratory research into the anti-inflammatory effects of various plant extracts.

Earlier German animal studies performed in 1989 found that ash produced anti-inflammatory,

analgesic (pain-relieving) and antipyretic (temperature-lowering) effects comparable with the strong anti-inflammatory effects of salicyl alcohol and indomethacin.

The leaves are also diuretic and mildly purgative. As such, ash is beneficial in treating gout, kidney stones, oedema and water retention.

In 1980 French scientists found that ash stimulated the immune response of mice inoculated with *Escherichia coli* bacteria.

Ash is a tonic and an infusion of ash leaves mixed with leaves of blackcurrant, meadowsweet and mint makes a refreshing drink.

The bark has long been used to reduce fevers and also possesses astringent properties.

Cultivation

Ash should be planted in well-drained neutral to alkaline soil.

CAUTIONS

● No toxic effects have been reported even after prolonged use.
● However, you should take medical advice if using ash while also taking pharmaceutical drugs for pain relief.

PREPARATION AND DOSAGE
For internal use
TO TREAT kidney stones, rheumatism, gout, oedema, water retention and obesity
INFUSION Put 10-20g of dried leaves into 1 litre of boiling water. Infuse for 10 minutes and strain. Drink 0.5-1 litre a day.
CAPSULES (300mg) Take 2 capsules three times a day with a large glass of water.

TO TREAT fever
TINCTURE Put 50 drops into a glass of water. Take three times a day.
DECOCTION Put 50g dried bark into 1 litre of boiling water. Boil for 10 minutes and strain. Take 3-4 cups a day.

IF SYMPTOMS PERSIST, CONSULT A DOCTOR

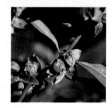

Ashwagandha

Withania somnifera Solanaceae **Also called** Withania

A native of tropical India, ashwagandha forms a bush that can reach 1.2m in height. The plant has been used in traditional Indian medicine for more than 2000 years. Its Sanskrit name means 'the thing that has the smell of a horse' – a reference to the horse's strength and vitality rather than its odour. It is also said to be an aphrodisiac and beneficial in infertility. Its yellowy green flowers give way to gleaming red berries.

Parts used
Roots
● These are harvested in autumn, dried, then cut up for use in decoctions, capsules of the powder, tinctures, and liquid or dry extracts.

Constituents
The ashwagandha root is notable for a steroid called withanolide, which is anti-inflammatory. It also contains alkaloids, particularly withasomnine, that supply sedative qualities.

Medicinal uses
Ashwagandha has traditionally been prescribed as a tonic. This use was supported by a paper published in the *Journal of Ethnopharmacology* in 2000, which described how the plant helps the body to cope with stressful situations. It also lowers blood pressure, slows the heart rate and boosts the immune system. In Indian medicine ashwagandha is commonly prescribed to help convalescing patients to overcome fatigue. The plant is also used to treat anxiety and nervous problems and in large doses can induce sleep.

Research performed in America in 1991 found that ashwagandha contains components that act in the same way as the main inhibitory neurotransmitter in the central nervous system. It is this that is likely to account for its sedative qualities.

Painful rheumatic joints respond to its anti-inflammatory properties and its high iron content makes it useful in the treatment of anaemia.

Cultivation
Plant in dry, stony soil, preferably in the sun or light shade.

CAUTIONS
● Do not use if pregnant or breastfeeding.
● Avoid taking barbiturates and other tranquillisers when using ashwagandha.
● Do not use if you have an overactive thryroid gland.
● Avoid ashwagandha if you have severe kidney or liver disease.

PREPARATION AND DOSAGE
For internal use
TO TREAT fatigue, rheumatic joints
DECOCTION Allow 1-2g of root per cup of water. Boil in a saucepan for 15 minutes, leave to infuse for 10 minutes, then strain. Take 2 cups a day.
TINCTURE (1:3 in 45% alcohol) put 20 drops into a glass of water. Take three times a day.

TO TREAT insomnia, anxiety, nervous problems
CAPSULES (250mg) Take 2-3 capsules, twice a day.

IF SYMPTOMS PERSIST, CONSULT A DOCTOR

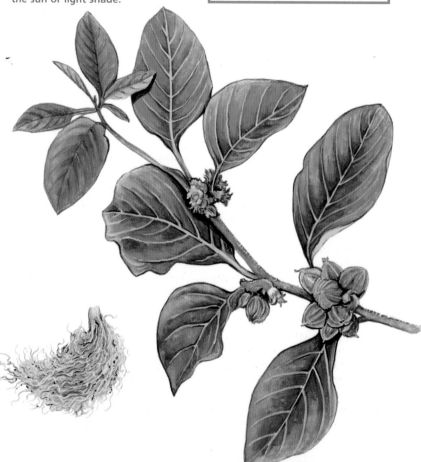

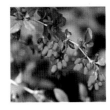

Barberry

Berberis vulgaris Berberidaceae

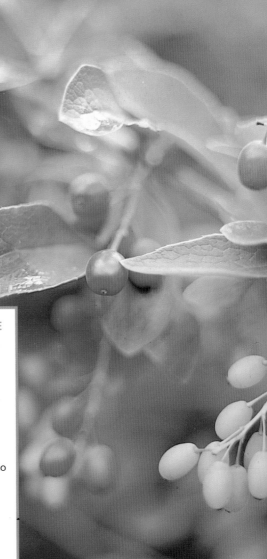

This thorny deciduous shrub is seen throughout Europe in gardens, hedgerows and on scrubland. The ancient Egyptians used barberry as a cure for fevers. It grows to a height of about 3m and has grooved yellow-grey bark, yellow wood and a yellow root. It bears bright yellow flowers in spring followed by elongated berries in shades of pink or red.

Parts used

Leaves, berries, root and stem bark
• The leaves are collected in May and June and the ripe berries in August or September.
• The root and stem bark are collected in spring or autumn and dried for use in powders, tinctures, decoctions and other extracts.

Constituents

The whole plant contains alkaloids, which are believed to possess anticancer properties. Some of the alkaloids are yellow, hence the plant's brightly coloured wood. The alkaloids berbamine and berberine are both antibacterial; the root bark contains up to 3 per cent berberine.

Medicinal uses

Berberine accounts for several of the plant's properties. Animal studies have shown that the alkaloid reduces muscle spasms, which may explain why bitter-tasting barberry can help to aid digestion.

Because berberine is also a highly effective antibacterial, barberry is used to combat infections such as *Helicobacter pylori*, which is associated with gastritis and peptic ulcers, and to treat yeast infections, such as thrush (*Candida albicans*).

Berberine also acts on the gall bladder to stimulate the secretion of bile, which carries waste products away from the liver. This supports the traditional use of barberry to combat liver disorders such as jaundice and gallstones.

Externally, barberry's anti-inflammatory properties make it a useful treatment for sore, swollen eyes, eczema, psoriasis, rheumatism, hepatitis and other inflammatory disorders. Recent laboratory studies in Bulgaria have confirmed the anti-inflammatory effect of berberine extracted from the barberry root.

Cultivation

Barberry prefers neutral or alkaline soil and can be grown in direct sunlight or light shade. It can be grown from seeds or from cuttings taken in summer. However, it is not advisable to cultivate it for use in homemade herbal preparations.

PREPARATION AND DOSAGE

Barberry should only be taken internally on the advice of a medical herbalist.

For external use
TO TREAT swollen eyes, skin inflammation
TINCTURE (1:3 in 25% alcohol)
Add 20 drops to a glass of water. Soak a cloth in this and squeeze out the excess. Apply to the closed eye for 15 minutes two or three times a day.

IF SYMPTOMS PERSIST, CONSULT A DOCTOR

CAUTIONS

• Barberry should never be taken except under supervision and for no longer than a period of 4-6 weeks.
• Barberry should not be taken during pregnancy.
• Do not take barberry to treat food poisoning or chronic heartburn.
• If using as an antibacterial, avoid vitamin B_6 and the amino acid L-histidine as they suppress barberry's efficacy.
• Berbamine and berberine have an anaesthetising effect, which can cause low blood pressure.

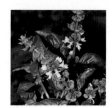

Basil

Ocimum basilicum Lamiaceae or Labiatae

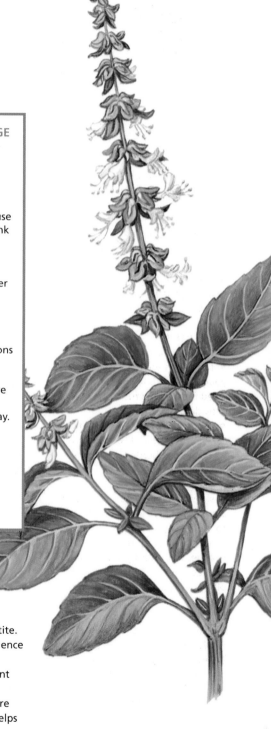

Although it is native to southern Asia, basil has long been grown in Europe as a culinary and medicinal herb. Its common name comes from the Greek word 'basilikon', which means royal, perhaps because it was prized as a king among herbs. Basil is an annual plant, growing to a height of about 40cm. Its square stems and soft leaves are hairy and aromatic. Its flowers are white, crimson or multicoloured and form whorls on the plant's flower spike.

Parts used

Leaves and flowerheads
- The leafy, flowering stems are harvested when the flowers first appear in summer right through to autumn.
- The leaves and flowerheads are then dried and blanched for use in infusions or decoctions.
- Alcoholic extracts taken from fresh flowerheads are an ingredient in ointments used to heal wounds.

Constituents

Basil contains an essential oil (up to 7ml a kg), whose major chemical constituents differ according to where the plant has been cultivated. The essential oil of the variety grown on the islands of the Indian Ocean has an estragole content of 65-85 per cent. The variety that is cultivated in southern Europe and Egypt produces an essential oil whose main component is linalool. Basil also contains tannins.

CAUTIONS
- Women who are pregnant or breastfeeding should avoid medicinal doses of basil.
- Basil should not be administered to babies or young children.
- Do not take medicinal doses of basil for long, unbroken periods.

PREPARATION AND DOSAGE

For external use

TO TREAT indigestion, loss of appetite, flatulence, bloating
INFUSION Put 4-6g of dried leaves into 250ml of boiling water. Cover and leave to infuse for 10 minutes and strain. Drink 1 cup without sugar a day.
In cases of chronic bloating, drink 2-5 cups a day between meals. Stop the treatment after a week and then re-start it a week later.

TO TREAT inflamed throats
DECOCTION Boil 2 dessertspoons of dried leaves in 250ml of water in a covered pan for 10-15 minutes. Strain and leave to cool. Use the liquid as a gargle two or three times a day.

For external use
TO TREAT wounds, cuts
OINTMENT Apply to affected area two or three times a day.

IF SYMPTOMS PERSIST, CONSULT A DOCTOR

Medicinal uses

Basil is known above all for its capacity to relieve spasms, especially stomach spasms. The leaves help digestion and improve the appetite. They are also used to treat flatulence and stomach bloating.

Externally, the plant's astringent qualities make it a useful cold remedy: in a gargle it relieves sore throats and as an inhalation it helps to clear the sinuses and air passages. As an ointment it can help to heal wounds and cuts, and is often combined with mint and caraway. The essential oil combats worms and germs. Indian clinical trials published in 1985 have demonstrated its antibacterial effects in acne sufferers.

Cultivation

Basil should be grown in rich, light soil that is well drained. It is also suited to dry soil. It needs a warm, sunny position in the garden, but can also be grown in a pot on a sunny kitchen windowsill.

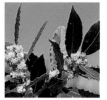

Bay

Laurus nobilis Lauraceae **Also called** Bay tree, Sweet bay, Laurel

This Mediterranean tree was much revered in Roman times. It was dedicated to Apollo and leafy twigs were made into the laurel crowns worn by emperors. Male and female flowers are carried on separate trees, which can reach 20m tall. In Britain, however, bay trees rarely reach more than 8m in height. The tough, oval leaves are pleasantly aromatic and used as a culinary flavouring. The flowers are yellow and the fruit is a black berry containing one seed.

Parts used
Leaves and berries
• The leaves are gathered from young branches in summer and then dried for use as infusions. They also provide an essential oil.
• The berries are collected when ripe in October and November and produce an oil called bay butter.

Constituents
Besides tannins and other active constituents, the leaves contain up to 3 per cent essential oil, which is composed of up to 70 per cent cineole. This oil is found in the berries which also contain lauric, oleic, palmitic and linoleic acids.

Medicinal uses
The oil of the bay tree has antiseptic, antifungal and stimulant properties. Externally, the oil is excellent as a rub for easing aches and pains, rheumatism, sprains and bruises. It also helps to soothe mouth ulcers and inflammation. It can be used (under medical supervision) to treat fungal infections.

When taken by mouth, the plant is traditionally used to treat digestive disorders, such as colic and stomach bloating. Studies published in 1997 in the *Journal of Ethnopharmacology* found that the seeds helped to prevent the formation of certain types of stomach ulcers in rats.

Cultivation
Bay grows best in well-drained soil in sun or light shade.

CAUTIONS
• Women who are pregnant or breastfeeding should avoid medicinal doses of bay.
• The essential oil should not be taken internally.
• External use may result in an allergic reaction. If it does, seek advice from a doctor or herbalist.

PREPARATION AND DOSAGE
For internal use
TO TREAT stomach disorders
INFUSION Put 5-10g of dried leaves into 1 litre of boiling water. Leave to infuse for 10 minutes and then filter. Drink 2-3 cups a day.

For external use
TO TREAT inflammation of the mouth and mouth ulcers
ESSENTIAL OIL Dilute, allowing 1 drop to 10ml of carrier oil. Apply three or four times a day.

TO TREAT rheumatism and general aches and pains
BAY BUTTER Apply to affected area two or three times a day as instructed on the label.

IF SYMPTOMS PERSIST, CONSULT A DOCTOR

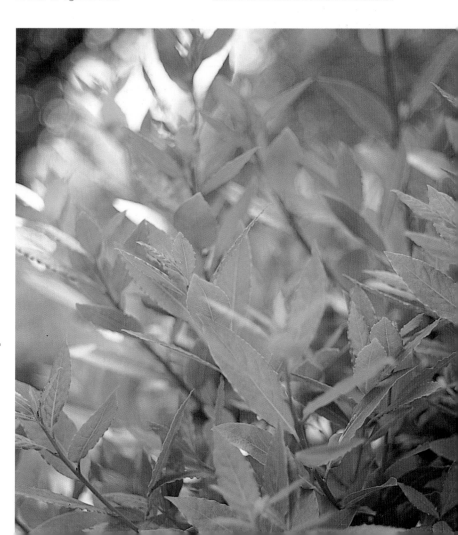

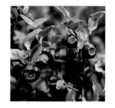

Bilberry

Vaccinium myrtillus Ericaceae **Also called** Whortleberry, Blaeberry

Preferring the damp, acidic soils of heaths, woods and moorland, bilberry is found throughout Europe. It is a low-growing shrub with oval, serrated leaves. Its white or pinkish flowers give way to purplish black, edible berries. Each berry is the size of a small pea and, when ripe, has a clearly visible depression at the top.

Parts used
Leaves and berries
- In summer the leaves are stripped from their branches, collected and then dried.
- The berries are gathered when ripe and usually used fresh.
- Both leaves and berries are used in infusions, powders and dry or liquid extracts.

Constituents
The berries contain anthocyanins, which strengthen and protect the capillaries, and vitamin C. Polyphenols (catechin) and tannins are also present. The leaves contain phenolic acids (caffeic acid) as well as tannins and iridoids.

Medicinal uses
Bilberry is often prescribed for vein and lymphatic disorders and to strengthen the capillaries. Studies performed in 1976 revealed that the beneficial effect on the small blood vessels is due to the anthocyanins in the berries, which increase the strength of the capillaries while reducing their permeability.

Anthocyanins are antioxidants and so, along with vitamin C, protect against damage from free radicals (present in the atmosphere and in food). Bilberry has been shown to be useful in treating eyesight problems. For example, it can improve the eye's ability to adapt to darkness. A clinical trial published in 1989 found that anthocyanins from bilberry plus vitamin E improved the symptoms of cataracts in older people.

Bilberry has been used to treat diarrhoea and inflammation of the digestive tract, as well as other inflammatory conditions. The leaves have been indicated in the treatment of diabetes.

Cultivation
The plant is commonly harvested from the wild and seldom cultivated. It grows in moist, acid soil in sun or light shade.

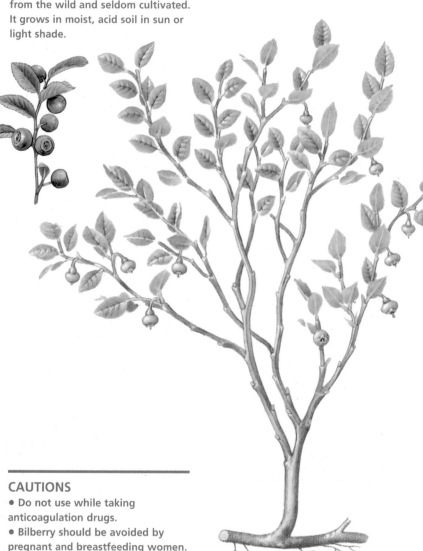

PREPARATION AND DOSAGE

For internal use
TO TREAT vein disorders, eyesight problems
TABLETS (60mg bilberry extract)
Take 1-3 tablets a day with water.
LIQUID EXTRACT Take 50 drops in a glass of water before meals.

IF SYMPTOMS PERSIST, CONSULT A DOCTOR

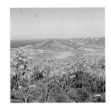

Bitter fennel

Foeniculum vulgare var. *vulgare* Umbelliferae/Apiaceae **Also called** Wild fennel

This tall perennial herb with feathery leaves is native to the Mediterranean and was cultivated in the ancient world. All parts of fennel smell strongly of aniseed and it has long been a popular culinary herb. Its tiny greenish yellow flowers grow in large, flat heads. The small, yellow-brown, flattened seeds have an aromatic odour and taste.

Parts used
Seeds
● The seeds are collected in autumn when they turn yellow.
● They are used whole or essential oil may be extracted from them.

Constituents
The essential oil makes up about 6 per cent of the seed and contains mainly anethole plus estragole and fenchone. The seeds contain phytosterols, flavonoids and coumarins.

Medicinal uses
Bitter fennel is traditionally used to ease problems of the digestive system such as constipation, spasms, irritable bowel, acid stomach, colic and flatulence, and the seeds may help to dissolve kidney stones.

Chewing the seeds is a remedy for bad breath and since fennel also has anti-inflammatory and antimicrobial properties, it is frequently used in natural toothpaste products.

Fennel is further reputed to help those wishing to lose weight by suppressing the appetite while stimulating the metabolism. It is also thought to relieve motion sickness and other types of nausea.

Bitter fennel has also been used to soothe inflamed eyes (in an eyewash) and sore throats. It is also an expectorant and because of its antispasmodic action can be used effectively to treat coughs.

It is believed to mimic oestrogen, which may explain why Indian women used it to stimulate lactation.

Cultivation
Plant in well-drained soil in full sun.

CAUTIONS
● Fennel may induce periods in menopausal women.
● Pregnant and breastfeeding women should not consume greater amounts than that found in food.
● Women with breast or uterine cancer should avoid fennel.
● Those allergic to carrots, celery or mugwort may have an adverse reaction when using fennel.
● Fennel may induce nausea and vomiting, fluid in the lungs and may cause sensitivity to sunlight.
● Avoid fennel if taking hormone replacement therapy.

PREPARATION AND DOSAGE

For internal use
TO TREAT digestive ailments
FENNEL WATER Take 5-15 drops in water once a day.
LIQUID EXTRACT Take 10-40 drops in water once a day.
INFUSION Add ½ teaspoon of crushed seeds to a cup of boiling water; cover and infuse for 10 minutes. Strain. Drink 1 cup three times a day.
CAPSULES (300mg) Take 2 capsules before meals.

For external use
TO TREAT eye irritation
EYEBATH A cold infusion of fennel (see above) may be used but it must be sterile. Otherwise use a commercial preparation.

IF SYMPTOMS PERSIST, CONSULT A DOCTOR

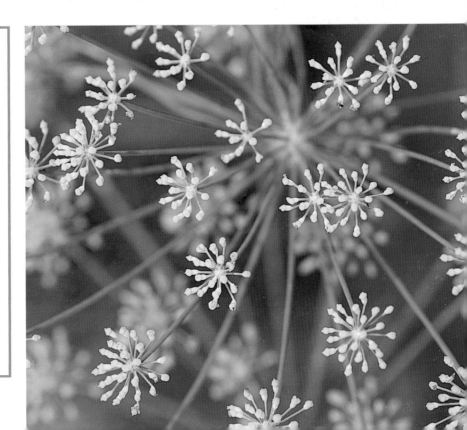

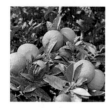

Bitter orange

Citrus aurantium Rutaceae **Also called** Seville orange

A native evergreen of India, bitter orange is now cultivated throughout the Mediterranean region. It can grow to a height of 10m. Its dark green leaves are shiny and tough, and have a distinctive winged leafstalk. Groups of sweet-smelling, white flowers emerge at the point where the leafstalks join the stem. The fruit is similar to a sweet orange, only smaller.

Parts used

Leaves, flowers and fruits (peel)
● The bitter-tasting leaves are gathered, then dried in the open air. They are mainly used for infusions.
● The strongly scented flowers are picked in the morning before they have fully opened, then dried out of direct sunlight. They are used to prepare orange flower water.
● The peel, which has a strong smell and very bitter taste, is taken from the fruit when it is not quite ripe and then dried in the open air. The essential oil and flavonoids are extracted from the peel, which is also rich in vitamin C.

Constituents

The leaves contain a small quantity of an essential oil called petitgrain. The essential oil from the flowers is called neroli. The oil from the peel is composed of 90 per cent limonene.

Medicinal uses

Bitter orange flowers are used to treat nervous agitation and minor sleeping difficulties. In 2002 Brazilian scientists showed that essential oil from the leaves enhanced the effects of barbiturates in prolonging sleep. The bitter leaves stimulate digestion and the flowers are antispasmodic and so relieve digestive disorders. The fruits have been used to treat headaches and heart palpitations.
   Bitter orange is also antibacterial, antifungal and anti-inflammatory, and has a diuretic action.

Cultivation

Plant in a sheltered, sunny spot in well-drained, nutrient-rich soil. The tree requires a good supply of water.

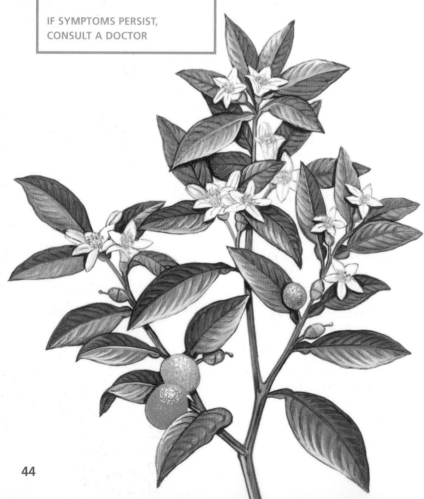

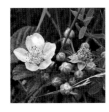

Blackberry

Rubus fructicosus Rosaceae **Also called** Bramble

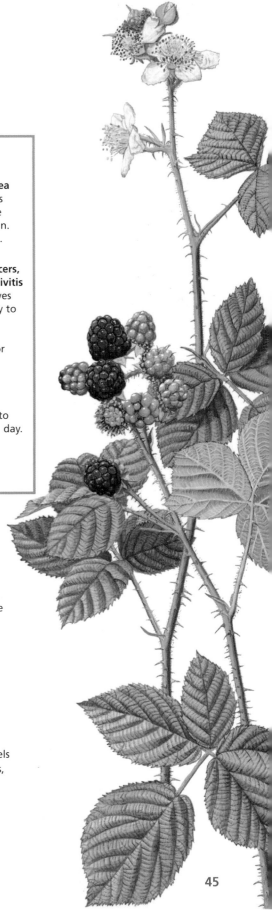

This sprawling perennial shrub with long flexible, thorny stems grows wild in hedgerows throughout Europe. Its leaves are made up of oval leaflets with serrated edges. Each leaflet has a vein running down the centre that is covered with fine prickles. Its white to pale pink flowers form clusters at the end of their stalks in summer. The sweet berries turn black as they ripen.

Parts used

Leaves and occasionally roots and berries

- Young tender leaves are gathered in spring before flowers appear.
- The leaves are dried and crushed into fragments for use in infusions and decoctions.
- Sometimes fresh leaves are used for external applications.
- The roots are collected in summer.
- The berries are collected as they ripen in autumn.

Constituents

The blackberry leaf is rich in tannins, organic acids, especially citric and isocitric acids, pentacyclic triterpenes and flavonoid glycosides of quercetin and kaempferol. The leaves and berries also contain vitamin C.

Medicinal uses

Blackberry has astringent, antiseptic, antifungal and tonic properties. The wealth of tannins provides its astringent qualities. It strengthens capillaries and is antibacterial. Blackberry leaves are taken internally to treat minor cases of diarrhoea.

CAUTIONS

- Blackberry leaves have no known adverse side effects when used in the prescribed therapeutic doses.
- Pregnant or breastfeeding women should avoid blackberry leaves.

PREPARATION AND DOSAGE

For internal use

TO TREAT minor cases of diarrhoea
INFUSION Put 1.5g of dried leaves into a cup of boiling water. Leave to infuse for 10 minutes and strain. Take 3 cups a day between meals.

For external use

TO TREAT sore throats, mouth ulcers, inflammation of the mouth, gingivitis
DECOCTION Put 10g of dried leaves into 100ml of water. Bring rapidly to the boil and leave to infuse for 15 minutes. Strain, sweeten with honey and use as a mouthwash or gargle twice a day.

TO TREAT skin ulcers, wounds
COMPRESS Soak a cloth in the decoction (see above) and apply to the affected area once or twice a day.

IF SYMPTOMS PERSIST, CONSULT A DOCTOR

Blackberry is also indicated for vaginal discharge and is reputed to have expectorant properties. The fragrant tea is prescribed for flu, colds and coughs.

Externally, a decoction of blackberry leaves is used as a gargle for sore throats, mouth ulcers and inflammation of the mouth and gums. It is also used to dress skin ulcers and wounds that are slow to heal. For these purposes blackberry leaves can be combined with agrimony, witch hazel and carob.

Research published in *Planta Medica* in 1980 showed that blackberry reduces blood sugar levels in both normal and diabetic rabbits, an effect partly due to its ability to stimulate the release of insulin.

Cultivation

Blackberry grows best in moist, well-drained soil.

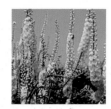

Black cohosh

Cimicifuga racemosa (Actaea racemosa) Ranunculaceae

The Native Americans have long known about the medicinal properties of black cohosh. They call it squaw root and use it to alleviate menstrual problems and the pain of childbirth. The plant originates from eastern North America where it can be seen growing on hillsides and in shady places on the edge of woods or hedgerows. The plant reaches about 2-3m in height.

Parts used
Root
• In autumn, after the fruits have ripened, the root is dug up, then cut and dried.
• The dried root is used for powder and tinctures, and to make dry and liquid extracts.

Constituents
The root is rich in compounds that mimic the effects of oestrogen. Anti-inflammatory and antioxidant triterpenoid glucosides are also present as well as salicylic acid, which acts in a similar way to aspirin. The root contains tannins, which are antibacterial and aid wound healing.

Medicinal uses
Black cohosh is prescribed for gynaecological problems, including periods (absent, painful or heavy), and to soothe premenstrual tension.

In 1998, a German review documented the benefits of black cohosh in the treatment of menopausal problems such as hot flushes and depression. In a 1987 trial, tablets containing black cohosh extract improved menopausal symptoms significantly, but whether this is due to oestrogenic action is not clear.

In 1998 Japanese scientists demonstrated the effects on blood vessels and arteries of piscidic acids – found in black cohosh – *in vitro* (laboratory tests). In earlier clinical studies in 1962 Italian researchers discovered that the plant could cause dilation of blood vessels without adversely affecting blood pressure levels.

In traditional Chinese medicine black cohosh is used to treat inflammation, pain and fever. The plant's anti-inflammatory properties, which suggest its potential use in the treatment of rheumatism, were reported in Planta Medica in 2000. Black cohosh also has a sedative effect and is beneficial in the treatment of anxiety. The plant has also been used to remedy coughs.

Cultivation
Grow in moist, rich soil, ideally in a lightly shaded position.

CAUTIONS
• In most studies, black cohosh has been shown to be safe, although there have been a few reports of adverse affects on the liver so it is important to take it only as prescribed by a medical herbalist.
• It should not be taken by women who are pregnant or breastfeeding.
• Women who have a history of breast cancer and other oestrogen-related cancers should also avoid it.
• Black cohosh should not be taken with other drugs that lower blood pressure, except on the advice of a medical herbalist.
• It should not be taken if you are allergic to aspirin.

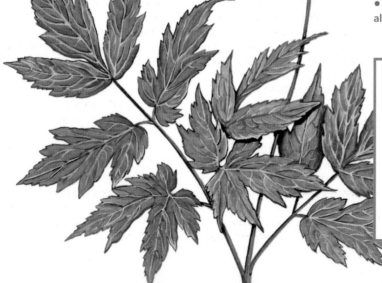

PREPARATION AND DOSAGE
Whether used in the form of a dry or liquid extract, a powder or in any other pharmaceutical preparation, a treatment based upon black cohosh should only ever be used in consultation with a medical herbalist.

IF SYMPTOMS PERSIST, CONSULT A DOCTOR

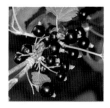

Blackcurrant

Ribes nigrum Grossulariaceae

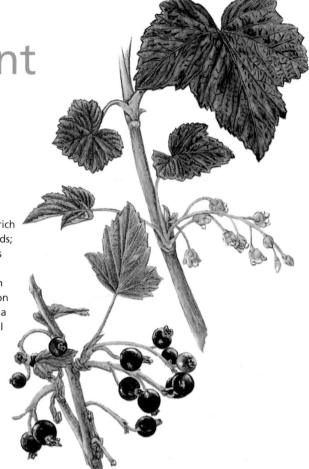

Found throughout Europe, except in the most northerly parts, blackcurrant is widely grown for its sweet black berries. A deciduous shrub, it can reach a height of 1.3m. Its aromatic leaves are coarsely toothed and have yellow oil-containing glands on their undersides. Small, green flowers form loose, hanging bunches in spring followed by the edible, sweet-smelling fruit.

Parts used

Fruit and leaves

- The leaves are gathered during April and May before flowering takes place.
- The berries are harvested during summer when they are ripe and dried very carefully, because they tend to rot quickly.
- Blackcurrant is used as infusions, extracts and powders. The berries and leaves are used to flavour numerous pharmaceutical products.

Constituents

Blackcurrant berries are rich in sugars and organic acids; they contain polyphenols (in particular, flavonoids and anthocyanins), which have a beneficial effect on veins. The leaves possess a small amount of essential oil and flavonoids. The anthocyanins and flavonoids are likely to account for the anti-inflammatory properties of blackcurrant and its ability to protect the blood vessels.

Medicinal uses

Blackcurrant has long been used to treat rheumatism and its anti-inflammatory effect has been demonstrated in research. In 1994 American researchers found blackcurrant seed oil to be a potentially effective treatment of rheumatoid arthritis. Scottish studies performed earlier in 1992 showed that the seed oil may help to treat inflammatory disorders. In the treatment of rheumatic pains, it can be used in combination with other herbal plants such as willow and devil's claw.

Blackcurrant can be used as a mouthwash for bleeding gums, or as a gargle for an inflamed mouth or throat.

Research has highlighted the protective effect of blackcurrant fruit on the capillaries, giving them elasticity and strength – the fruit is often prescribed for vein and arterial ailments, including varicose veins. Furthermore, blackcurrant is an ingredient in many medicines that improve blood circulation in the veins by keeping the blood thin.

Infections, including those of the urinary tract, can be treated with blackcurrant. Studies performed in 1976 found that anthocyanins in the fruit inhibit the growth of bacteria and in 2001 Japanese scientists found that they had an antiviral action on the influenza virus.

The berries are also rich in vitamin C which can help the body to fight off infections.

Cultivation

Plant in well-drained clay soil in a sunny or lightly shaded position.

PREPARATION AND DOSAGE

For internal use

TO TREAT vein and arterial ailments, urinary infections, rheumatic pains
INFUSION Put 5g of dried leaves into 1 litre of boiling water. Leave to infuse for 5 minutes, then strain. Drink 2-3 cups a day.
CAPSULES (340mg leaf powder combined with devil's claw and willow) Take 2 three times a day.
LEAF EXTRACT (combined with boldo and silver birch) Put 15-30 drops into a glass of water. Take two or three times a day.

IF SYMPTOMS PERSIST, CONSULT A DOCTOR

CAUTIONS

- When used in therapeutic doses, no toxic effects have been recorded.
- Do not use in combination with devil's claw if you have a gastric or duodenal ulcer.

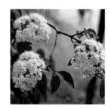

Black haw

Viburnum prunifolium Caprifoliaceae

This small tree, a native of the central and southern parts of the United States, is common in large forests and on dry, rocky slopes. From its bent trunk, which can reach 5m in height, grow stiff branches and downy twigs that are brilliant red when young but turn green as they age. The leaves are oval and sharply pointed. Black haw bears clusters of white flowers followed by blue-black berries.

Parts used

Trunk and root bark
● Bark is collected from the trunk and branches in spring and summer.
● Bark pieces about 1mm thick are used to make infusions, extracts and tinctures.
● The root bark is collected in autumn.

Constituents

The bark contains bioflavonoids, which keep capillary walls strong, antiviral and anti-inflammatory triterpenes and organic acids. It also contains tannins and the coumarin scopoletin, which acts as a relaxant on the uterus.

Medicinal uses

It has long been known that the bark of black haw has an antispasmodic effect on uterine muscle. It is therefore beneficial in treating period pains, heavy menstrual bleeding, colic and other abdominal cramps. Its anticoagulant and sedative properties are also helpful in this respect.

Other therapeutic properties include anti-inflammatory and anticlotting activity. It has been suggested that it can be used to remedy ulcers. The plant is prescribed for internal use to treat problems arising when

fragile skin capillaries are damaged, such as tiny haemorrhages just below the surface of the skin, as well as bruising and haemorrhoids.

The role of black haw in the treatment of cardiovascular ailments, particularly high blood pressure, is currently being investigated.

Cultivation

Suited to moist soil, black haw can be placed in sunny or slightly shady positions.

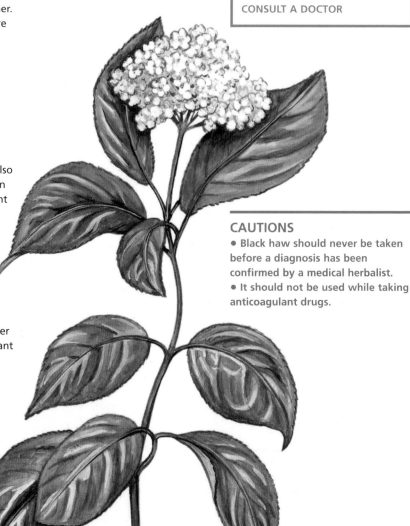

PREPARATION AND DOSAGE

For internal use

TO TREAT fragile skin capillaries, vein disorders, haemorrhoids, uterine spasms, painful periods

INFUSION Put 3 level teaspoons of bark into 500ml of boiling water. Leave to infuse for 10 minutes, then strain. Drink 2-3 cups a day.

TINCTURE (1:3 in 25% alcohol) Take 20 drops in a glass of water three times a day after meals.

LIQUID EXTRACT Put 20 drops into a glass of water. Take three times a day.

DRY EXTRACT Take 100-300mg three times a day.

IF SYMPTOMS PERSIST, CONSULT A DOCTOR

CAUTIONS

● Black haw should never be taken before a diagnosis has been confirmed by a medical herbalist.
● It should not be used while taking anticoagulant drugs.

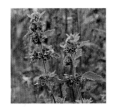

Black horehound

Ballota nigra Lamiaceae or Labiatae

Common in Europe, black horehound is distinguished by its unpleasant 'mouldy' smell. The Roman botanist Dioscorides recommended black horehound as an antidote for the bite of a mad dog. All parts of the plant are hairy, which probably accounts for its common name. In summer pinkish purple flowers are arranged in numerous whorls where the upper leaves meet the square, leafy stems.

Parts used

Flowers

● Collected in July and August, the flowers are dried, crushed into fragments and used for infusions, decoctions and tinctures.

● Black horehound is often combined with other sedative plants.

Constituents

The flowerheads contain phenyl-propanoids, especially verbascocide and forsythoside, which have sedative properties. Anti-inflammatory flavonoids are also found in black horehound.

Medicinal uses

Black horehound is recommended for nervous conditions, particularly insomnia (often combined with passionflower, lime and valerian), anxiety, irritability and nervous problems caused by the menopause.

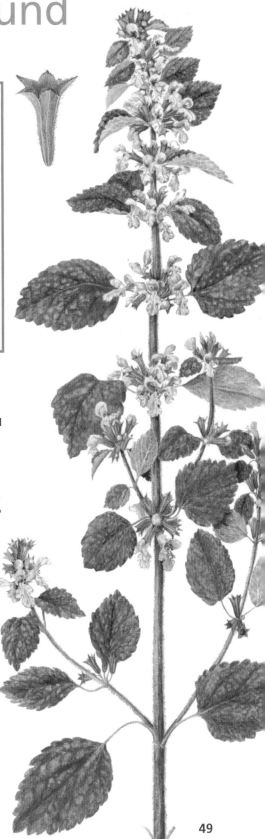

PREPARATION AND DOSAGE

For internal use

TO TREAT insomnia, anxiety, irritability, nervous problems caused by the menopause, coughing fits, whooping cough, stomach cramps and ringing in the ears

INFUSION Put 15-30g of black horehound flowers into 1 litre of boiling water. Leave to infuse for 10 minutes, then strain. Take 3 cups a day before meals.

TINCTURE Take 30 drops in a glass of water three times a day.

IF SYMPTOMS PERSIST, CONSULT A DOCTOR

Research published in 2000 by a team from the University of Lille, France, has confirmed the sedative and antioxidant properties of several of the phenylpropanoids found in black horehound.

Black horehound is antispasmodic and soothes coughing fits and stomach cramps. Preparations with a base of black horehound are used to treat whooping cough. The herb is also used to relieve nausea and vomiting, and ringing in the ears.

Cultivation

Prefers well-drained soil in sun or shade. The plant is harvested during flowering in summer.

CAUTIONS

● Black horehound contains furane and labdane derivatives which may damage the liver, and therefore the plant has to be used with the utmost care.

● It should not be used by women who are pregnant or breastfeeding.

● People with liver ailments should not use black horehound.

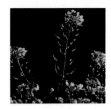

Black mustard

Brassica nigra Brassicaceae

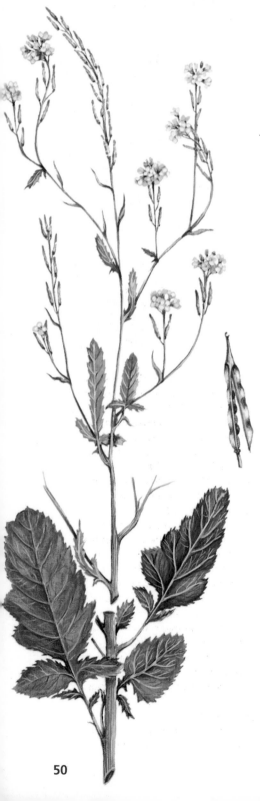

This annual herb is widespread in both Europe and Asia, where it has been grown as a condiment and for medicinal purposes for over 2000 years. The leaves at the base of its stem are serrated; those at the top are unserrated and narrower. Its flowers are yellow and the fruits are long seedpods, which contain little, spherical, blackish seeds.

Parts used

Flowerheads and seeds

• The flowerheads are harvested in early summer before they have bloomed fully. They are dried, crushed and used for infusions.
• The seeds are harvested in late summer, then dried and crushed. The black mustard powder that results is used in poultices.

Constituents

Mustard seeds contain lipids that are rich in unsaturated fatty acids, such as erucic, oleic and linoleic acids. The seeds also contain glucosinolates, especially sinigrin, as well as different kinds of mucilage.

Medicinal uses

Black mustard seed has a warming effect since it improves the circulation by dilating the blood vessels. In the same way it is able to relieve pain caused by inflammation. These properties lead to its use externally in poultices for the treatment of bronchitis, rheumatic and joint pains, and influenza.

When used internally, black mustard is recommended in small doses to restore lost appetite and cure indigestion. The glucosinolates in black mustard are currently being investigated for their potential as agents that inhibit the development of cancer. But it is not yet known if they are as effective as those present in other plants of the brassica family such as broccoli.

Cultivation

Plant in well-drained, nutrient-rich soil in a sunny location.

CAUTIONS

• Use poultices with care: if they are applied with too high a dosage or for too long a time they can cause intense pain, blisters and irreversible damage to skin tissue.
• Mustard must not be used on broken skin or near the eyes.
• Patients with serious circulatory problems, respiratory diseases or vein disorders such as varicose veins should not use these preparations.
• Mustard preparations are not recommended for children.

PREPARATION AND DOSAGE

For internal use

TO TREAT loss of appetite, indigestion

INFUSION Put 1 teaspoon of flowerheads (1.5g) into a cup of boiling water. Leave to infuse for 5 minutes, then strain. Take 3 cups a day.

For external use

TO TREAT bronchitis, rheumatic and joint pains, influenza

POULTICE Mix 50g of fresh black mustard powder with 200g of flax powder. Add enough lukewarm water to make a thick paste, then wrap in a cloth. Place the poultice on the affected area for about 10 minutes.

IF SYMPTOMS PERSIST, CONSULT A DOCTOR

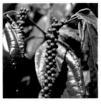

Black pepper

Piper nigrum Piperaceae

This woody perennial climber originates in South-east Asia, where its culinary and medicinal properties have been known for 4000 years. Its leaves are unlobed, thick and shaped like spearheads. The small lateral branches sprout roots, which enable the plant to grip as it climbs. Its small white flowers form long spikes and are followed by green fruits that ripen to reddish brown.

Parts used

Fruits

● The fruits are picked when ripe from plants that must be at least three years old. After drying in the sunshine, they turn black.

● A pungent essential oil is extracted from the seeds. It is the oil that is usually employed medicinally although the seeds can also be used.

Constituents

As much as 2.5 per cent of the black pepper seed consists of the pungent, greeny yellow essential oil. The seed is rich in the alkaloid piperine (5 to 9 per cent).

PREPARATION AND DOSAGE

For internal use

TO TREAT sluggish digestion
INFUSION Put 3g of pepper seeds into 150ml of boiling water. Flavour with mint. Leave to infuse for 5-10 minutes, then strain. Take two or three times a day.

For external use

TO TREAT rheumatism
CREAM (with a base of essential oil) Rub into the painful areas two or three times a day.

IF SYMPTOMS PERSIST, CONSULT A DOCTOR

Medicinal uses

Black pepper stimulates digestion and in Europe it is taken orally to treat sluggish digestion, flatulence, bloating and lack of appetite. Its antispasmodic properties make it useful for treating stomach cramps.

CAUTIONS

● Black pepper seeds present no immediate dangers although excessive intake can have an adverse effect on the liver.

● Pure essential oil must only be taken on a doctor's prescription.

● Seek medical advice before using black pepper when taking other drugs. For example, it should not be taken with blood-thinning agents.

● It is not recommended for pregnant or breastfeeding women.

Black pepper has long been used to soothe rheumatic pains, a use that is supported by Indian research in 1990, which showed that piperine inhibits inflammation. Applied externally, black pepper produces a warming and reddening of the skin (and considerable temporary irritation), which eventually leads to an anaesthetic effect.

In 2000, UK researchers found that black pepper had antibacterial properties since it was shown to effectively combat the bacteria responsible for food poisoning.

Piperine can strengthen the effect of numerous other medicines, herbal remedies and spices. Therefore it is important to seek advice from a doctor or qualified herbalist before taking medicinal doses of black pepper in addition to other drugs.

Cultivation

The plant thrives in rich, moist soil and temperatures above 15°C.

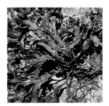

Bladderwrack

Fucus vesiculous Fucaceae **Also called** Kelp

Found in abundance on the rocky coastlines of cold and temperate seas, bladderwrack is characterised by its brownish green fronds that bear numerous fluid-filled bulges or 'bladders'. The fronds can be up to 1m long.

Parts used

Frond or thallus
• Bladderwrack is collected from the coasts of the English Channel and the Atlantic in early to midsummer.
• It is dried for use in powders, capsules, tablets, suspensions, gels and massage creams.

Constituents

The main component of bladderwrack is alginic acid. The salts, called alginates, produce a sticky solution in water. Bladderwrack also contains polysaccharides, minerals (notably iodine) and a wide range of trace elements, including chromium.

Medicinal uses

Bladderwrack is an appetite suppressant and has long been used to treat obesity. Its iodine content supports the function of the thyroid gland, which needs iodine to make its hormone thyroxine.

Bladderwrack possesses anti-inflammatory properties and is used to treat inflammatory bladder conditions, as well as rheumatism. The alginates in bladderwrack have a protective effect on the mucous membrane of the stomach lining and help to reduce acid reflux.

Used externally, bladderwrack moisturises dry skin and is reputed to possess antibacterial qualities. In 2002 Japanese researchers found that a daily application of seaweed extract improved the thickness and elasticity of the skin.

Cultivation

Bladderwrack is gathered from the wild but it should not be collected from polluted shores. Commercially sustainable harvesting is important to protect the plant.

CAUTIONS
• Prolonged use can lead to intolerance, the main symptom being the painful dilatation of the thyroid gland. This should disappear once you stop taking bladderwrack.
• Bladderwrack can aggravate acne.
• It should not be used during pregnancy or breastfeeding, nor by children under the age of 12.
• Do not take with aspirin and other blood-thinning preparations.
• Consult a medical herbalist before taking bladderwrack if you have a thyroid problem.

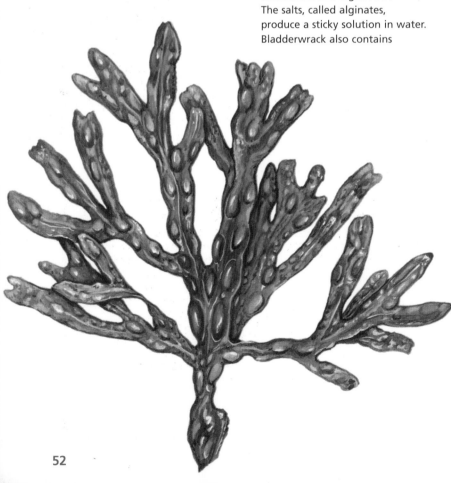

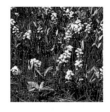

Bogbean

Menyanthes trifoliata Menyanthaceae **Also called** Buckbean

*As its name suggests, bogbean
thrives in wet places – by ponds
and lakes, and in ditches and
marshes throughout Europe. It has
short, soft, creeping stems and thick,
scaly rhizomatous roots. Its leaves
are made up of three oval leaflets
and its pink-and-white star-shaped
flowers form funnel-shaped spikes.
The fruit is a round capsule
containing bright yellow oval seeds.*

Parts used
Leaves
● Bogbean leaves are collected at
the beginning of the flowering
season in May and June.
● The leaves can be used fresh
or are dried for use.

Constituents
The plant contains numerous active
components, including bitter
phenolic acids, flavonoids and
tannins.

Medicinal uses
Traditionally bogbean is used to
stimulate the appetite and promote
digestion as its bitter taste
encourages gastric and salivary
secretions. Research published in
Planta Medica in 1986 confirmed
that the phenolic acids in bogbean
has confirmed this effect. Bogbean
is also a laxative and diuretic.

The anti-inflammatory properties
of the plant mean that it is indicated
in the treatment of rheumatic
conditions. Research has also
confirmed its anti-inflammatory
activity and explored the way it
works on the body's metabolism.

The plant's capacity to regulate
the menstrual cycle, for which it has
been traditionally used, has been
the subject of many studies. As yet
researchers have not been able to
produce any convincing results.

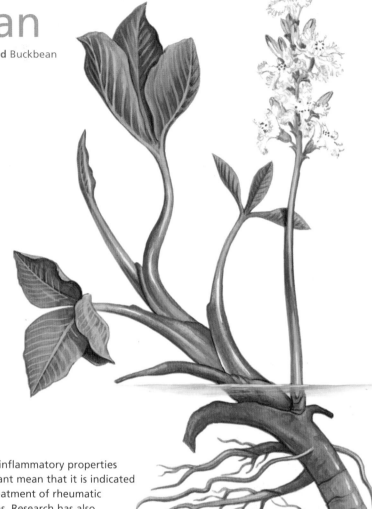

CAUTIONS
● In large amounts bogbean could
cause vomiting. Never take more
than 6g – 15 (400mg) capsules – in
the course of one day.
● It is not recommended if you
have diarrhoea, or an infection or
inflammation of the intestine.
● Bogbean is not suitable for
women who are pregnant or
breastfeeding.

Cultivation
This aquatic plant prefers to be
planted in shallow, acidic water or
wet soil. A sunny location is best.

PREPARATION AND DOSAGE
For internal use
**TO TREAT loss of appetite,
constipation, sluggish digestion**
INFUSION Put 1-2g of dried leaf
into 500ml of boiling water and
leave to infuse for 15 minutes.
Drink 3 cups a day.
**CAPSULES (350-400mg of
powder)** Take 3-6 at intervals
throughout the day to a
maximum of 15 a day.

IF SYMPTOMS PERSIST,
CONSULT A DOCTOR

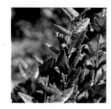

Boldo

Peumus boldus Monimiaceae

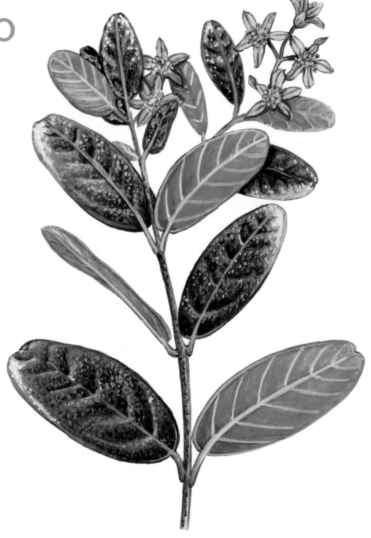

This evergreen shrub, a native of Chile, is now cultivated in Italy and North Africa, particularly Morocco. It grows to 4-5m in height and has rough, brittle, greyish green leaves, which give off a camphor-like smell when crushed. Clusters of pale yellow flowers are followed by small black berries.

Parts used

Leaves and bark
- The leaves are dried and crushed and taken as infusions.
- Boldo leaves are also used in various pharmaceutical products that stimulate bile secretion.
- The bark is collected for boldine, the alkaloid substance it contains.

Constituents

The leaves are rich in the volatile oils ascaridole, cineole and camphor – which gives it its distinctive aroma. Both leaves and bark contain flavonoids – cancer-fighting antioxidants; and various alkaloids, the main one being boldine.

Medicinal uses

Boldo is widely used in herbal medicine to treat gallstones and for various liver, stomach and digestive disorders. The active constituent, boldine, stimulates bile secretion and reduces gall-bladder inflammation.

Boldo has a soothing effect on the lining of the bladder, and antiseptic properties, and so can help cystitis sufferers. In Chile the herb has long been utilised as a cure for syphilis and gonorrhoea and is also used to get rid of parasitic worms. In Brazil, the herb is taken to eliminate gas and bloating, for digestive and liver complaints and as a diuretic. It has also been used traditionally to treat ailments including rheumatism, gout, jaundice, colds and earaches.

Boldo has been clinically proven to aid digestion and is often combined with other plants such as fumitory and rosemary to treat dyspepsia.

Cultivation

Plant in sandy well-drained soil. The shrub prefers a sunny position and an acidic soil.

CAUTIONS

- Boldo should not be used during pregnancy as it may be associated with a risk of miscarriage.
- To date no toxicity or undesirable side effects have been recorded.
- Do not use boldo if you have kidney or liver disease or gallstones.

PREPARATION AND DOSAGE

For internal use

TO TREAT dyspepsia
INFUSION Put 1 teabag (2g) into 200ml of boiling water. Leave to infuse for 10 minutes. Take up to 3 infusions a day.
LIQUID EXTRACT Take 1 teaspoon diluted in a little water in the mornings on an empty stomach and at night just before going to bed.

IF SYMPTOMS PERSIST, CONSULT A DOCTOR

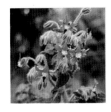

Borage

Borago officinalis Boraginaceae

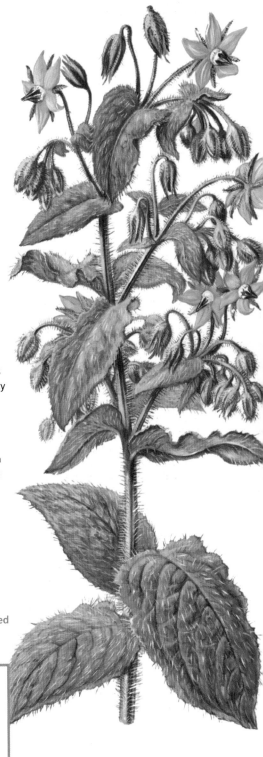

A rampant herbaceous annual, borage is the bane of many a gardener. It tends to grow on rough ground or at the roadside – but it loves flowerbeds too. The whole plant is covered with prickly hairs and grows up to 60cm tall. In summer, bright blue flowers appear followed by little nut-like fruits, each containing a seed.

Parts used

Flowers, leaves and seeds
- The flowers contain a diuretic.
- The seeds are commercially harvested and crushed for their oil.
- The fresh leaves, which have a mild cucumber-like taste, can be used to flavour summer punches.

Constituents

Both leaves and flowers are rich in diuretic minerals. The plant also contains a substance called mucilage. This is a demulcent, which means it soothes and relieves the pain of inflamed mucous membranes. The oil, extracted from the seeds, is rich in unsaturated fatty acids.

However, the leaves and flowers have been found to contain pyrrolizidine alkaloids, substances thought to damage the liver and cause cancer. The European Commission is currently considering banning the sale of all species of borage that contain these alkaloids.

Medicinal uses

Traditionally, borage flowers were used for their sweat-inducing, soothing and diuretic effects. In 1989, Canadian researchers found that borage reduced the effect of stress on the cardiovascular system. It is also said to soothe the throat and possess expectorant properties.

Polyunsaturated fats found in borage seed oil are believed to be beneficial for some skin ailments, such as the loss of elasticity and dryness that result from ageing. The seed oil may also have anti-inflammatory properties: it contains g-linolenic acid, an unsaturated fatty acid, which was shown in 1993 by US researchers in Pennsylvania, to be an effective treatment for rheumatoid arthritis. The oil may help to combat lung disease, too: in 1997 American scientists found that borage oil in combination with fish oil helped to prevent inflammation caused by acute lung injury in rats.

Cultivation

This hardy plant grows best in a sunny location from seeds planted in spring and will then self-sow in the same spot. However, it should only be taken medicinally as directed by a medical herbalist.

CAUTIONS
- Do not use borage without consulting a doctor or medical herbalist, as it contains potentially harmful pyrrolizidine alkaloids.
- Do not use borage as an infusion.
- Borage should not be taken when pregnant or breastfeeding.
- People suffering from epilepsy schizophrenia, or those taking phenothiazine tranquillisers should not use borage.
- The hairy leaves and stems may cause contact dermatitis.

> ### PREPARATION AND DOSAGE
> **Borage preparations should only be used in consultation with a qualified medical herbalist.**
>
> IF SYMPTOMS PERSIST, CONSULT A DOCTOR

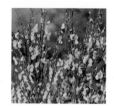

Broom

Cytisus scoparius Leguminosae-Papilionoideae **Also called** Common Broom, Scotch Broom

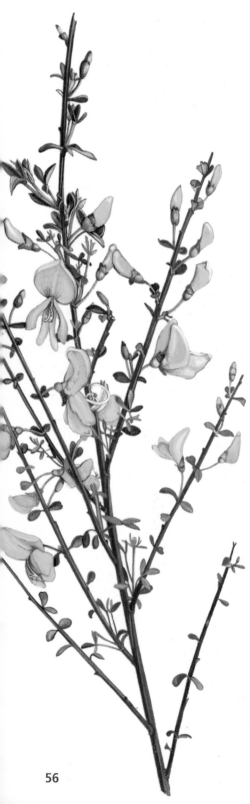

Growing wild all over Europe, broom is a tough perennial shrub that thrives on scrubby moorland. Long, flexible branches grow in bundles from its stems – a fact that made it useful for broom-making, hence the name. Sweetly scented flowers bloom in May and June, followed by downy seedpods. On hot July days you may hear loud crackling as hundreds of pods snap open to fling their seeds away.

Parts used

Flowerheads

- Blooms are gathered just as they open in May and June.
- Flowers are dried carefully to stop them from turning black and losing their active constituents.
- Dried broom is used in infusions, tinctures or liquid extracts.
- Broom is often combined with other plants.

Constituents

The flowers are rich in carotenoids and flavonoids – both of which are antioxidants, known to help to prevent cardiovascular disease and fight cancer. The flowers also contain small amounts of powerful alkaloids including a sedative called sparteine, dopamine and tyramine.

CAUTIONS

- Use broom under medical herbalist supervision: it can have toxic effects.
- Do not use during pregnancy or if breastfeeding.
- Do not use if you have high blood pressure.
- An overdose may cause dizziness, vomiting, diarrhoea and palpitations.
- The alkaloid tyramine can trigger a harmful interaction if used with certain antidepressants, particularly monoamine oxidase inhibitors.

Medicinal uses

The flavonoids in broom are diuretic making the plant useful for treating oedema – in which body tissues swell due to water retention. Broom can also be used to improve or re-establish urine flow that has been reduced by illness (oliguria).

The sedative, sparteine, has a documented effect on the heartbeat, and broom is used to treat mild cases of irregular heartbeat (medically known as arrhythmia). A 1995 study in Canada found that patients taking sparteine had a reduced risk of ventricular fibrillation – a life-threatening weakness in the heartbeat that can follow a heart attack or an electric shock.

The tyramine in broom constricts blood vessels; preparations made using a combination of broom, black haw and juniper are used to treat varicose veins and poor circulation.

Cultivation

Sow ripe seeds in well-drained soil in a sunny position. Prune immediately after flowering.

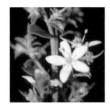

Buchu

Agathosma betulina Rutaceae **Also called** Round buchu

A native of the mountainous regions of South Africa, the round buchu is a small, bushy shrub. Its bright, greeny yellow oval leaves are covered in little depressions that hold the plant's aromatic essential oil. White or pink flowers and egg-shaped fruits appear when the leaves drop in autumn.

Parts used
Leaves
● The leaves are harvested in summer.
● They can be used alone or with other diuretic plants.

Constituents
The essential oil from round buchu leaves is rich in pulegone and diosphenol, colloquially known as 'buchu camphor'. These give it its strong, distinctive aroma, reminiscent of blackcurrant, but also similar to a combination of rosemary and peppermint. The oil also contains flavonoids and mucilage.

Medicinal uses
Round buchu is mainly used to treat bladder problems and urinary tract infections such as cystitis, urethritis and prostatitis. The leaf also contains mucilage, which soothes inflamed mucous membranes, making it good for soothing the inflamed airways of chronic bronchitis. It is also used to treat rheumatism and gout.

The leaf oil is well known for its diuretic and antiseptic qualities, which are attributed to the volatile oil, diosphenol.

Buchu can help to ease digestive problems: UK research in London demonstrated its antispasmodic properties in laboratory animal studies in 2001. In traditional medicine, the leaf is used as a carminative, to expel wind from the gut. It also relieves the bloating associated with premenstrual syndrome. It is usually combined with other plants such as barberry, yarrow or marsh mallow.

Cultivation
Propagate buchu from seeds or cuttings. Plant established shrubs in a well-drained, sunny position ideally in an acid soil. Water on very hot days and during dry spells.

CAUTIONS
● Do not use buchu if you have a history of serious kidney disease.
● Pulegone, a constituent of the essential oil, is toxic in large doses.
● Avoid buchu if pregnant – pulegone is a uterine stimulant.
● Do not use buchu if you are taking blood-thinning agents such as Warfarin.
● Diuretics cause potassium loss, but this can be offset by eating plenty of fresh fruit and vegetables.

PREPARATION AND DOSAGE
For internal use:
TO TREAT cystitis
INFUSION Place 1 sachet (2g) into a cup of boiling water. Drink 1 cup up to three times a day before meals.
CAPSULES (350g) Take 1 capsule with a large glass of water twice daily at meal times.
TINCTURE Take 40 drops in a glass of water three times a day before meals.

IF SYMPTOMS PERSIST, CONSULT A DOCTOR

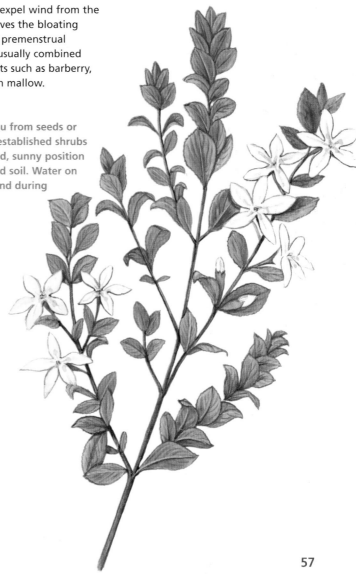

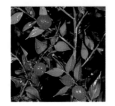

Butcher's broom

Ruscus aculeatus Ruscaceae **Also called** Knee holly

Found throughout southern England and Wales, butcher's broom is a low woody shrub. Butchers used to sweep their blocks with bundles of its branches, hence its name. The evergreen 'leaves' are not true leaves but a widening of the stem. A tiny white flower appears in the middle of each leaf in spring, followed in autumn by a red, cherry-like berry. Each leaf is tipped with a spike and, because the plant reaches about knee-height, has been nicknamed knee holly.

Parts used

Rhizome
• Knotty rhizomes, grey and ringed with grooves, are dug up in autumn.
• Once dried, they are ground into powder or made into extracts.
• They are used in tablets, capsules, drinkable solutions and creams.

Constituents

The active components of butcher's broom are substances known as steroidal saponins. These have beneficial effects on the veins, improving blood circulation, and also possess anti-inflammatory properties.

Medicinal uses

When taken orally, the saponins in butcher's broom have the effect of contracting superficial blood vessels (the veins near the skin's surface).

Studies on human patients have shown that butcher's broom improves poor circulation in the veins of the lower limbs and reduces haemorrhoids. The plant is therefore recommended as a treatment for stiff, aching legs, varicose veins and piles. It can be combined with other plants that help to protect veins and capillaries, such as witch hazel.

Butcher's broom is a good remedy for oedema (swelling). German clinical trials published in 2002 found that extracts of butcher's broom reduced lower leg oedema in women who suffered chronic vein problems as a result of poor circulation. The study authors concluded that this was a safe and effective treatment for this condition. In 1988, Italian researchers reached the same conclusion, also highlighting the plant's beneficial effects on veins in the lower limbs. Butcher's broom can also help to combat vein problems associated with premenstrual syndrome and taking oral contraception.

The rhizome is a mild laxative and a cure for cramp. It also has diuretic and anti-inflammatory properties.

Cultivation

Butcher's broom is very hardy. It thrives in sun and shade and likes a dryish soil. It is grown from seed or by dividing the roots in autumn.

DOSAGE

For internal use
TO TREAT premenstrual syndrome, stiff, aching legs, varicose veins, haemorrhoids, cramp, oedema
CAPSULES (50mg) Take 1 capsule with a large glass of water three times a day at mealtimes.

For external use
TO TREAT stiff, aching legs varicose veins
CREAM Massage into the legs, as directed, once a day, starting at the ankles and moving up to the thighs.

IF SYMPTOMS PERSIST, CONSULT A DOCTOR

CAUTIONS

• Do not use if pregnant or breastfeeding.
• Overdose may cause vomiting and low blood pressure.
• Do not use if taking monoamine oxidase inhibitors (antidepressants), or drugs for high blood pressure or an enlarged prostate gland.
• No adverse effects have been reported, but it is recommended that you consult your medical herbalist before using.

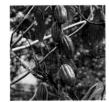

Cacao

Theobroma cacao Sterculiaceae **Also called** Chocolate tree

Reaching an average height of 4-5m, the cacao tree is a native of central America. It bears leaves, flowers and fruit all year round. Its small reddish flowers grow on the surface of the trunk and branches, and the pods grow directly on the bark. They contain white pulp and 20-40 seeds – the cacao beans.

Parts used

Beans

• The beans are processed by roasting and crushing, so as to extract the cacao.

• Most cacao is used in chocolate and other foods.

• Some derivatives, such as cocoa butter, are used in pharmacology and in the cosmetics industry.

Constituents

The beans are made up of between 40 to 60 per cent solid fat – the cacao butter. This is composed of fatty acids (palmitic, stearic and oleic acids) and triglycerides. The levels of these compounds vary according to where the cacao is grown. The beans also contain the stimulants theobromine and caffeine, plus proteins, flavonoids, minerals (mainly magnesium), and polyphenols and procyanidins, both of which combat excessive free radicals. Fermenting the beans releases their aroma.

CAUTIONS

• Susceptible individuals may find that cacao triggers migraines.

• Cacao may cause constipation.

• Consult a doctor before using cacao if you are taking prescribed drugs, especially monoamine oxidase inhibitors (antidepressants) and theophylline, a bronchiodilator.

• Do not use if you suffer from an inflammatory bowel condition or heart disorder.

Medicinal uses

Although regarded mainly as a delicious food, cacao is also a tonic – it appears to boost serotonin and endorphin levels in the brain, which has an uplifting effect.

The beans contain polyphenols – antioxidants that help to prevent cancer, heart disease and wrinkles. Japanese research in 2000 showed the ability of polyphenols to inhibit the oxidation of harmful low density lipoprotein (LDL) cholesterol; high levels of LDL often indicate a higher risk of heart disease.

The flavonoids in cacao also benefit the circulatory system. In 2000, American scientists showed that they help to combat the formation of blood clots and have a blood-thinning aspirin-like effect.

The anti-inflammatory action of procyanidin was illustrated by an *in vitro* study published in the *Journal of Nutrition* in 2000.

Used externally, cacao butter is recommended as a treatment for rough skin, sore nipples (caused by breastfeeding) and chapped lips.

Cultivation

The cacao tree thrives only in hot climates, where it prefers a fertile, well-drained moist soil and a shady position.

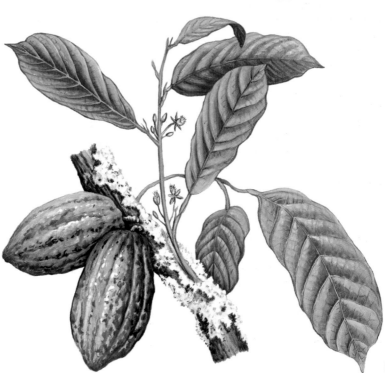

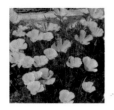

Californian poppy

Eschscholzia californica Papaveraceae

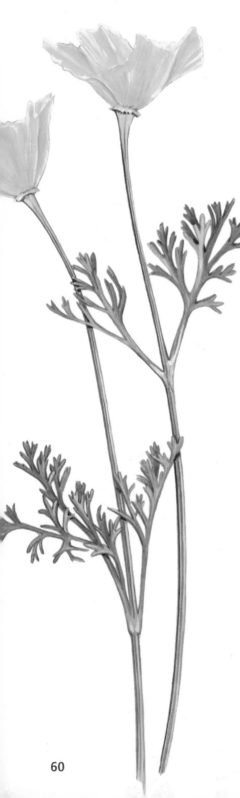

A perennial in its native United States, Californian poppy grows as an annual or biennial in Europe, where it has been cultivated since its introduction in 1790. Its attractive flowers have made it a favourite with gardeners. The erect stem grows to a height of 60cm and is covered in long, serrated, bluish green leaves, and crowned with a solitary orange, yellow, pink or red flower in summer. The fruit, a lined capsule, splits itself open when ripe, scattering the seeds.

Parts used

Stems, leaves and flowers

● The aerial parts – stems, leaves and flowers – are collected from July to September.

● These are then dried and broken into fragments to be used for making infusions, liquid extracts, capsules and tinctures.

● Californian poppy is often combined with other sedative plants, such as passionflower and valerian, in herbal preparations.

PREPARATION AND DOSAGE

For internal use

TO TREAT sleeping problems, nervous exhaustion, bedwetting

INFUSION Put 1 teaspoon of the dried plant into a cup of boiling water. Leave to infuse for 10 minutes. Strain. Drink 1-2 cups in the evening.

LIQUID EXTRACT Take 1-2ml in a glass of water in the evening.

CAPSULES (50-75mg dry extract) Take 1-2 capsules just before going to bed.

TINCTURE (1:4 in 45% alcohol) Take 10 drops, three times a day in a little cold water after meals, and up to 20 drops at bedtime.

IF SYMPTOMS PERSIST, CONSULT A DOCTOR

Constituents

The Californian poppy, like all members of the Papaveraceae family of plants, contains a large number of alkaloids. It is also rich in flavonoids, including the various carotenoids, that are responsible for the bright colours of its flowers.

Medicinal uses

Californian poppy preparations are widely recommended for the treatment of nervous disorders and for repeated bedwetting in children. Taken orally, they have long been used to help to induce sleep and to facilitate a deeper level of sleep – actions supported by animal research published in *Planta Medica* in 1991. The plant is used either on its own or in conjunction with valerian, passionflower and olive tree.

Californian poppy is also reputed to have anti-inflammatory and antispasmodic properties.

Cultivation

A hardy plant, the Californian poppy can be grown easily from seed, planted either from spring to early summer, or towards the end of summer. It thrives in well-drained, sandy soil and prefers to be placed in a warm, sunny position.

CAUTIONS

● It is advisable to consult a medical herbalist before taking the plant.

● Because of the sedative effect of Californian poppy, you should avoid operating machinery or driving a car while taking it.

● Californian poppy preparations should not be taken when pregnant.

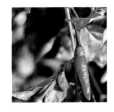

Capsicum

Capsicum fructescens Solanaceae **Also called** Cayenne, Chilli, Hot pepper, Tabasco pepper

Native to tropical America, the capsicum is now grown successfully as an annual in temperate parts of the world. This little perennial shrub is no taller than 70cm. Slender branches shoot out from the main stem, bearing oval leaves. The long, thin fruits, known as peppers, can reach a length of 50cm in certain varieties. The peppers are green at first, progressing to orange then bright red as they ripen.

Parts used

Fruit (pepper)
● The peppers are harvested from June to September, when ripe.
● They are dried at a temperature below 35°C, then used to make tinctures, powders and capsules, poultices and ointments.

Constituents

The hot spicy taste is imparted by capsaicinoids, particularly capsaicin – first isolated from the plant in 1876. Carotenoids constitute 0.3-0.8 per cent of the pepper, and are responsible for its bright colour.

The peppers are also rich in vitamin C and contain saponins, which are thought to be able to kill bacteria.

CAUTIONS

● Capsicum should not be taken at the same time as drugs for lowering blood pressure or certain types of antidepressants. Take medical advice before using it.
● Avoid capsicum when pregnant or breastfeeding.
● Take care that capsicum does not come into contact with sensitive areas, such the lips, mouth and eyes.
● Do not apply to broken skin.
● Consult a doctor or medical herbalist if suffering from gastric problems, before using capsicum.

Medicinal uses

Taken internally, capsicum stimulates the digestive system, and is used to treat indigestion, flatulence, colic and constipation.

Capsaicin acts to reduce pain and inflammation when capsicum is used externally for conditions such as lumbago, arthritis, general muscle and joint pain, and skin irritations. The capsaicin in capsicum improves the circulation, which promotes healing by helping to remove toxins from and deliver nutrients to the affected area. Capsicum is also applied to the scalp in poultices with the aim of preventing hair loss.

Because of the antiseptic and anti-inflammatory effects of its saponins, capsicum is also used in a gargle to treat laryngitis.

Cultivation

Capsicum grows best in a greenhouse or sunny site, at temperatures above 18°C. Plant the seeds in well-drained soil that is rich in nutrients.

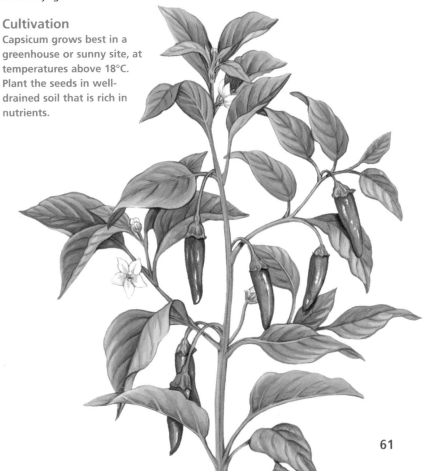

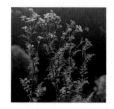

Caraway

Carum carvi Apiaceae

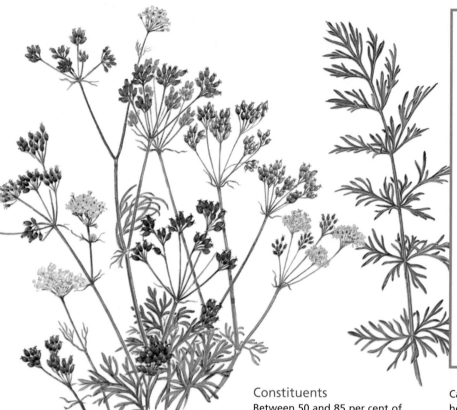

With its feathery leaves and umbrella-like clusters of tiny white flowers, caraway is a pretty and popular garden herb. It grows to about 1m in height and bears deep brown seeds with a distinctive smell. Caraway is used to flavour digestive liqueurs and spirits such as the German Kümmel.

Parts used
Seeds
• Caraway seeds are gathered in July and August just before they ripen.
• The seeds are often confused with cumin seeds.
• Caraway is used in herbal medicine throughout Europe in infusions and as essential oil.

Constituents
Between 50 and 85 per cent of caraway's volatile essential oil is carvone, which is antiseptic and gives the seed its distinctive flavour. Limonene makes up another 20 per cent and there are also flavonoids.

Medicinal uses
People have used caraway as a digestive herb for thousands of years. It stimulates the secretion of gastric juices and encourages the expulsion of wind. In Europe, caraway has long been combined with fennel and anise in an infusion to treat intestinal cramps, bloating and other uncomfortable ailments such as flatulence.

Research published in 1985 found evidence for caraway's helpful effect on painful gut cramp: it proved that caraway oil relaxed intestinal muscle. It also has this effect on uterine muscles, and so relieves period pains.

Carvone's antibacterial properties help to fight off gut infections. In traditional Arabic medicine, caraway is a treatment for incontinence in children. As an expectorant, caraway can ease a chesty cough. And its oil has been applied to clear up scabies.

Cultivation
Sow seeds or plant seedlings in a well-drained soil in the sun.

CAUTIONS
• The essential oil should be used as directed by a medical herbalist.
• No toxic effect has been recorded to date, so caraway seeds can be used without medical supervision.
• Like other plants in this family (coriander, cumin, dill), caraway may cause an allergic reaction such as a runny nose, watering eyes or diarrhoea. If you notice any side effects, stop using it.

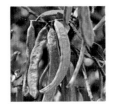

Carob

Ceratonia siliqua Caesalpiniaceae **Also called** St John's bread, Locust bean

The 'locusts' on which John the Baptist survived in the desert are thought to be carob beans, hence the popular name, St John's bread. The large evergreen carob tree grows in the Mediterranean region and can reach 20m in height. Its flowers are small, reddish, have no petals and form gleaming clusters. The bean is a large purple-brown pod in which 8-12 seeds lie in a fleshy pulp.

Parts used

Pod and the seeds

• The seeds are soaked to soften them, then the outer coating and the germ are removed.
• What remains, the albumen, is ground to make carob gum – also known as locust bean gum.
• Carob flour is made by drying and grinding the pulp of the seedpods.

Constituents

Carob is largely made up of sugars and tannins. Almost 90 per cent of the bean is composed of sugar-type compounds and soluble fibre. It is also rich in mucilage, which soothes inflamed mucous membranes.

The pulp in the seedpods is high in soluble sugars, too (40 to 50 per cent), as well as being rich in tannins.

Medicinal uses

Carob preparations are used to treat diarrhoea, indigestion and heartburn. Carob flour is mixed with sunflower seed and rice flours to make an absorbent preparation gentle enough to treat diarrhoea in babies. Tests in Belgium in 1989 found that infants suffering with

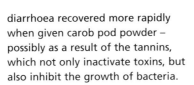

diarrhoea recovered more rapidly when given carob pod powder – possibly as a result of the tannins, which not only inactivate toxins, but also inhibit the growth of bacteria.

In a Turkish teaching hospital study in 1998 carob bean juice was found to effectively combat diarrhoea in children. Carob helps to sooth intestinal irritation. The mucilage and gum are also both used as a treatment for vomiting in mild preparations, which are suitable for babies and pregnant women.

Carob bean gum is used in slimming foods and as a chocolate substitute. It lacks absorbable nutrients and thus makes food more substantial but not more fattening. Research published in 2002 showed that carob may improve lipid levels in overweight people.

CAUTIONS

• To date, there have been no reported toxic effects from using therapeutic doses of preparations based on carob.

PREPARATION AND DOSAGE

For internal use

TO TREAT diarrhoea
CAROB FLOUR Take 20-30g a day mixed with lukewarm water or milk. So as to avoid irritating the throat, add a teaspoon of flour to the mixture. Consult a doctor before treating a baby with diarrhoea – hydration with a high electrolyte fluid is vital.

TO TREAT vomiting
CAROB GUM For an adult Put 1 tablespoon of gum in a glass of water. Drink in the evening.

IF SYMPTOMS PERSIST, CONSULT A DOCTOR

Cultivation

The carob can only be cultivated outdoors in a warm Mediterranean-like climate and can tolerate dry soil.

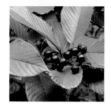

Cascara

Rhamnus purshiana Rhamnaceae

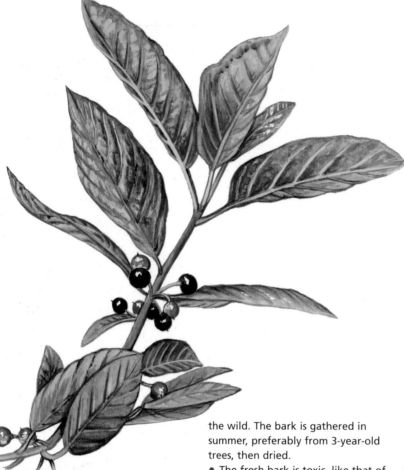

This evergreen tree is native to the west coast of the USA but is now cultivated in East Africa, where the climate is similarly hot and dry. The cascara grows to a height of 3-12m and has oval, pointed leaves with numerous straight veins. Its fruit is a black poisonous berry with a stone that contains a black seed. The bark is brownish and scattered with whitish pores.

Parts used

Bark

• Only cultivated trees are harvested, never those that grow in the wild. The bark is gathered in summer, preferably from 3-year-old trees, then dried.

• The fresh bark is toxic, like that of alder buckthorn, a related species.

• After drying and fragmentation, the bark is used in infusions and pharmaceutical preparations.

Constituents

The active principles in cascara bark are hydroxyanthraquinone glycosides, known as cascarosides, which exert a laxative effect.

Medicinal uses

Cascara bark has a laxative or purgative effect according to how much is taken. These effects are due to the way the plant affects the absorption of water and electrolytes and stimulates contractions within the intestine. Cascara bark is prescribed to treat the symptoms of occasional bouts of constipation and must be taken strictly as prescribed by a doctor or medical herbalist.

Cascara may also be beneficial in the treatment of liver disorders. Studies by Chinese scientists in 2000 found that the glycoside emodin reduced the development of fibrosis in the livers of rats.

Cultivation

Propagated by ripe seed, green-wood cuttings or layering, this species should be grown in well-drained soil in sun or light shade.

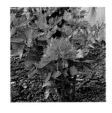

Celery

Apium graveolens Umbelliferae/Apiaceae **Also called** Smallage, Wild celery, Chinese celery

A biennial plant with a ridged, shiny stem, celery can grow to a height of 45cm. The stalks of the wild plant have an unpleasant taste and should not be confused with those of the cultivated variety. The plant has indented, aromatic leaves and small, white flowers. The small, brown seeds have a characteristic celery odour and taste.

Parts used
Seeds
● The seeds are collected during summer and autumn.

Constituents
The seeds contain 1.5 to 3 per cent essential oil, mainly limonene. Phthalides present in the oil impart celery's characteristic odour. The seeds also contain coumarins, flavonoids and furanocoumarins.

Medicinal uses
Celery seeds have traditionally been used to treat rheumatism and tests performed in 1998 confirmed celery's anti-inflammatory and pain-killing qualities. Celery is also useful in treating arthritis and gout, perhaps as a result of its diuretic action, which may help to remove the toxins associated with these conditions.

The diuretic and antiseptic qualities of the seeds indicate their use in the treatment of cystitis and other urinary infections. The seeds are also reputed to expel trapped wind and so remedy flatulence. Celery is thought to lower blood pressure, and calm anxiety and tension. Studies published in *Fitoterapia* in 1985 document the sedative and antispasmodic effects of the phthalide compounds present in the essential oil.

Celery has also been used to treat coughs, bronchitis, asthma, muscle spasms, hiccups and bad breath.

Cultivation
Grow from seed sown in spring, in damp, nutrient-rich soil in a sheltered location.

PREPARATION AND DOSAGE

For internal use
TO TREAT rheumatism, arthritis and digestive problems
INFUSION Put 1 teaspoon of seeds into a cup of boiling water. Infuse for 5-10 minutes, strain and drink 1 cup a day.
TINCTURE Take 30 drops in water three times a day.
LIQUID EXTRACT (diluted 1:1 in 90% alcohol) Take 0.5-2ml three times a day.

IF SYMPTOMS PERSIST, CONSULT A DOCTOR

CAUTIONS
● Celery seeds are thought to stimulate the uterus, and so are not recommended for pregnant women.
● Celery is also inadvisable for people with an acute renal disorder.
● The furanocoumarins present may induce sensitivity to sunlight.
● Celery may sometimes provoke an allergic reaction.

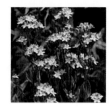

Centaury

Erythraea centaurium Gentianaceae **Also called** Feverwort

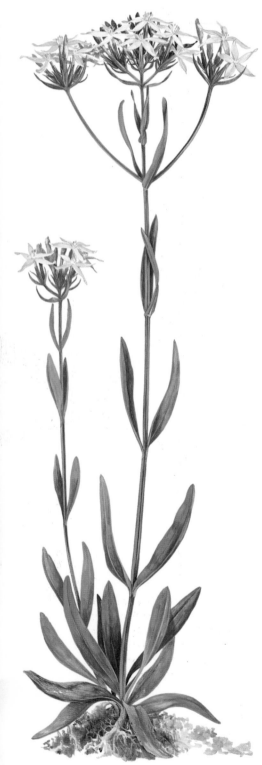

The ability of this elegant little biennial to cure fever has long been known, hence its other common name, feverwort. Found in grassy places across Europe, centaury grows to a height of 10-60cm. Its spindly stems are crowned in summer by clusters of pink, star-shaped flowers. Its long, pale leaves grow in a dense rosette around the base, but in pairs higher up the stem.

Parts used

Leaves, stems and flowers
• The aerial parts are gathered just as the flowers come into full bloom, in June, July and August.
• They are dried and crushed for use in infusions, decoctions, powders and tinctures.
• Centaury is often combined with other herbs that stimulate the appetite, such as gentian and mugwort.

Constituents

The aerial parts of centaury are rich in phenolic acids, flavonoids and xanthone derivatives. It also contains bitter principles, including a number of secoiridoids.

Medicinal uses

The bitter secoiridoids stimulate the appetite by increasing the flow of gastric juices. Centaury is also taken to treat chronic digestive problems

CAUTIONS

• A course of treatment involving centaury should last no longer than ten days, as the plant can irritate the lining of the stomach.
• Centaury is not suitable for people who suffer from peptic ulcers or inflammation in any part of the digestive tract.
• Do not use centaury preparations when pregnant or breastfeeding.

and flatulence. It is diuretic and stimulates bile flow, so is used to help to eliminate toxins and treat liver and gall-bladder disorders. The plant is often prescribed as a tonic in combination with anise, chamomile, peppermint and fennel, for cases of extreme fatigue and during convalescence.

Experiments have shown that an aqueous extract of centaury helps to fight fever and is anti-inflammatory. These properties are believed to be due to the phenolic acids.

Centaury is also used as an active ingredient in lotions to combat head lice and prevent hair loss.

Cultivation

Plant in sandy, neutral to alkaline soil, in a sunny spot.

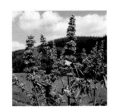

Chaste tree

Vitex agnus-castus Verbenaceae **Also called** Monks' pepper

A native of the Mediterranean, chaste tree now grows in all the subtropical zones of the world. It reaches a height of 3-5m and each of its graceful leaves is made up of between five to nine long, thin leaflets. Purple flower-clusters are followed by a mass of red-and-yellow berries in autumn. These taste like a blend of sage and pepper, which is why the plant is sometimes called monks' pepper.

Parts used

Berries

● The berries are picked when ripe, in September and October.

● They are dried, then used to make liquid and dry extracts, which must contain at least 0.2 per cent of the active components to be effective.

Constituents

The chaste tree berry contains an essential oil, labdanes (diterpenic), iridoids, flavonoids, alkaloids, vegetable steroids and fatty acids.

Medicinal uses

Chaste tree is used to treat problems that arise from malfunctions of the pituitary gland, which secretes some of the hormones that are involved in controlling the menstrual cycle and in stimulating ovulation and the production of sperm. The plant can therefore be helpful in treating various menstrual problems, including premenstrual tension, absence of periods, pain and infertility due to poor or a total absence of ovulation.

Research has recently provided scientific backing for the medicinal powers of chaste tree berries. In Germany and the Czech Republic, scientists have demonstrated their effectiveness in easing the symptoms of premenstrual syndrome, including breast pain. Also, further controlled trials of a homeopathic chaste tree preparation, involving women who were experiencing fertility disorders characterised by very light or no menstrual bleeding, resulted in the restoration of the menstrual cycle in most participants, and pregnancy.

Cultivation

Suited to rich, moist to dry soil, the chaste tree prefers to be placed in a warm, sunny location.

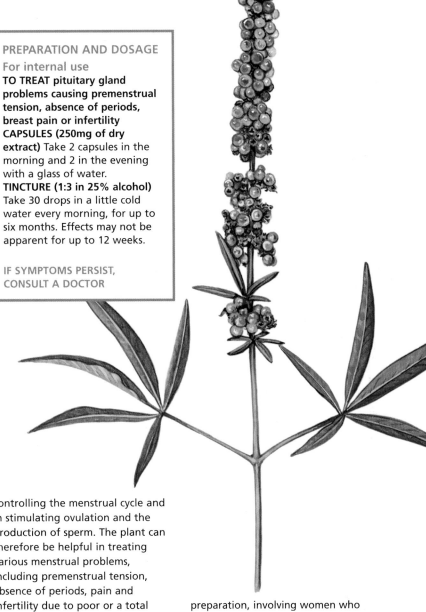

CAUTIONS

● Chaste tree can trigger allergic reactions. If this occurs, see a doctor.

● Do not use when pregnant or breastfeeding.

● Excessive use of chaste plant preparations may affect the nervous system, causing a prickling sensation across the skin.

● Do not use at the same time as antipsychotic drugs that block the action of the neurotransmitter dopamine or drugs (for conditions such as Parkinson's disease) that boost dopamine levels.

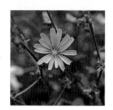

Chicory

Cichorium intybus Compositae/Asteraceae

Valued by the ancient Romans, who cultivated it as a vegetable, wild chicory is a common sight on waste ground and roadsides in Europe. Growing up to 1m tall the hardy perennial has deeply indented leaves crowding around erect stems that are downy on the underside. Flowerheads appear between June and September. Most are bright blue, but can be pink or white.

PREPARATION AND DOSAGE

For internal use

TO TREAT liver and kidney problems, bloating, belching, sluggish digestion, flatulence

DECOCTION Put a 15-30g mixture of root, leaves and flowers into 1 litre of water. Boil for 5 minutes. Strain and drink 1 cup before the midday and evening meals.

INSTANT DRINK PREPARATION Add 1 heaped teaspoon of instant chicory to a cup of boiling water. Add milk and sweeten to taste.

IF SYMPTOMS PERSIST, CONSULT A DOCTOR

Parts used

Leaves, flowers and roots

- The leaves are gathered when the plant is in flower and are used to prepare infusions.
- The flowers and roots may be harvested at any time of the year if they are to be used fresh, or in September if they are to be dried. Roots are chopped up into small pieces before drying in the sun.
- Chicory roots are sometimes roasted and ground for use as a coffee substitute.

Constituents

The entire chicory plant contains a milky sap, of which the main constituent – about 45-60 per cent – is inulin. Phenol acid is also found in the flowers, and in the roots there are bitter sesquiterpene lactones.

Medicinal uses

For centuries it was known that chicory had anti-inflammatory and antiseptic powers, and it was applied in poultices to ease swelling. This is due to the phenol acid, which also acts as a diuretic, remedying any bloating caused by fluid retention. More recently, it has been shown that chicory will ease inflammation caused by rheumatism and gout.

The inulin encourages the growth of bacteria needed for the intestines to work properly. Chicory, therefore, can help to prevent and treat problems such as sluggish digestion, gastric ulcers and flatulence. It has also been shown that the inulin can lower levels of blood cholesterol.

Both inulin and the sesquiterpene lactones are bitter principles which stimulate the flow of digestive juices, including that of bile from the gall bladder. This allows the liver to work more efficiently; in 1998 scientists in India confirmed that the root had this protective effect.

Cultivation

Chicory grows easily in almost any type of soil, especially if it is rich and well drained. The plant prefers a sunny location.

CAUTIONS

- People suffering from an intestinal blockage or inflammation of the intestines should consult a medical herbalist before using chicory.
- No adverse side effects have been reported to date.

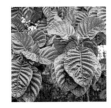

Cinchona

Cinchona succiruba Rubiaceae

A native of South America, cinchona grows to over 20m tall. It has long, elliptical leaves, with reddish undersides, and bright pink flowers. The outer bark layer is brownish grey, while the inner is reddish brown. Jesuit missionaries discovered its antimalarial properties in the 17th century and had for years a monopoly on the drug, which was known as 'Jesuit's bark'.

Parts used
Bark
● The bark is collected in autumn from trees that are over six years old.
● Once dried, the bark is broken up and used for tinctures, dry extracts decoctions and medicinal wine.

Constituents
Alkaloids, mostly quinine and quinidine, make up 5-15 per cent of cinchona bark. It also contains about 8 per cent tannins and considerable amounts of the bitter quinovin.

Medicinal uses
C. succiruba is a species of cinchona from which quinine, a potent antimalarial, is extracted. Quinine and quinidine are antispasmodic, making the bark potentially useful for treating muscle cramps as well. Recent Australian research, however, stresses that this use may cause bleeding under the skin. The alkaloid quinidine is used in conventional medicine for heartbeat irregularities.

CAUTIONS
● Never take cinchona at the same time as anticoagulant drugs, as it reinforces their effect.
● Do not take while pregnant or if allergic to quinine and quinidine.
● Cinchona can reduce the effectiveness of antacids and drugs used for peptic ulcers.

PREPARATION AND DOSAGE
For internal use
TO TREAT indigestion, lack of appetite, nervous exhaustion
TINCTURE (1:5 in 25% alcohol) Add 2-4ml to a glass of water. Drink three times a day.
MEDICINAL WINE Drink 1-2 tablespoons, three times a day.

TO TREAT fevers, influenza
DECOCTION Put 0.5g of finely cut bark into a cup of water. Boil for 3 minutes, then infuse for 10 minutes and sweeten to taste. Drink 3 cups a day, half an hour before meals.

For external use
TO TREAT scabs, bedsores and stabilised wounds
DECOCTION Put 30g chopped bark into 1 litre water. Boil for 5 minutes. Use to wash affected areas once or twice a day.

IF SYMPTOMS PERSIST, CONSULT A DOCTOR

The bitter quinovin in cinchona bark stimulates gastric secretions and helps to improve the appetite. This tonic effect makes cinchona useful for treating nervous exhaustion, fevers and flu. It is often combined with other fever-fighting plants such as willow and meadowsweet.

Cinchona bark is also antibacterial and its tannins help to heal broken skin. It is used externally for healing scabs, bedsores and wounds.

Cultivation
Cinchona should be grown in a greenhouse in the UK or as a pot plant on a sunny windowsill.

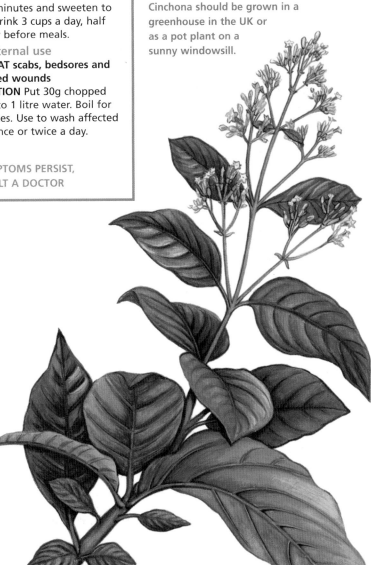

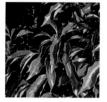

Cinnamon

Cinnamomum zeylanicum and *C. cassia* Lauraceae

This evergreen tree grows to a height of 5-8m. It has tough leathery leaves and clusters of small flowers followed by acorn-like berries. The varieties most used are Ceylon cinnamon (Cinnamomum zeylanicum) and Chinese cinnamon (C. cassia). Cinnamon is an important element in Ayurveda – a traditional medicine practised in India for more than 5000 years.

Parts used

Bark
- Trees that are eight years old or older are harvested every two years.
- The tubes of dried bark are used for infusions, tinctures and powders.
- A distillate of the bark produces an essential oil with a smell like pepper.

Constituents

Ceylon and Chinese cinnamon have constituents that vary slightly. Both types of bark contain up to 2 per cent essential oil, largely made up of cinnamic aldehyde. But Ceylon cinnamon also contains a small amount – 1 per cent – of eugenol, while only a trace of this substance occurs in Chinese cinnamon.

Medicinal uses

The properties of the Ceylon and the Chinese varieties are very similar. Cinnamon bark is antispasmodic; it also stimulates the salivary glands and the mucous membranes of the stomach. It is used to treat a range of digestive problems including indigestion, poor appetite, trapped gas, nausea, belching, flatulence, diarrhoea and intestinal spasms.

The liquid extract has a soothing effect on gastro-duodenal ulcers. In 1989 Japanese scientists found that two compounds in Chinese cinnamon acted as antiulcer agents in rats. The compounds improved gastric blood flow, thereby increasing the numbers of defensive blood cells reaching the site of the ulcer. However, in 2000, clinical trials in Israel found that cinnamon extract had no effect on *Helicobacter pylori*, the bacterium that causes most ulcers.

The oil is used externally to ease cramps, joint pains, rheumatism and neuralgia. The analgesic and anti-inflammatory properties of Chinese cinnamon are key constituents of tiger balm, a soothing liniment. And in 1994, Chinese scientists isolated the constituent cinnamophilin as an effective anti-inflammatory.

Cinnamon is antifungal: in 1995, Indian research showed cinnamic aldehyde to be potent against certain fungal organisms that cause respiratory tract infections.

The spice is a warming stimulant and can combat fatigue. It is good for the circulation and it stimulates the respiratory system, the uterus and the production of oestrogens.

Cultivation

Cinnamon trees cannot survive at temperatures below 15°C. They need a well-drained soil and a sunny spot.

PREPARATION AND DOSAGE

For internal use

TO TREAT gastritis, digestive problems, loss of appetite, minor cases of fatigue
INFUSION Put 1g Chinese cinnamon bark or 0.5-1g Ceylon cinnamon bark into a cup of boiling water. Leave to infuse for 10 minutes, then strain. Drink 3 cups a day.
POWDER Take 0.3-1g three times a day with food.
LIQUID EXTRACT Dilute 0.5-1ml in a glass of water and take three times a day.

IF SYMPTOMS PERSIST, CONSULT A DOCTOR

CAUTIONS

- The essential oil can trigger skin allergies and inflammation of the mucous membranes.
- Use cinnamon oil only under medical herbalist supervision.
- If pregnant or breastfeeding do not consume more cinnamon than is normally present in food.

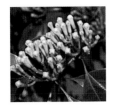

Clove

Syzygium aromaticum Myrtaceae

A native of the Spice Islands, this tall, slender evergreen can reach a height of 20m. Its flowers grow in clusters and, if allowed to bloom, open into red-and-white bells. However, mature trees are not often in full bloom as the flower buds are picked for use as cloves. The tree does not produce these cloves until it is 20 years old. It then remains productive for about 50 years.

Parts used
Flower buds
- Buds are harvested twice a year, in summer and winter.
- Cloves are the dried flower buds.

Constituents
Clove oil consists largely of eugenol, an anaesthetic and antiseptic substance. Cloves also contain tannins and flavonoids – cancer-fighting antioxidants that also strengthen the walls of the veins.

Medicinal uses
Herbal practitioners use cloves to treat digestive complaints and oil of cloves for toothache.

The eugenol contained in cloves is their main active constituent. It is known to combat inflammation and bacterial and fungal infections, as well as being analgesic. Clove oil is the active ingredient in several mouthwashes and over-the-counter pain-relief remedies for toothache.

A paper published in 1999, in the *International Journal of Antimicrobial Agents*, reports on cloves' efficacy against both bacteria and yeasts: Chinese physicians have long used the herb to treat athlete's foot – a yeast (fungal) infection.

Studies performed in Taiwan showed that eugenol reduces blood clotting and is also an effective anti-inflammatory. Research published in 1985 found clove oil to have a

potent relaxant effect on the smooth muscle of both lungs and intestines. But because of this powerful sedative effect, an overdose of eugenol could have a depressive effect on the central nervous system.

Cloves are often combined with other plants to treat bloating, gastritis, dyspepsia and rheumatic pains. They are also incorporated into various remedies to combat infections of the ear, nose and throat, and genito-urinary infections.

Cultivation
The tree needs a tropical or glasshouse environment to thrive.

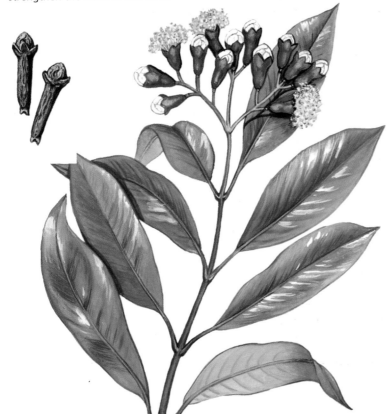

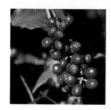

Coffee

Coffea arabica Rubiaceae

A native of Ethiopia, the evergreen coffee tree has dark green glossy leaves and can grow to 10m tall. Its clusters of decorative white flowers are delicately perfumed with the scents of coffee and jasmine. The fruits are called cherries because they turn red as they ripen. Each cherry contains two coffee beans.

Parts used

Seeds (coffee beans)
- The cherries, picked when ripe contain green, odourless raw seeds – used in homeopathic medicine.
- The seeds are roasted and gain their distinctive coffee-bean aroma.
- Caffeine is used in many medicines.

Constituents

Phenolic acids constitute up to 5 per cent of coffee beans; they possess stimulant and antiseptic properties. The caffeine content ranges from 0.6 to 3 per cent: caffeine stimulates activity in all the major organs of the body. Roasting reduces caffeine content and adds pigments and aroma. Coffee beans also contain small amounts of theobromine, tannin and trigonelline.

CAUTIONS
- Classed as a stimulant, caffeine in preparations should be avoided by those involved in competitive sports.
- Avoid if you are pregnant or breastfeeding.
- May aggravate or induce peptic ulcers and reflux problems.
- Not recommended for people with cardiovascular disease or those receiving electro convulsive therapy.
- Side effects can include increased heart rate, headache, increased urination, insomnia and agitation.
- Expect caffeine withdrawal headaches if you quit drinking coffee.

PREPARATION AND DOSAGE

For internal use
TO TREAT fatigue, nausea, obesity
CAFFEINE TABLETS (50mg) Take 1-2 tablets as directed. Do not exceed 2 tablets in one hour or 12 in 24 hours.

For external use
TO TREAT excess weight gain
CREAM Apply a caffeine-containing cream in the morning and early evening.

IF SYMPTOMS PERSIST, CONSULT A DOCTOR

Medicinal uses

Caffeine, the main active constituent in coffee, causes people to feel more alert. One study published in 1987 in *Psychopharmacology* reported that a caffeine dose smaller than that found in a cup of coffee increased hearing and visual performance.

An Australian clinical study in 1996 demonstrated that coffee lessens the fall in blood pressure that normally occurs after eating. The researchers concluded that this stimulant action on the cardiovascular system was particularly beneficial for elderly individuals.

Because caffeine increases the metabolic rate, it maximises the painkilling effect of analgesics like aspirin or paracetamol, and is often added to them in 'ultra' versions.

Caffeine can alleviate nausea and vomiting, and treat headaches and migraines. As a stimulant, it is vital in preventing coma following collapse through narcotic poisoning. Other constituents of coffee also play a role. Trigonelline, for example, may relieve migraine, while theophylline has stimulant, diuretic and cardio-vascular properties. Research in 2002, at Imperial College, London, showed that theobromine relieves coughing.

Externally, caffeine-containing creams can stimulate lipolysis – the destruction of body fats – and are a useful part of a slimming regime.

Cultivation

Coffee will not survive where the temperature falls below 10°C. It likes well-drained soil and partial shade.

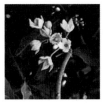

Cola

Cola nitida Sterculiaceae

A native of West Africa, the cola tree is widely cultivated in the tropics. Cola nitida, C. acuminta and other species may be used. The cola fruit is made up of five seedpods that form a star shape. Each pod contains five or six large seeds – the cola nuts. These harden when dry and turn reddish inside. Their smooth outer surface is dark mahogany brown.

Parts used

Seeds (cola nuts)

- Seeds are harvested unripe.
- The pods are opened and the pulpy outer coating of the seeds is removed.
- They are used as powders or extracts in various pharmaceutical products: capsules, granules, massage gels and drinkable solutions.
- In regions where the cola tree grows, the caffeine-rich seed is chewed as a stimulant.

Constituents

The seeds contain caffeine, theophylline and tannins. A dried cola nut can contain as much as 2.5 per cent caffeine.

Medicinal uses

Cola helps to maintain alertness and intellectual sharpness, mainly because of its caffeine content.

CAUTIONS

- If large amounts of cola are taken, excess caffeine in the body may cause rapid heartbeat, headache, agitation, insomnia and trembling.
- Caffeine is on the list of banned stimulants for competitive sports.
- Do not take if you have heart disease or high blood pressure.
- Avoid if you are pregnant or breastfeeding.
- Do not give to children under 14.

Caffeine is used to treat exhaustion and can help during convalescence. It raises blood pressure slightly and opens coronary blood vessels as well as increasing heartbeat and respiratory rates. Caffeine is slightly diuretic and helps to dissolve lipids (fats). But the effects of cola seed cannot simply be equated with those of caffeine, since the effects of caffeine are modified by its combination with tannins.

Cola nuts contain theophylline, which stimulates the appetite and respiratory rates, and can be used to treat diarrhoea. The body develops a tolerance to cola and, over time, requires larger amounts in order to produce the same results.

Cultivation

Likes sun or light shade and a rich soil and – ideally – a tropical climate.

PREPARATION AND DOSAGE

For internal use

**TO TREAT exhaustion, through overwork or following illness
POWDER (or powder in capsule form)** Take up to 3g a day with plenty of water.
LIQUID EXTRACT Take 5 drops in water twice a day.

IF SYMPTOMS PERSIST, CONSULT A DOCTOR

Coltsfoot

Tussilago farfara Asteraceae

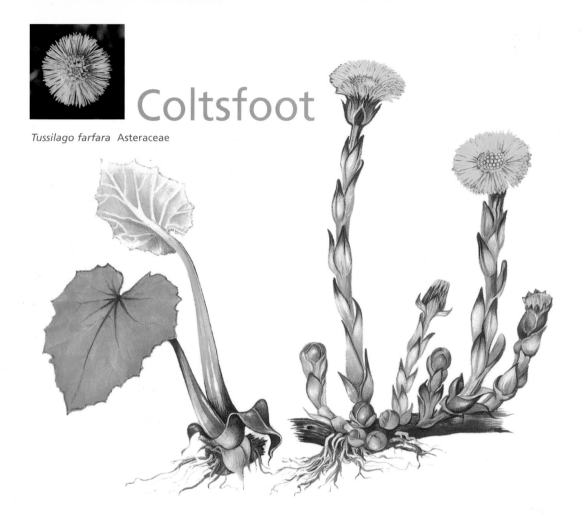

A native of Europe and Asia, coltsfoot is a perennial that grows no taller than 30cm. In spring, well before there are any leaves, yellow flowers start to appear upon the plant's scaly stems. The delicate, heart-shaped leaves that follow are covered on their underside by a fine, white down.

Parts used
Flowers and leaves
● Harvesting takes place between February and May. The flowers are then dried for use in infusions and pharmaceutical preparations.

CAUTIONS
● Because of the pyrrolizidine alkaloids present, coltsfoot should only be taken in consultation with a medical herbalist, and for no longer than three to four weeks.
● Coltsfoot must not be used during pregnancy or when breastfeeding.

Constituents
Between 6 to 10 per cent of the coltsfoot flower is made up of mucilage and about 5 to 10 per cent of tannins. Other components include flavonoids, carotenoids, triterpenes, phytosterols and traces of pyrrolizidine alkaloids.

Medicinal uses
The tannins have antiseptic properties, while the mucilage helps to boost immunity and has the power to reduce inflammation and loosen phlegm.

Coltsfoot's mix of flavonoids and phytosterols also gives the plant anti-inflammatory properties, while the flavonoids on their own help to reduce muscle spasms. This variety of properties makes coltsfoot preparations useful in treating asthma, bronchial inflammation, dry coughs, and mouth and throat irritations.

A coltsfoot ointment or poultice can be highly effective in soothing cuts and skin irritations, killing any bacteria and reducing inflammation.

Cultivation
Coltsfoot is grown from seeds. Plant in moist, neutral or alkaline soil, in a sunny or lightly shaded spot. Do not use for making home preparations.

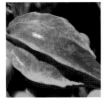

Condurango

Marsdenia condurango (Gonolobus condurango) Asclepiadaceae

A native of the South American rain forest, the vine-like condurango grips onto tree trunks, as it climbs in search of sunlight. In the Andes, its heart-shaped leaves are still used to treat snake bites. The greeny white, bell-shaped flowers grow in umbrella-like clusters, while its 10cm-long fruits resemble shuttles.

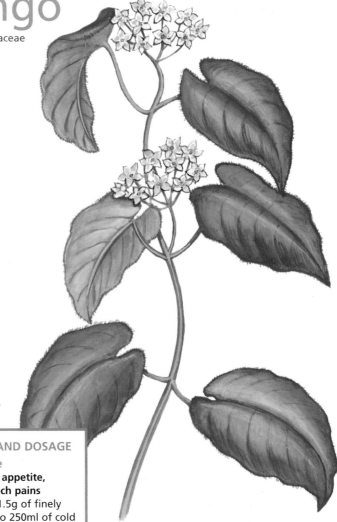

Parts used

Bark

● Collected during spring and early summer or during autumn, the bark is dried, and then either broken or cut into fragments, or crushed to make a powder.

● The cut or crushed bark is used to prepare decoctions, and in capsules, liquid extracts, tinctures and medicinal wines.

Constituents

Condurango bark contains glycosides of condurangogenins, which are bitter principles related to saponosides, phytosterols and flavonoids.

Medicinal uses

The combination of chemicals found in condurango helps to stimulate the appetite, improve digestion and relieve gastritis. It is therefore used in preparations for treating stomach disorders and is combined with centaury, juniper and gentian to boost the appetite of people who are convalescing.

Condurango has also been used to treat fluid retention and bleeding, and recent animal studies suggest that it may help to stop or inhibit the growth of cancerous tumours.

Cultivation

Condurango can be grown from seed in a partially shaded plot of sandy soil, that is rich in humus.

PREPARATION AND DOSAGE

For internal use

TO TREAT loss of appetite, dyspepsia, stomach pains

DECOCTION Put 1.5g of finely chopped bark into 250ml of cold water and bring to the boil. Cool completely, then strain. Drink 1 glass 30 minutes before every meal.

CAPSULES (100mg of dry extract) Take 1-2 capsules three times a day, 30 minutes before meals.

LIQUID EXTRACT Put 20 drops into 300ml water and drink before each meal.

TINCTURE Take 25 drops in 300ml of water, three times a day.

MEDICINAL WINE Drink 1-2 tablespoons 30 minutes before each meal.

IF SYMPTOMS PERSIST, CONSULT A DOCTOR

CAUTIONS

● If using other drugs, see a medical herbalist before taking condurango.

● Avoid condurango when pregnant or breastfeeding, or if you suffer from a liver disorder.

● Do not drive or operate machinery while taking condurango.

● Overdoses can produce side effects including excessive salivation, vomiting, diarrhoea, coordination problems, rapid pulse and breathing, and general weakness.

● Ingesting the bark has also been known to bring on seizures, leading to paralysis.

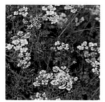

Coriander

Coriandrum sativum Apiaceae

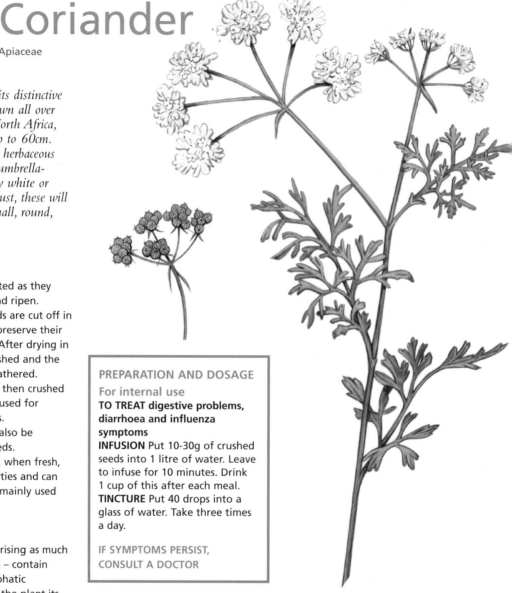

Easily recognised by its distinctive scent, coriander is grown all over Europe, India and North Africa, reaching heights of up to 60cm. In early summer, this herbaceous annual is covered in umbrella-shaped clusters of tiny white or pink flowers. By August, these will have given way to small, round, wrinkled seeds.

Parts used

Leaves and seeds

• The seeds are collected as they start to turn yellow and ripen.

• Coriander seed heads are cut off in the early morning to preserve their beneficial properties. After drying in the sun, they are threshed and the individual seeds are gathered.

• The seeds are dried, then crushed to a powder, which is used for infusions and tinctures.

• An essential oil can also be extracted from the seeds.

• The aromatic leaves, when fresh, have antiseptic properties and can aid digestion, but are mainly used in cooking.

Constituents

Very oily fruits – comprising as much as 25 per cent fatty oil – contain phenolic acids and aliphatic aldehydes, which give the plant its scent. The essential oil extracted from the seeds contains a large quantity of linalool, which is antibacterial and controls spasms.

CAUTIONS

• Coriander can cause abdominal pain, poor appetite and an enlarged liver. See a doctor if you experience any abnormal symptoms.

• Avoid coriander if pregnant or breastfeeding.

• Never use pure extracted coriander essential oil internally.

PREPARATION AND DOSAGE

For internal use

TO TREAT digestive problems, diarrhoea and influenza symptoms

INFUSION Put 10-30g of crushed seeds into 1 litre of water. Leave to infuse for 10 minutes. Drink 1 cup of this after each meal.

TINCTURE Put 40 drops into a glass of water. Take three times a day.

IF SYMPTOMS PERSIST, CONSULT A DOCTOR

Medicinal uses

Various studies have shown that nearly all of coriander's medicinal properties are due to the essential oil in the plant's seeds, which can help to regulate gastric secretions and to release trapped wind. The seeds are therefore effective in treating digestive problems, and are also recommended for common forms of diarrhoea due to infections such as gastroenteritis.

Animal studies in India in 1997 demonstrated that preparations made from coriander seeds could help to lower blood cholesterol. The seeds are also believed to fight off bacterial and fungal infections.

Externally, coriander seed oil can be applied to help to soothe the pain of haemorrhoids and joints affected by rheumatism.

Cultivation

Coriander seeds can be sown in any type of light, well-drained soil, during warm weather, from late March to the end of April. The plant grows best in a sheltered position, exposed to plenty of sunlight.

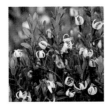

Cranberry

Vaccinium macrocarpon Ericaceae

Native to peat bogs and forests in North America, the cranberry is a slow-growing shrub. Now widely cultivated, the dark green leaves are topped by pinkish white flowers towards the end of May. The fruit – used in folk remedies since the 16th century or earlier – is a small greenish berry, that turns dark red as it ripens.

Parts used
Fruits
• The berries are gathered when ripe in September.
• They are consumed fresh, dried, or as juice and are also used to make capsules and tablets.

Constituents
Cranberry berries contain glucose and fructose, many essential minerals and several organic acids, including vitamin C. They are also rich in antioxidant anthocyanins and proanthocyanins.

Medicinal uses
Cranberry is recommended to complement the use of antibiotics in the treatment of repeated urinary infections. Scientific tests have demonstrated that it is the proanthocyanins, along with the fructose, in cranberry juice that prevent bacteria such as *E. coli* from colonising the cells of the bladder and urinary tract. It has been noted that cranberry reduces the odour of urine – an asset for elderly people who suffer from incontinence.

Cranberry juice is also used to prevent the bacterial build-up on teeth, which leads to plaque and tooth decay.

Its vitamin C, along with various antioxidant minerals can help to ward off colds and flu.

Cultivation
Cranberries can be grown from cuttings or seeds, and are best suited to damp, acidic soil. Although the plant can become dormant to survive extreme cold, frosts will kill off any buds. Warmth and sunny conditions are needed to ripen the fruit fully.

CAUTIONS
• When using to treat a urinary infection, it is advisable to combine cranberry preparations with conventional pharmaceutical remedies, such as antibiotics.
• People suffering from an enlarged prostate gland or from an obstruction of the urinary tract should consult their doctor before using any cranberry preparations.
• Do not use cranberry preparations if taking anticoagulants.

PREPARATION AND DOSAGE
For internal use
TO TREAT recurrent urinary infections
DRY EXTRACT (400mg capsules or tablets) Take 1 capsule twice a day with plenty of water.
FRESH UNDILUTED JUICE Drink 500ml twice a day. This treatment must be prolonged.
TO PREVENT plaque and tooth decay
JUICE Make up a solution of 3 parts cranberry juice to 7 parts water. Drink 0.5-1 litre a day.

IF SYMPTOMS PERSIST, CONSULT A DOCTOR

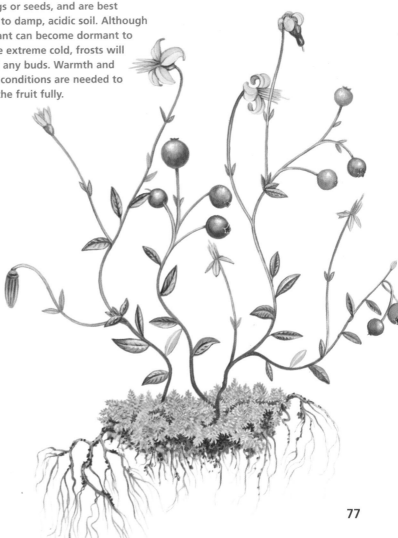

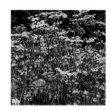

Cumin

Cuminum cyminum Apiaceae

Native to Egypt and Asia, cumin is a herbaceous annual that grows to a height of about 30cm, its slender stem divided into long, slim secondary stalks. Narrow, ridged seedpods, about 5mm long, contain the cumin seeds.

Parts used

Seeds

• Cultivated in India and the Near East, the seedpods appear in summer and are gathered by hand.

• The seeds are used, whole or ground, in infusions. Its essential oil is colourless or pale yellow with a characteristic musky smell and a bitter, aromatic taste.

• In addition to its medicinal uses, cumin is an ingredient in many renowned spice mixtures, including Madras curry and ras-el-hanout – a combination of Moroccan spices.

Constituents

The essential oil constitutes 2 to 5 per cent of the seed and contains around 40 per cent cuminaldehyde. Cumin also contains flavonoids, which are beneficial in treating minor circulatory disorders and also possess anti-inflammatory properties.

Medicinal uses

Used internally, cumin is considered to be highly effective in the treatment of indigestion, bloating and stomach infections. It can help to relieve flatulence and to relax the intestine. Research performed in India in 1999 validated the use of cumin as a food preservative, disinfectant and astringent by demonstrating its action against various types of bacteria.

Cumin is available as an essential oil for external use and it is a constituent of various medicinal products that are used for massaging painful joints.

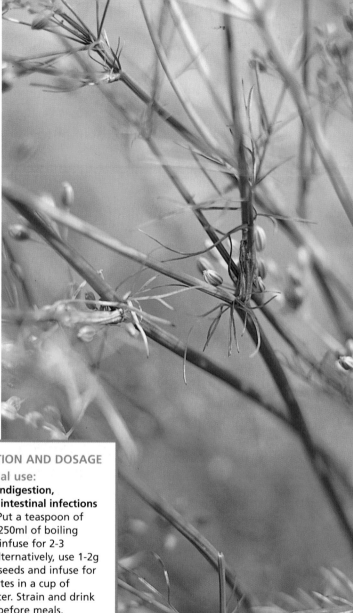

PREPARATION AND DOSAGE

For internal use:

TO TREAT indigestion, flatulence, intestinal infections

INFUSION Put a teaspoon of seeds into 250ml of boiling water and infuse for 2-3 minutes. Alternatively, use 1-2g of ground seeds and infuse for 10-15 minutes in a cup of boiling water. Strain and drink half a cup before meals.

For external use:

TO TREAT painful joints

GELS, OINTMENTS Rub in slowly once or twice a day as directed.

IF SYMPTOMS PERSIST, CONSULT A DOCTOR

In 1989 Danish scientists found that cumin extracts inhibited platelet aggregation and the generation of inflammatory mediators. These findings suggest that cumin might be beneficial in the treatment of thrombosis and inflammation.

Cumin is sometimes prescribed for breast engorgement during breastfeeding. It can also stimulate menstruation and lactation. In addition, cumin is reputed to have aphrodisiac properties.

Cultivation

In spring scatter seeds in a well-drained sunny spot. Harvest the seeds at the end of summer.

CAUTIONS

• Large doses of the essential oil have caused nervous tension.

• The essential oil is used externally and should be avoided in pregnancy.

• Cumin can reduce blood sugar levels so diabetics should monitor their blood glucose carefully.

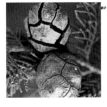

Cypress

Cupressus sempervirens Cupressaceae **Also called** Italian cypress

A tree typical of Mediterranean countries, the cypress has reddish grey bark and small, triangular, opposed leaves that overlap and cover the whole branch. The female flowers produce fruits (cones), made of round, soft scales, which turn yellowy grey when ripe. Both the ancient Egyptians and Romans dedicated the tree to their gods of death and the underworld, which may explain why it is often planted in cemeteries.

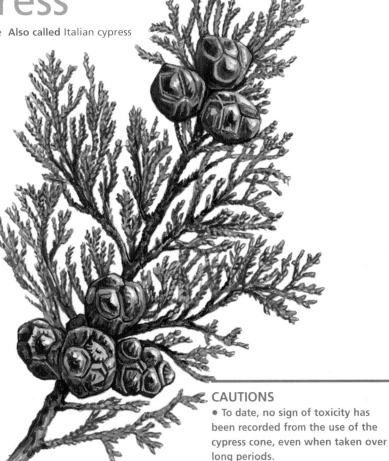

Parts used

Cones

● These are gathered while still green, and used to make infusions, powders or extracts for capsules, tablets and drinkable solutions.

● Cypress is also used in gels and ointments for external use.

Constituents

Cypress cones are composed mainly of dimeric proanthocyanidins, which have a strengthening effect on the veins improving blood circulation particularly in the hands and feet. The cones contain a small quantity of essential oil and diterpenic acids.

Medicinal uses

As it can effectively treat all kinds of vein disorders, cypress is commonly prescribed for haemorrhoids and varicose veins. Formulations often combine cypress with horse chestnut and witch hazel.

    Cypress is antiseptic, sedative and diuretic, and also has an antispasmodic action, which may explain why it is sometimes used to ease coughs.

Cultivation

Grow in well-drained, acid or alkaline soils in full sunlight and away from shelter and excessive wind.

CAUTIONS

● To date, no sign of toxicity has been recorded from the use of the cypress cone, even when taken over long periods.

● Caution should be taken by pregnant or breastfeeding women.

PREPARATION AND DOSAGE

For internal use

TO TREAT varicose veins, haemorrhoids

INFUSION Put 1 dessertspoon of crushed cones into a cup of boiling water. Drink 4-5 cups a day, before or between meals.

DRINKABLE SOLUTIONS Put 40-60 drops into a little water to dilute. Take two to three times a day before meals.

For external use

TO TREAT varicose veins

GELS, OINTMENTS Gently apply to the affected areas. Massage-in working upwards. Do this in the evening just before going to bed, or as directed.

AROMATHERAPY Dilute 2-4 drops in a carrier oil and massage into affected area.

IF SYMPTOMS PERSIST, CONSULT A DOCTOR

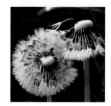

Dandelion

Taraxacum officinale Asteraceae

Common to fields and roadsides in Europe and parts of Asia, the dandelion, a herbaceous perennial, grows to about 10-30cm high. Deeply indented leaves spring up from around its base, with single yellow flowers appearing in April and May. These are followed by seeds, each topped by a tuft of soft hairs, that catch the wind, helping to disperse the plant far and wide.

Parts used

Root and leaves
- The root is collected in May, June, and autumn.
- Young leaves are gathered in spring.
- Both are dried for use in infusions, drinkable extracts and capsules.

Constituents

The root and leaves are rich in fructose and inulin and also contain bitter principles (sesquiterpene lactones), phenol acids and sterols. The leaves also contain flavonoids, potassium salts and coumarins.

Medicinal uses

The bitter principles give dandelion strong diuretic powers – the old English name for it was 'piss-a-bed'.

Dandelion is therefore widely used to stimulate urination in cases of water retention, kidney disorders, cellulite and obesity. It also contains potassium to replace that which is lost when urine production is increased. In addition, the root is also diuretic and a mild laxative.

Animal studies have confirmed the diuretic effects of dandelion. The sterols in the leaves also act on the gall bladder and liver, and stimulate the secretion and excretion of bile, all of which can help to cleanse the body of toxins and waste matter.

Because of this, preparations made from dandelion leaves are given to help to dissolve gallstones, and are believed to be beneficial for skin problems and rheumatism.

In an exciting new development, animal studies in 2001 demonstrated that a herbal preparation containing dandelion could lower blood sugar levels, suggesting its potential for treating diabetes.

Cultivation

Sow by seed in spring in moist to dry, neutral to alkaline soil.

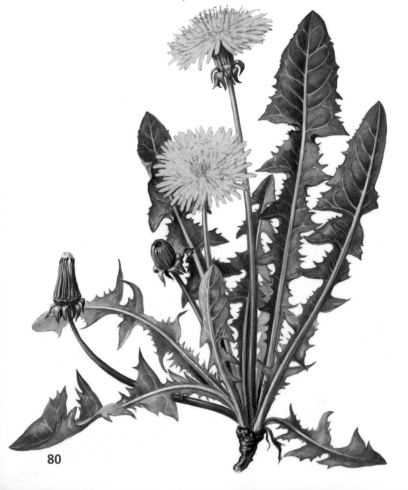

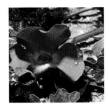

Devil's claw

Harpagophytum procumbens Pedaliaceae **Also called** Grapple plant

A native of southern Africa, where it has been used for centuries to treat a variety of ailments from indigestion and fever to skin cancer, devil's claw gets its name from its strange capsule-like fruits that are covered in what look like miniature grappling hooks. In summer, this creeping perennial bears stunning deep red, trumpet-shaped flowers.

Parts used
Tubers
● The tubers, or swollen roots, are dug up in autumn, dried and cut into small round pieces.
● They are used for infusions, powders and drinkable solutions and in ointments, gels and creams.
● Only wild plants are used in herbal medicines, which could potentially endanger the survival of the species.

Constituents
The major constituents are iridoids (monoterpenic glucosides), which make up 0.5 to 3 per cent of the dried drug. Harpagoside is the most active of these medicinally; therefore it is best to choose preparations that contain at least 1.5 to 2 per cent harpagoside. Phytosterols and flavonoids are also present.

Medicinal uses
Studies have demonstrated that devil's claw can help to relieve pain and in some cases improve mobility in people suffering from osteoarthritis or degenerative rheumatism. The anti-inflammatory powers conferred by harpagoside and the phytosterols are responsible for this, and the plant is often recommended for treating less serious cases of rheumatism. It is also used externally for joint pain.

The bitter principles help to stimulate the digestive system, and the plant is used to treat indigestion.

Cultivation
This species has proved impossible to cultivate outside its native habitat.

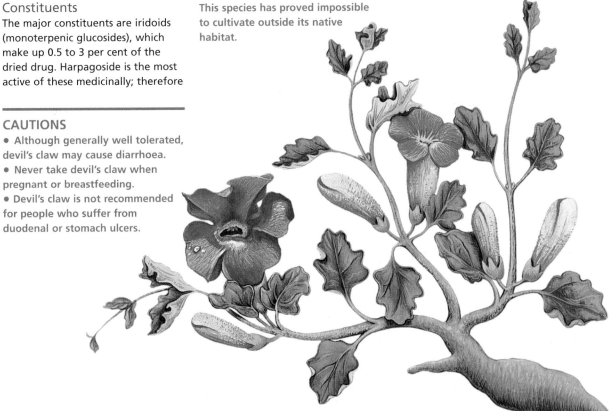

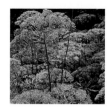

Dill

Anethum graveolens Umbelliferae/Apiaceae

Native to the Mediterranean, where it still grows wild, the dill plant sports a flourish of feathery leaves that fan out from the hollow, ridged stem. In midsummer it bears tiny yellow flowers in umbrella-shaped clusters, to be followed by large quanties of flat oval winged seeds, that are scattered on the wind.

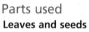

Parts used
Leaves and seeds
- The leaves are used in poultices and compresses.
- The seeds are harvested when fully ripe, then dried in a shady place, so that their constituent compounds remain active.
- They are used in infusions, tablets, tinctures and powders. An essential oil is also extracted from them.

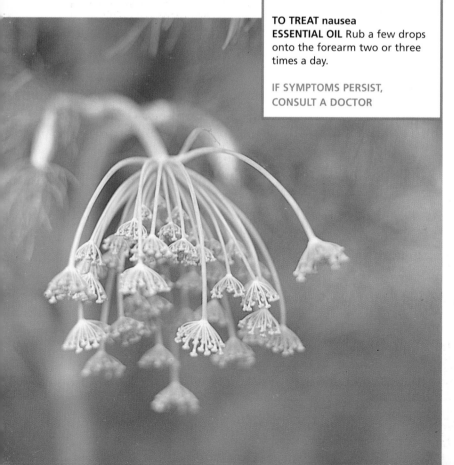

Constituents
Dill seeds contain tannin and mucilage, resinous substances, aleurone and albuminoid fats. They are also rich in essential oil.

Medicinal uses
Dill was traditionally used to treat swelling and pain, and as a sedative. It has long been known that dill can also relieve flatulence and aid digestion, which partly explains its centuries-long culinary use.

   Dill seeds are effective for treating indigestion and hiccups, particularly in infants and young children – probably because of their high concentration of essential oil. Research has also established that the essential oil has antibacterial properties, which inhibit the growth of harmful intestinal bacteria.

   Essential oil rubbed onto the skin can stop feelings of nausea, and dill seed preparations, applied externally in a poultice, can be used to treat bruises and gum infections.

Cultivation
Dill can be grown by planting the seeds in well-drained, neutral to acid soil. The plant prefers a position in direct sunlight.

CAUTIONS
- The essential oil must only be taken in small doses, due primarily to the presence of myristicin.
- The oil should not be taken when pregnant or breastfeeding.
- Dill naturally contains high levels of salt, therefore any dried plant material or the water extract are not recommended for people who need to follow a salt-restricted diet.

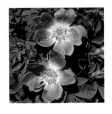

Dog rose

Rosa canina Rosaceae **Also called** Common briar

A bushy shrub, the dog rose grows wild in most temperate regions of the world. It can reach a height of 1-3m, and from May to early July bears pretty bright pink or whitish flowers on its thorny branches. Once the petals have fallen, the flower's receptacle starts to ripen, becoming red and pulpy; this is the rosehip. Seedpods are found in its pulp.

Parts used

Rosehip

• Ripe rosehips are gathered from June to September, then dried and broken into fragments or crushed into powder.
• Both fragments and powder are used to make infusions, decoctions, tinctures or dry extracts.
• Dog rose is often combined with other tonic plants, such as stinging nettle and echinacea.

Constituents

Rosehips are rich in vitamins C and B_2 and contain substantial amounts of pectins, some organic acids – particularly malic and citric – and tannins. It also contains proanthocyanidines, which have a protective antioxidant effect.

Medicinal uses

Because rosehips have such a high vitamin C content, preparations with a base of rosehip have a tonic effect and can help to boost the immune system. They are given as a general pick-me-up during illnesses and convalescence, and to help to increase resistance to infections such as colds and influenza.

CAUTIONS

• **Preparations made with a base of dog rose are not recommended for women who are pregnant or breastfeeding.**

PREPARATION AND DOSAGE

For internal use
TO TREAT chills, influenza, vitamin C deficiency, general fatigue
INFUSION Put 2-2.5g of fragmented rosehips into a cup of boiling water. Leave to infuse for 10 minutes and then filter. Drink 3-4 cups a day.
CAPSULES (with a dose of 50-200mg of dry extract) Take 1-2 capsules with a large glass of water three times a day before meals.
TINCTURE Put 30 drops into a glass of water. Take three times a day before meals.

TO TREAT diarrhoea
DECOCTION Put 30-50g of fragmented rosehips into 1 litre of boiling water. Boil gently for 5 minutes. Leave to infuse for 15 minutes and filter. Take regularly, particularly at breakfast.

IF SYMPTOMS PERSIST, CONSULT A DOCTOR

In addition, the tannins confer astringent powers that ease diarrhoea, particularly if caused by fever; the pectins and organic acids have a diuretic effect, and the organic acids help to stimulate the gastric juices, relieving gastritis.

Recent research also suggests that rosehip might help to ease the pain and improve the mobility of joints affected by arthritis.

Cultivation

Dog rose can be grown from a cutting in moist, well-drained ground that is rich in nutrients. It is best suited to a neutral to mildly acidic soil and should be placed in a sunny spot.

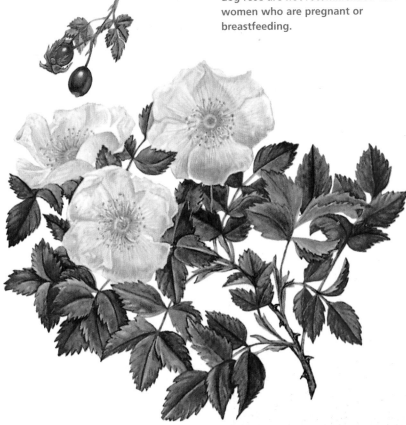

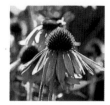

Echinacea

Echinacea augustifolia, E. purpurea, E. pallida Asteraceae/Compositae **Also called** Coneflower

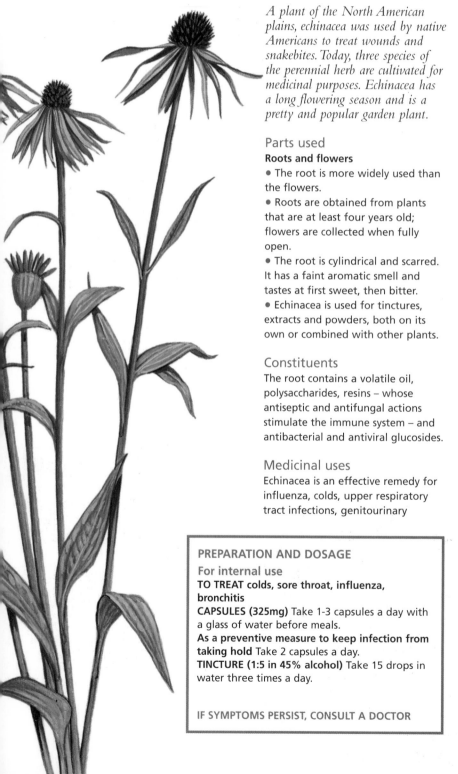

A plant of the North American plains, echinacea was used by native Americans to treat wounds and snakebites. Today, three species of the perennial herb are cultivated for medicinal purposes. Echinacea has a long flowering season and is a pretty and popular garden plant.

Parts used
Roots and flowers
- The root is more widely used than the flowers.
- Roots are obtained from plants that are at least four years old; flowers are collected when fully open.
- The root is cylindrical and scarred. It has a faint aromatic smell and tastes at first sweet, then bitter.
- Echinacea is used for tinctures, extracts and powders, both on its own or combined with other plants.

Constituents
The root contains a volatile oil, polysaccharides, resins – whose antiseptic and antifungal actions stimulate the immune system – and antibacterial and antiviral glucosides.

Medicinal uses
Echinacea is an effective remedy for influenza, colds, upper respiratory tract infections, genitourinary infections and other diseases. It is widely used to combat the common cold: it restores the body to health quickly while helping the immune system to fight off other infections.

In 2002, Canadian scientists showed that, *in vitro*, echinacea was an effective antiviral agent against herpes simplex. In 1988, German researchers discovered that the herb produced a noticeable increase in phagocytosis, a process by which foreign bodies are engulfed by the body's immune cells.

Echinacea strengthens the body's immune system and increases resistance to infection, particularly to influenza. This makes the herb especially useful for those with weakened immune systems. It may, therefore, be valuable as a supplementary treatment when the immune system is suppressed by drugs, for example, as a result of anticancer chemotherapy. However, this should only be considered in consultation with a doctor.

Cultivation
Plant in a sunny spot in rich, well-drained soil.

PREPARATION AND DOSAGE
For internal use
TO TREAT colds, sore throat, influenza, bronchitis
CAPSULES (325mg) Take 1-3 capsules a day with a glass of water before meals.
As a preventive measure to keep infection from taking hold Take 2 capsules a day.
TINCTURE (1:5 in 45% alcohol) Take 15 drops in water three times a day.

IF SYMPTOMS PERSIST, CONSULT A DOCTOR

CAUTIONS
- **Talk to your doctor before taking echinacea if you have an auto-immune illness such as lupus, or a progressive disease such as multiple sclerosis or tuberculosis.**
- **If you are allergic to flowers of the daisy family, you may be allergic to echinacea as well.**
- **Do not use to replace prescribed treatments: antibiotics and other medicines may be needed, too.**
- **No toxic properties or adverse side effects have been reported to date.**
- **Prolonged use weakens the herb's beneficial effect.**

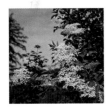

Elder, common

Sambucus nigra Caprifoliaceae **Also called** Elderberry

A native of Europe and North America, the deciduous elder tree can grow as tall as 10m. Large flat clusters of small creamy flowers bloom in May, filling the hedgerows with a sweetly pungent scent. They are followed by small, black berries filled with dark purple juice.

Parts used

Flowers, berries and inner bark
● The flowers are picked in late spring, when in full bloom.
● They are dried and used to make infusions and decoctions.
● The berries are picked when ripe in early autumn.
● The fresh inner bark, revealed when the blackish outer coating is peeled away, is less frequently used.

Constituents

Elderflower contains tannins, potassium, mucilage, phenols and flavonoids. The bark contains sambucine, an alkaloid-like substance. The berries, often used in syrups, jams and wines, are rich in anthocyanins, folic acid and vitamins A and C. They also contain flavonoids and cyanidin glucosides, which are poisonous in large doses.

Medicinal uses

Elderflowers and berries are expectorant and also promote sweating, thus helping to reduce high temperatures, and to rid the body of toxins. These combined effects make elder a good choice for treating colds and flu.

In 1990 Bulgarian scientists found elderflowers to have antiviral action against herpes simplex type I (the virus responsible for causing cold sores) and influenza types A and B. And recent clinical evidence from Israel also showed elderberry extract effectively inhibiting various strains of flu virus. If taken early enough in infection, elder can greatly improve recovery times from influenza.

A French study published in 1983 found that elderflower preparations were diuretic. The berries are known to be mildly laxative.

An elderflower decoction makes a good anti-inflammatory mouthwash or gargle for swollen painful gums and sore throats.

The roots appear to be insecticidal – badgers rub their bodies vigorously against them to kill lice infestations in their fur, and it is possible that a decoction used topically might help to eradicate an infestation of head lice.

CAUTIONS

● Do not eat raw fruit: it can cause nausea and vomiting.
● Do not use elder if pregnant or breastfeeding.
● Excessive or prolonged causes excess potassium loss via the urine.
● To date, there are no reported adverse side effects, despite the presence of small amounts of cyanidin glucosides.

PREPARATION AND DOSAGE

For internal use
TO TREAT influenza, colds, catarrh
INFUSION Put 2-5g dried flowers into a cup of boiling water. Infuse for 5-10 minutes and strain. Drink at least three cups a day.
TINCTURE (1:5 in 25% alcohol) Take 20 drops in a glass of water, three times a day after meals.

For external use
TO TREAT sore throat, inflamed gums (gingivitis) or mouth
DECOCTION Put 50g flowers into 1 litre boiling water. Boil for 5 minutes, then leave to cool. Use as a gargle or mouthwash four to six times a day, particularly after meals.

IF SYMPTOMS PERSIST, CONSULT A DOCTOR

Cultivation

Elder likes a rich damp soil and a sunny or lightly shaded location.

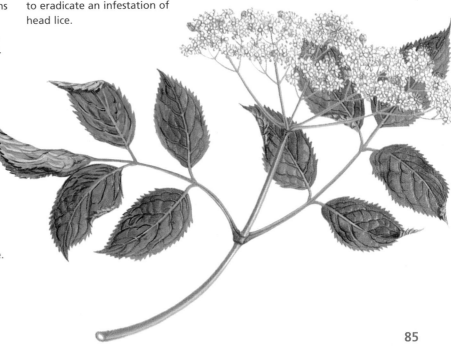

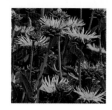

Elecampane

Inula helenium Asteraceae **Also called** Scabwort

Native to central Europe and Asia, elecampane has been renowned for its healing powers for thousands of years. By the Middle Ages, it was cultivated across much of Europe. A hardy perennial, it can grow up to 3m high. Long oval leaves shoot out from the strong, branched stem, and from June to August its large golden flower heads can be seen across damp meadows and along woodland fringes. The tough, thick root has many buds and a dense, spreading network of strong rootlets.

Parts used

Root

• The roots are dug up in September and October, then cut up and dried at a temperature of at least 40°C.
• Decoctions, tinctures and extracts are prepared from the dried root, which is also used in an ointment for treating skin infections.

Constituents

The elecampane root is composed mainly of inulin – about 44 per cent. It also contains mucilage and a small amount of essential oil. Antolactone (that can sometimes irritate the mucous membranes) and helenin are found in this oil.

Medicinal uses

Preparations made from elecampane root are prescribed to treat a wide range of respiratory problems. The mucilage acts as an expectorant, soothing coughs caused by infection and inflammation, and elecampane extract is known to significantly inhibit the growth of the bacteria responsible for tuberculosis. Research has shown that the alantolactone is largely responsible for these antibacterial powers. When mixed with other plants extracts, elecampane is also a highly effective treatment for bronchitis and asthma.

The helenin has anti-fungal properties, and is particularly effective against the *Microsporum* and *Trichophyton* types of fungi. The plant root is therefore used externally in ointments to treat certain fungal skin infections.

Elecampane is also known to act as a diuretic, helping to eliminate toxins, and to stimulate the secretion of bile by the gall bladder, easing digestive problems.

CAUTIONS

• High doses of elecampane may cause vomiting, diarrhoea and abdominal pains.
• As a result, it should not be used if pregnant or breastfeeding.
• Elecampane can sometimes cause an allergic reaction, when used in an ointment to treat skin infections.

PREPARATION AND DOSAGE

For internal use
TO TREAT coughs, inflammation of the respiratory system
DECOCTION Put 10-15g of dried root into 1 litre of water. Leave to boil for 10 minutes and then filter. Take 1 tablespoon every 2 hours.

For external use
TO TREAT fungal skin infections
OINTMENT (50% elecampane) Apply several times a day.

IF SYMPTOMS PERSIST, CONSULT A DOCTOR

Cultivation

Elecampane grows easily from root cuttings. Plant these in moist, clay soil that contains plenty of leaf mould, preferably in the shade.

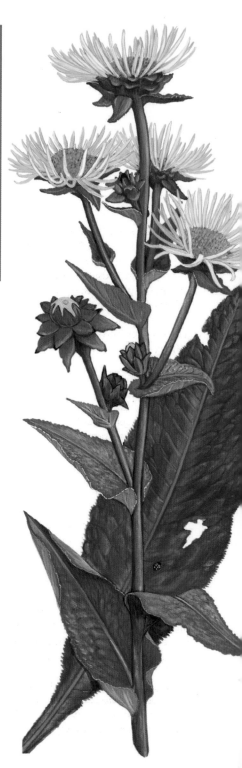

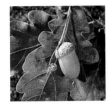

English oak

Quercus robur Fagaceae

Venerated by the Druids, the oak was well known for its medicinal powers in the ancient world. The long-lived tree can grow to over 50m tall, with boughs spreading to a circumference of nearly 100m. In spring, dense clusters of oval, lobed leaves appear along with dangling male flowers, or catkins. Female flowers are barely visible, turning to the familiar brown, egg-shaped fruits, or acorns, by autumn.

Parts used

Bark from young branches
• The bark is collected in April and May, then cut up or crushed.
• It is used in infusions, decoctions, tinctures and compresses, and may be added to foot and hand baths.
• Oak bark also used in combination with other astringent plants, such as bilberry and witch hazel.

Constituents

Tannins make up about 10 to 20 per cent of oak bark. These include epicatechin, gallocatechin and catechin. The highest concentration of tannins is found in trees that are about 10 years old.

Medicinal uses

Oak bark is known for its ability to combat various viruses, and the tannins give it astringent properties. For these reasons, when taken internally in small doses, it can help to relieve non-specific, acute diarrhoea and indigestion.

Applied externally, it can treat inflamed or chapped skin, chilblains, wet eczema and minor bleeding. It can also be added to baths to combat foot odour.

Gargles and mouthwashes made with oak bark are used to soothe inflammation of the gums and lining of the mouth, as well as sore throats.

Tests have recently shown that the tannins in oak are able to limit tissue damage in people suffering from rheumatic disease. This discovery may herald a new medicinal use for the bark of the oak.

Cultivation

Plant acorns in well-drained soil in sun or partial shade, or propagate by grafting in autumn or late winter.

CAUTIONS

• Oak bark preparations should not be taken internally for more than four weeks at a time.
• Do not use oak bark baths on skin that is cut or affected by dermatitis. Also avoid them if you have an infectious illness or feel feverish.
• Make sure an oak bark bath does not come into contact with the eyes.

PREPARATION AND DOSAGE

For internal use
TO TREAT non-specific acute diarrhoea
INFUSION Put 10g of bark powder into 1 cup of boiling water. Drink 4-5 cups a day.

For external use
TO TREAT foot odour, inflamed or chapped skin, chilblains, wet eczema, light bleeding
BATHS AND COMPRESSES Put 100g of bark powder into 1 litre of water. Boil for 20 minutes and filter. Bathe the feet or hands three or four times a day. Alternatively, apply soaked compresses to the area affected.
TINCTURE (diluted to 10% strength) Add to a bath or apply on a compress three or four times a day.

IF SYMPTOMS PERSIST, CONSULT A DOCTOR

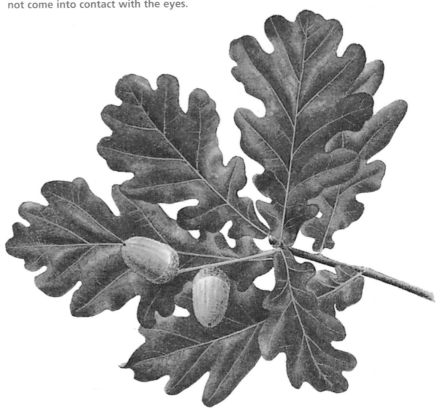

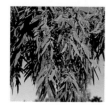

Eucalyptus

Eucalyptus globulus Myrtaceae **Also called** Blue gum, Tasmanian blue gum

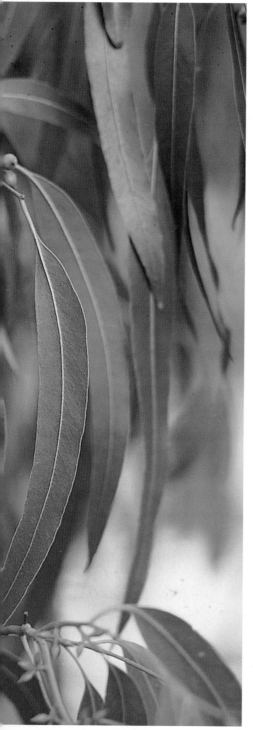

Native to Australia, the eucalyptus is a giant evergreen tree, usually 30-100m tall, with a smooth, grey-blue trunk. The German botanist, Ferdinand von Müller, was the first European to recognise the medicinal powers of the fragrant oil in the long, narrow, leathery leaves growing on branches that are more than five years old.

Parts used
Leaves
● Aromatic leaves from the older branches are collected, usually in summer.
● The leaves are either dried or distilled for their essential oil.
● The dried leaves are ground to a powder or used in infusions and tinctures. The oil is used in syrups, balms and ointments.

Constituents
The leaves contain flavonoids, and also large amounts of essential oil, that is rich in cineole and eucalyptol.

Medicinal uses
A number of studies have shown that eucalyptus can combat certain bacteria, and that it has antifungal and antiviral powers. Its antiseptic action, along with its ability to act as a decongestant, stems from the eucalyptol in the essential oil, making eucalyptus an effective treatment for respiratory ailments such as coughs and colds. For its antiseptic action, it is used to treat cuts and wounds, and has also been shown to be effective for burns.

The flavonoids in eucalyptus are known to help to lower blood sugar levels – an effect demonstrated in various clinical trials. One study has also shown its ability to ease aching muscles by increasing the blood flow to them.

Cultivation
Eucalyptus prefers a warm climate, but can grow at temperatures as low as –15°C. Plant seeds in a sunny position, in well-drained, fertile, acid to neutral soil.

CAUTIONS
● Eucalyptus should not be used by children under 3 years old, women who are pregnant or breastfeeding, or people suffering from digestive or liver disorders.
● Never use eucalyptus preparations if you are taking any drugs to lower blood sugar levels.
● The essential oil can cause kidney problems if taken internally. Also the cineole in the oil can sometimes induce seizures in children.

PREPARATION AND DOSAGE
For internal use
TO TREAT bronchial ailments, sore throats, coughs
POWDER Take 4-10g a day in capsule form or with water.
TINCTURE Put 50 drops into a glass of water. Take four to six times a day.

For external use
TO TREAT bronchial ailments, sore throats, coughs
BALM AND OINTMENT Rub into the chest and throat once or twice a day.
ESSENTIAL OIL Rub into the chest and throat once a day.

TO TREAT colds, blocked noses
INHALATIONS Prepare an infusion of leaves and essential oil. While hot inhale the steam through the nose or mouth, under a towel, for 10 minutes twice a day. Use as needed.

IF SYMPTOMS PERSIST, CONSULT A DOCTOR

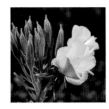

Evening primrose

Oenothera biennis Onagraceae

Although a native of North America, the biennial evening primrose is also very common in Europe. Its large, short-lived yellow flowers appear clustered in spikes from June to September, and open only in the evenings, hence the name of the plant. Each fruit contains about 600 small seeds.

Parts used
Seeds
- The seeds are collected when ripe.
- Oil is extracted from them and put into capsules for pharmaceutical use.
- The oil is also occasionally used as a food flavouring.

Constituents
Twenty-five per cent of each seed is made up of an oil rich in essential fatty acids, including linolenic acid and gammalinolenic acid. The seeds also contain proteins, fibre and mineral materials rich in calcium.

Medicinal uses
Evening primrose oil has long been used as a treatment for premenstrual syndrome and works especially well in relieving breast pain. This is because its fatty acids, mainly gammalinolenic acid, play an important role in the body's synthesis of substances called prostaglandins (PGEs). PGEs are important because they help to regulate the action of several hormones – oestrogen, progesterone and prolactin – that are associated with the menstrual cycle. A good supply of the fatty acids found in evening primrose oil ensures a good supply of the PGEs that make sure these hormones perform correctly.

PGEs also help to maintain the suppleness and elasticity of the skin by controlling the secretion of sebum, an oil that protects skin tissues. Evening primrose oil is therefore used in cosmetics to help to prevent skin ageing.

In addition, research has shown that prostaglandin E_1 controls the dilation of blood vessels and is anti-inflammatory. Evening primrose oil could therefore be useful for acne, eczema and rheumatoid arthritis.

Cultivation
The plant does well in well-drained soil and sunny locations, and will self-sow in good conditions.

CAUTIONS
- Evening primrose oil should not be taken by people who suffer from any form of epilepsy or schizophrenia or who are taking phenothiazine tranquillisers.
- Do not use evening primrose oil if pregnant or breastfeeding.
- Taking the oil may cause weight gain in some people.

PREPARATION AND DOSAGE
For internal use
TO TREAT premenstrual syndrome (PMS)
SOFT CAPSULES (500mg) Take 2 capsules three times a day during the last 10 days of the menstrual cycle.

TO TREAT eczema, rheumatoid arthritis
SOFT CAPSULES (500mg) Take 2 capsules three times a day, with a glass of water at mealtimes.

TO TREAT ageing skin
SOFT CAPSULES (500mg) Take 1-2 capsules a day, with a glass of water at mealtimes.

IF SYMPTOMS PERSIST, CONSULT A DOCTOR

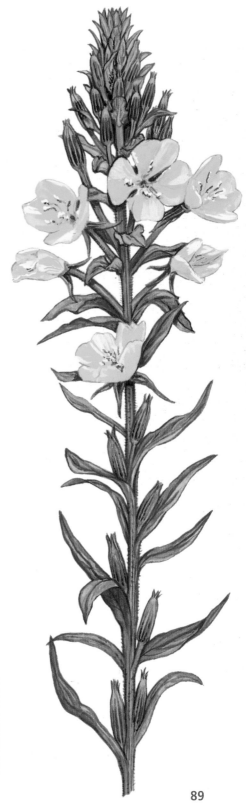

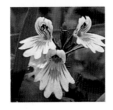

Eyebright

Euphrasia officinalis Scrophulariaceae **Also called** Eufragia, Euphrasia

Found on chalky grasslands and meadows, eyebright has long been used in remedies for sore eyes — hence its name. This little plant has downy leaves and small, lipped flowers whose white petals are tinged with mauve and yellow. It is widespread in Britain and Europe.

Parts used

All parts above ground
● Plants are collected when they begin to flower in July and August.
● The plant is cut off just above the root and then dried.
● Eyebright is used in decoctions, tinctures, infusions and eye lotions.

Constituents

Eyebright contains tannins (making it astringent), antimicrobial substances called iridoids that have anti-inflammatory properties, phenols (known to inhibit bacterial growth), an essential oil, flavonoids and resins.

Medicinal uses

The plant's astringent properties are known to be useful for treating eye problems. A compress soothes styes (infected eyelash follicles), inflamed cornea and conjunctivitis. It also cools tired and watering eyes and is often an ingredient in eye lotions prescribed for these ailments.

In Icelandic medicine, juice squeezed from the plant is used for a variety of eye problems. And Scottish Highlanders used to make an infusion of eyebright in milk and paint it onto sore and irritated eyelids with a feather.

In 1994 Spanish researchers demonstrated the anti-inflammatory properties of the iridoids in eyebright. Tannins in the herb improve resistance to infection by drying and contracting the body's tissues, while phenols help by inhibiting the growth of bacteria.

An infusion of eyebright taken internally complements any topical eye treatment. It is also anti-

catarrhal, making it useful for clearing runny noses, middle ear infections and painful sinuses.

Eyebright is a constituent of British Herbal Tobacco. Smokers with bronchitis may find that smoking this anti-inflammatory preparation soothes their irritable airways.

Cultivation

This hardy plant is semi-parasitic: it will thrive only if it is planted among grasses whose roots provide it with water and nourishment. Sow seed in a wild area of the garden.

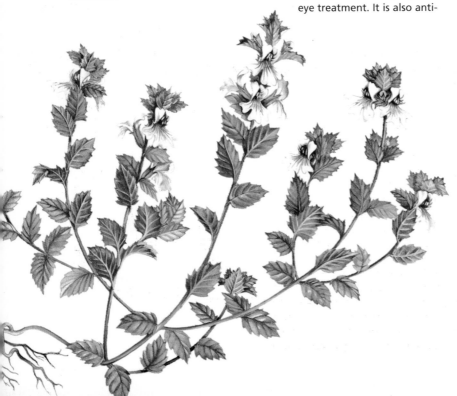

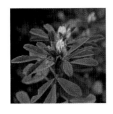

Fenugreek

Trigonella foenum-graecum Fabaceae/Leguminosae

Originally found beside the Black Sea, fenugreek is a widely grown annual in India, north Africa and the United States. The plant grows to a height of about 50cm and is strongly aromatic. It has oval leaves and triangular flowers, which range in colour from yellow to bright purple. The long curved seedpods contain many brown seeds, used in Indian cooking as a pungent curry spice.

Parts used
Seeds
- The seedpods are picked when ripe in August and September.
- The pods are stripped away and the seeds are made into a liquid extract or tincture, or ground and sold as powder or in tablet form.

Constituents
The main constituent of fenugreek is mucilage, a soluble fibre that soaks up water, forming a jelly-like substance. The seeds also contain coumarins, steroidal saponins (which have a hormone-mimicking effect), a volatile oil that gives the seeds their aroma, and alkaloids.

Medicinal uses
Fenugreek has a tonic effect that helps to combat tiredness and speeds convalescence. And because it is rich in mucilage, which protects mucous membranes from irritants, it soothes painful digestive disorders. Mucilage gives stools bulk and lubricates the bowel, so easing constipation.

In 2001 researchers in Jaipur, India, noted that fenugreek lowers blood sugar levels in Type 2 diabetes mellitus, reducing insulin resistance and removing excess triglycerides in the blood. Research published in the *Journal of Ethnopharmacology* in 2002 identified anti-ulcer properties.

Medical herbalists prescribe fenugreek to treat anorexia, but its bulking effects can also aid dieting by making the stomach feel full. The fibre and saponin in fenugreek reduce cholesterol and blood lipids, while its hormonal qualities can combat loss of virility in men.

Externally, a poultice of fenugreek powder reduces skin inflammation and relieves pain.

Cultivation
Plant seeds in a well-drained fertile soil in a sunny position.

PREPARATION AND DOSAGE
For internal use
TO TREAT fatigue, weight loss
POWDER Take 2g in a little water three times a day.
TINCTURE (1:3 in 25% alcohol) Put 20 drops in a little cold water. Take three times a day. (The solution tastes bitter.)
TABLETS (500mg) Take 1 tablet four times a day.
For external use
TO TREAT skin inflammation
POULTICE (using the powder) Apply to the affected part, changing the compress every 3-4 hours.

IF SYMPTOMS PERSIST, CONSULT A DOCTOR

CAUTIONS
- Fenugreek is not toxic and is considered completely safe.
- It contains steroid compounds and should not be taken by children before they reach puberty.
- Pregnant and breastfeeding women should not take more of the spice than is normally found in food.
- Diabetics should consult a medical herbalist before using fenugreek. Do not use if taking anticoagulants.

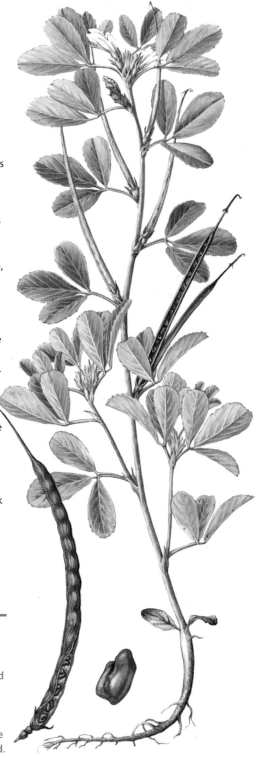

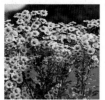

Feverfew

Tanacetum parthenium Asteraceae/Compositae

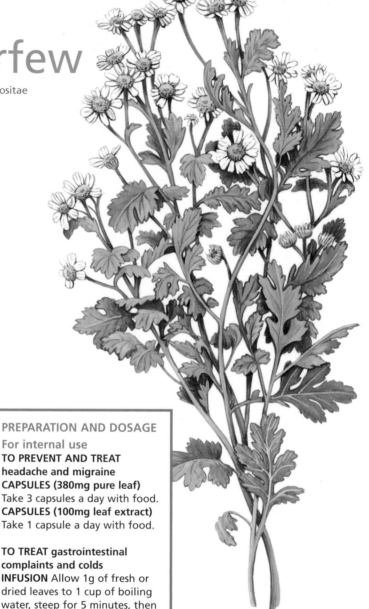

A hardy perennial herb, feverfew is native to Anatolia. The plant grows to a height of 60cm and looks like a cross between a daisy and chamomile. Its leaves and flowers exude a strong, quite bitter aroma. Feverfew was once planted near homes to ward off disease.

Parts used

Aerial parts
- Plants are collected in summer when in full flower.
- They are dried and stored away from sunlight and damp to prevent decomposition and loss of efficacy.
- Fresh leaves can be picked and used when required.

Constituents

The main active constituents are substances called sesquiterpene lactones, which have anti-inflammatory and antispasmodic properties. The most important of these is parthenolide.

Medicinal uses

A staple of the herbal medicine chest, feverfew gives effective relief from headaches caused by dilatation

CAUTIONS

- No serious side effects have been recorded.
- Can cause stomach upsets in susceptible individuals.
- Avoid if pregnant or breastfeeding.
- Do not use if taking the contraceptive pill.
- To prevent allergic reactions, do not use for more than four months at a time; avoid if allergic to the plant family Compositae (eg chamomile and yarrow).
- Discontinue use gradually to avoid withdrawal symptoms such as joint pain, headaches or insomnia.

PREPARATION AND DOSAGE

For internal use

TO PREVENT AND TREAT headache and migraine
CAPSULES (380mg pure leaf)
Take 3 capsules a day with food.
CAPSULES (100mg leaf extract)
Take 1 capsule a day with food.

TO TREAT gastrointestinal complaints and colds
INFUSION Allow 1g of fresh or dried leaves to 1 cup of boiling water, steep for 5 minutes, then strain. Take 1-2 cups daily.
TINCTURE (2:5 in 25% alcohol)
Take 20 drops in water twice a day after food.

IF SYMPTOMS PERSIST, CONSULT A DOCTOR

---

or contraction of blood vessels. It is used for migraine, period pain, fever, asthma and other inflammatory disorders.

There has been much research into the plant's anti-inflammatory properties, and a compound called parthenolide appears to be its main active ingredient. Scientists in Canada, India and at King's College in the UK have all conducted experiments that demonstrate feverfew's anti-inflammatory effects.

Studies at Nottingham University in 1988 found that the plant was effective in reducing the frequency and the severity of migraine attacks.

Cultivation

You can grow the plant on a windowsill, or sow seeds in spring in a well-drained stony soil in a sunny spot. Established plants will come back year after year.

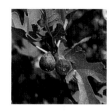

Fig

Ficus carica Moraceae

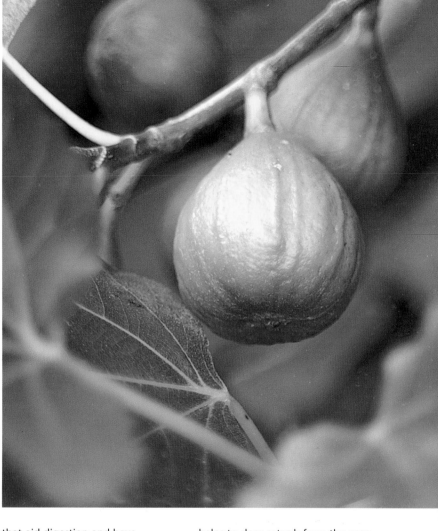

Often mentioned in the Bible, fig trees are found throughout the Mediterranean region. Athletes in ancient Greece gorged on figs, believing that they increased a man's speed and stamina. The deciduous tree can reach a height of 12m. It has large lobed leaves and its tiny flowers are hidden, clustered inside the green 'fruits', which ripen after fertilisation into fleshy figs.

Parts used

Fruit, leaves and, rarely, the sap

● Figs and fig leaves are used in tinctures and decoctions.
● The fruit is eaten fresh or dried.
● Fig syrup is used as a mild laxative.

Constituents

Fresh ripe figs contain up to 50 per cent sugar (glucose). They also contain flavonoids, which have an anti-inflammatory effect. Coumarins in the leaves are aromatic substances that aid digestion and have antiseptic properties. The coumarins include bergapten and psoralen, both photosensitising agents.

Medicinal uses

People have eaten this nutritious, sugar-rich fruit for thousands of years. The sugar and fibre in figs give them their famous laxative effect.

Flavonoids and coumarins in both the fruits and leaves contribute to fig's digestive, soothing, calming and anti-inflammatory effects. Fig also helps to clear catarrh from the nose and throat, and to remove poisons. Eating the fruit can ease coughs, sore throats and the pain of various inflammatory conditions.

Researchers have investigated the use of figs in treating diabetes. A Spanish clinical trial published in 1998 found that people with Type I (insulin-dependent) diabetes taking fig-leaf decoctions had lower blood sugar levels after eating meals.

In traditional medicine, the milky sap of the fig tree was applied externally to soothe minor aches, pains and insect bites, as well as to remove warts. However, the sap can burn and blister the skin and should be treated with caution.

Cultivation

Some varieties of fig do well against south-facing walls. Plant ready-bought young plants or cuttings in a well-drained, neutral to alkaline soil.

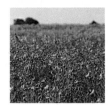

Flax

Linum usitatissimum Linaceae **Also called** Linseed

The slender, graceful flax is a herbaceous annual that is cropped throughout Europe. Its seeds, known as linseed, are widely used in herbal medicine and yield a valuable oil; the fibres of its stalks are used to make linen. Flax grows to about 1m in height and bears sky-blue flowers. The pea-sized fruits contain ten oily seeds.

Parts used

Seeds

● Flax is a major arable crop. It is harvested in late summer.

● The fruits are crushed to get the seeds which contain linseed oil.

PREPARATION AND DOSAGE

For internal use

TO TREAT chronic (long-term) constipation, disorders of the colon, inflammation of the gastric and intestinal mucous membranes

MACERATION Put 15-20g of seeds into 1 litre of cold water. Leave to soak overnight and strain. Drink 1 glass in the morning before eating and then 4-5 glasses during the day, but not at mealtimes.

WHOLE SEEDS Take 15-20 seeds with a glass of water three times a day.

For external use

TO TREAT spots and boils, itching, bruising, painful joints

POULTICE Slowly pour water onto flax meal stirring all the while until it has become a smooth paste. Warm this gently and spread it, still slightly warm, in a layer about 1cm thick onto a piece of gauze. Apply to the affected part one to three times a day.

IF SYMPTOMS PERSIST, CONSULT A DOCTOR

● Both whole and ground seeds are used in herbal medicine.

● The meal – what is left of the seeds once the seed oil has been extracted – is also used.

Constituents

The seed is made up of 35-45 per cent oil. Linseed oil is rich in omega-3 unsaturated fatty acids – which protect against heart and circulation problems and are anti-inflammatory. The seed also contains proteins, mucilage, cholesterol-lowering phytosterols, anti-inflammatory lignans and cyanogenic glycosides which are antispasmodic.

Medicinal uses

Flax seed is a gentle laxative. It is used to treat long-term constipation and colon disorders. It contains mucilage that lines and soothes the mucous membranes of an irritated digestive system and painful bowel.

The phytoestrogens in the seeds appear to have a beneficial effect on some breast and colon cancers. And a paper published in the *American Journal of Kidney Disease* in 2001 reported linseed's potential in the treatment of kidney disorders.

US research in New Jersey, in 1993, showed that flax seed reduced blood cholesterol in patients with high blood cholesterol levels. And a 2000 American paper suggested the seeds benefited those with atherosclerosis.

A paper published in *Obstetrics and Gynecology* in 2002 reported that taking flaxseed improved mild menopausal symptoms.

Flax meal has long been used as a poultice for skin disorders such as spots and boils, itching and bruising. It also helps to soothe painful joints.

Cultivation

Sow seeds in spring in well-drained soil in a sunny location.

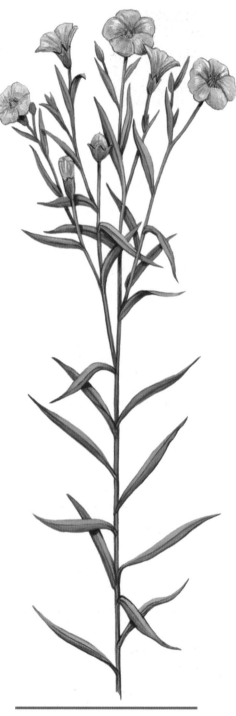

CAUTIONS

● No adverse effects or toxicity have been recorded to date.

● Do not use if you have prostate cancer or an intestinal blockage.

● Do not combine with other drugs, laxatives or stool softeners.

● Do not use flax if pregnant or breastfeeding.

● Do not use immature seeds, or meal past its sell-by date; its residual oil content causes it to go rancid.

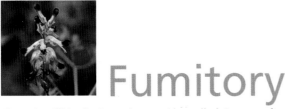

Fumitory

Fumaria officinalis Fumariaceae **Also called** Common fumitory

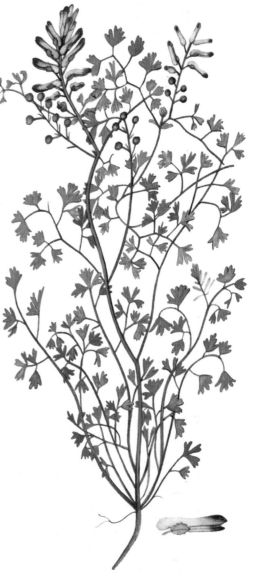

Colonising fields, banks, hedgerows and old walls, fumitory is found all over Britain. Clusters of deep pink or purple flowers bloom throughout summer. The delicate blue-green foliage has a whitish bloom, and its appearance, resembling smoke rising from the ground, is thought to be the source of the name: fumitory means 'smoke of the earth'.

Parts used

Whole plant above ground

- Plants are gathered in spring and summer, and dried.
- Fumitory is used as an infusion, a powder, a dry extract or a tincture.

PREPARATION AND DOSAGE

For internal use

TO TREAT digestive problems, gall-bladder problems, irregular heartbeat, high blood pressure, asthma, eczema, acne

INFUSION Put 2 teaspoons of dried flowers into 150ml of boiling water. Infuse for 10 minutes and strain. Drink 1 cup half-an-hour before meals, and between meals as required.

TINCTURE Put 30-50 drops into a glass of water and drink half-an-hour before meals.

CAPSULES (400mg powder) Take 3-6 capsules a day with a large glass of water.

CAPSULES (250mg dry extract) Take 3-4 capsules a day with a large glass of water.

For external use

TO TREAT psoriasis, eczema, the itching caused by scabies

COMPRESS Soak a cloth in an infusion of the dried flowers (see above) and apply it to the affected areas two or three times a day.

IF SYMPTOMS PERSIST, CONSULT A DOCTOR

Constituents

Fumitory contains some 30 alkaloids – substances which often have strong pharmaceutical actions. One alkaloid, protopine, seems to be fumitory's major active constituent. The plant also contains flavonoids (which are anti-inflammatory and good for the circulation), organic acids including fumaric acid, and mucilage.

Medicinal uses

Traditionally, fumitory has been used to treat skin problems such as acne and eczema. Its effectiveness may be due to its diuretic and purgative actions, which have a general cleansing effect on the whole body.

Fumitory is antispasmodic and reduces blood pressure. The plant's sedative properties are useful for treating a range of illnesses including irregular heartbeat (arrhythmia), high blood pressure and asthma.

A German article published in 1995 reviewed fumitory's beneficial actions on bile and urine flow – thus making it useful for gall-bladder and liver problems. It has also been used to remedy digestive disorders such as dyspepsia, flatulence and nausea.

In 1980 Russian research showed that fumitory alkaloids could help to restore healthy blood circulation after a cardiac arrest. And in 1986,

---

CAUTIONS

- To date, no adverse side effects or toxicity have been reported.
- Overdose can cause stomach upsets.
- Do not use when taking drugs prescribed to lower blood pressure or treat heart problems.
- Do not use if pregnant or breastfeeding.
- Do not use if you suffer from glaucoma or are prone to seizures.

German scientists noted that one of these alkaloids – protopine – has a beneficial effect on the functioning of the nervous system.

Fumitory is anti-inflammatory – or more specifically, protopine is anti-inflammatory, as observed in *Pharmacology Research* in 1997. Applied externally, it soothes psoriasis, eczema, scabies and other skin flare-ups. It may also be used as an eyewash to ease conjunctivitis.

Cultivation

Fumitory prefers sunny spots and is suited to light, well-drained soil.

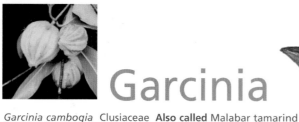

Garcinia

Garcinia cambogia Clusiaceae **Also called** Malabar tamarind

Native to South-east Asia and India, garcinia is a tropical shrub with glossy dark green leaves. It bears yellow, pumpkin-shaped fruits the size of an orange. The fruits are used in Thai and Indian cooking to impart a distinctive sour flavour, similar to tamarind.

Parts used
Fruit including rind
• The fruits are split in half and the seeds removed.
• The halves are dried and used to make dry extracts, drinks, chewing gum and tablets.
• Garcinia is also used in products for external use such as creams, ointments and lotions.

Constituents
Up to 50 per cent of the dry extract is made up of a fruit acid called hydroxycitric acid. This is the plant's main active ingredient, which is thought to help to control the formation of fat in the body. The fruit also contains other fruit acids that have antioxidant properties.

Medicinal uses
Garcinia has been used as a dietary aid for thousands of years in South-east Asia, where it has long been valued as an appetite suppressant.

This attribute seems to be due to the substance hydroxycitric acid (HCA). Researchers think that HCA somehow affects the absorption and synthesis of fats, so forcing the body to burn its own reserves.

In 2000 Japanese scientists found that hydroxycitric acid extracted from the rind of garcinia promoted lipid oxidation during exercise in mice. However, clinical trials have not supported its benefits in the treatment of obesity in humans. An American study published in the Journal of Physiological Behaviour in 2000 found that HCA failed to suppress the appetite. Another clinical study performed in New York in 1998 revealed that taking garcinia supplements produced neither significant weight loss nor loss of body fat.

Garcinia is reputed to benefit diabetics by regulating blood sugar levels, and to moderate blood cholesterol. Like all fruit acids, the hydroxycitric acid in garcinia can be used to treat wrinkles and acne.

Cultivation
Garcinia is grown from seed, but can be bought ready-grown. A tropical plant, it needs damp warmth and thrives in a heated greenhouse.

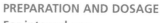

CAUTIONS
• No side effects or toxicity have been reported to date.
• Do not use if pregnant or breastfeeding.
• Do not give to children.

PREPARATION AND DOSAGE

For internal use
TO TREAT cases of mild obesity
CAPSULES (400mg dry extract)
Take 1 capsule with a glass of water 30-60 minutes before main meals, three times a day.

For external use
TO TREAT wrinkles, acne
CREAM, LOTION (containing 1-20% hydroxycitric acid) Apply once or twice a day.

IF SYMPTOMS PERSIST, CONSULT A DOCTOR

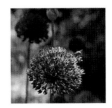

Garlic

Allium sativum Alliaceae

The long slender leaves of garlic give it its name, which means spear plant in Anglo-Saxon. Garlic is a small herbaceous perennial. Its grass-like leaves encase the main stem, which bears umbrella-shaped clusters of flowers. The garlic bulb is made up of 10-15 cloves, each enclosed in a whitish papery envelope. The cloves form the underground food storage system.

Parts used

Bulb

● Garlic is harvested in summer or autumn.
● A piece of the stem is left attached to each bulb so that the bulbs can be strung into bunches.
● Once the outer parts are dried, garlic bulbs are stored in a dry place.
● The bulbs are eaten as part of the diet or used pharmaceutically in powders, extracts and tinctures.

Constituents

The main active component is the sulphur compound allicin, which is released when fresh garlic is crushed. In turn this produces other sulphides, which occur after the crushed bulb has been oxidised by air. The bulb also contains phenols – antiseptic and anti-inflammatory when taken internally – and flavonoids, known to have anticancer properties.

CAUTIONS

● Individuals who are sensitive to garlic may experience heartburn.
● Those taking anticoagulant drugs should check with their doctor before taking garlic.
● Anyone scheduled for surgery should tell the surgeon if they are taking garlic supplements.
● Garlic is very safe and can be used freely as a food by pregnant and breastfeeding women.

Medicinal uses

Garlic has been used since Biblical times for treating parasitic worms, and respiratory and digestive problems. It was a vitally important antiseptic in the First World War.

Garlic can be used to prevent or treat infection: in 1999 Japanese scientists demonstrated its anti-bacterial action against E. coli, methicillin-resistant Staphylococcus aureus and Salmonella infections.

Garlic has an antiseptic effect on the digestive and respiratory systems. It is also an immune stimulant. It makes the breath smell because its sulphur compounds evaporate rapidly. (Eating parsley combats this.)

By reducing fatty deposits on blood vessel walls, garlic can help to prevent hardening of the arteries. It tones the circulation and reduces the formation of blood clots, helping to prevent heart attacks. Garlic may also dilate coronary blood vessels, helping to prevent angina and reduce blood pressure .

Cultivation

Plant cloves in a rich, well-drained soil in autumn or spring, in a sunny spot. Each clove will form a bulb by mid to late summer or early autumn.

PREPARATION AND DOSAGE

For internal use
TO TREAT intestinal worms
DRY EXTRACT Take 100-250mg a day.

TO TREAT digestive and respiratory infections and
TO PREVENT circulation problems
TINCTURE Take 40-50 drops three times a day.
CAPSULES, TABLETS (300mg, available in odourless form) Take 1-3 a day.

IF SYMPTOMS PERSIST, CONSULT A DOCTOR

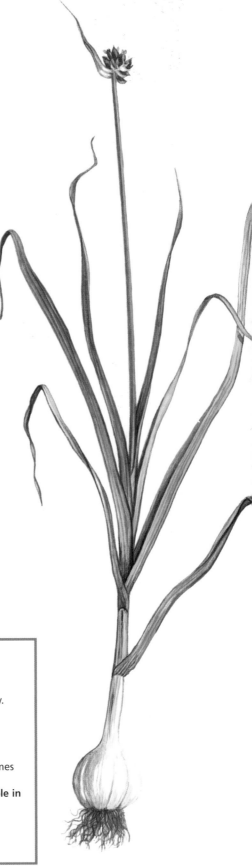

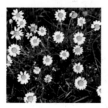

German chamomile

Matricaria recutita, formerly *Chamomilla recutita* Compositae/Asteraceae

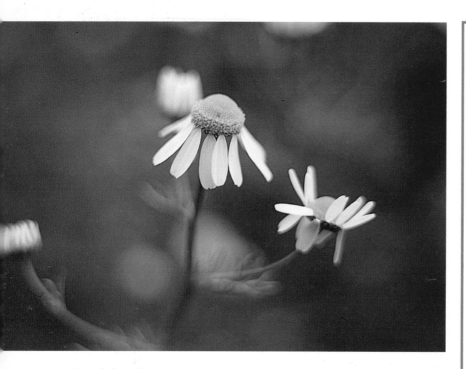

PREPARATION AND DOSAGE

For internal use

TO TREAT gastric or intestinal spasms, bloating, sluggish digestion, period pains, insomnia
INFUSION Put 1 sachet or 5-8g of loose chamomile into 1 cup of boiling water. Cover and leave to infuse for 10 minutes. Drink 3 cups a day before meals.

For external use

TO TREAT skin ailments, eye irritation, oral hygiene
OINTMENTS, EYE LOTIONS, PASTILLES, MOUTHWASHES Use as directed.

TO TREAT sinusitis, asthma
STEAM INHALATION Make an infusion as described above and inhale the rising steam.

IF SYMPTOMS PERSIST, CONSULT A DOCTOR

Found throughout Europe, German chamomile grows wild in fields and along roadsides, and is cultivated in gardens. It reaches a height of about 40cm and its daisy-like flowers have an aromatic scent.

Parts used

Flowers

● German chamomile grows wild and is also cultivated in the UK.
● The flowers are gathered in full bloom, then dried.
● The dried flowers have a strong smell and a very bitter taste.
● German chamomile is used in infusions, capsules and solutions. It is also a component of many pharmaceutical preparations and body and hair-care products.

Constituents

German chamomile's bitter taste is due to substances called sesquiterpenoid lactones. Its essential oil contains azulenes, bisabols and flavonoids. These active constituents give the herb its anti-inflammatory, antispasmodic and smooth muscle-relaxing properties – particularly in the gastrointestinal tract.

Medicinal uses

German chamomile has been used for centuries as a medicinal plant, mostly for digestive disorders. It is also a mild sedative, calming the nervous system. The essential oil has an anti-inflammatory effect on mucous membranes: a chamomile steam inhalation will help to ease sinusitis and asthma.

In 1979, German researchers found that bisabol was an anti-inflammatory, while French scientists in 1983 proved the herb's antiviral effects against polio and herpes.

The plant's anti-inflammatory and antispasmodic properties make it a good remedy for stomach aches and period pains. It also eases bloating due to excessive wind.

Externally, a German chamomile cream treats skin inflammation and promotes healing. It is recommended for eczema, nappy rash and cracked nipples. It is also used as an eye bath and in antiseptic mouthwashes.

Cultivation

Sow seeds in spring in well-drained, neutral to acid soil in a sunny spot.

CAUTIONS

● No toxic or adverse effects have been reported to date.
● Topical application may, in very rare cases, cause allergic reactions.
● Do not use if allergic to plants from the Asteraceae family (asters and chrysanthemums).
● Consult a doctor before use if taking anticoagulant drugs.

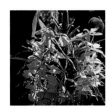

Ginger

Zingiber officinale Zingiberaceae

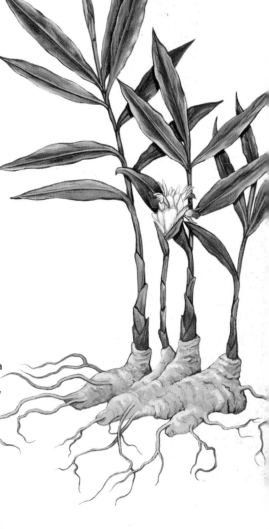

Originally from Asia, ginger is now cultivated in Africa, India, the West Indies and the USA. It is a tall, slender perennial with lance-shaped leaves and orchid-like flowers. The plant reproduces through its rhizome (rootstock) – the part used medicinally and in cooking. Ginger adds a spicy, hot and aromatic flavour to many Asian cuisines.

Parts used

Rhizome
- Rhizomes are gathered at least a year after planting but must be lifted carefully as they break easily.
- Root ginger is used fresh or dried.
- Dried ginger is used for infusions, extracts and tinctures and in many pharmaceutical products.

Constituents

Ginger is rich in aromatic volatile oils. These oils are its medically active constituents, and also give ginger its characteristic aroma and flavour. Ginger oil contains sesquiterpenes (known to be anti-inflammatory), particularly zingiberene. It also contains monoterpenes and aldehydes. These constituents have been shown by recent research to inhibit one of the most widespread common cold viruses. Pungent components called gingerols are thought to be responsible for ginger's antinausea effect.

CAUTIONS
- To date, no toxic or adverse side effects have been recorded.
- Overdose can cause stomach upsets and drowsiness.
- Ginger can help pregnant women with morning sickness, but consult your doctor before using.
- Do not use ginger if taking anti-coagulant (blood-thinning) drugs.

Medicinal uses

Ginger is a strong circulatory stimulant. It has an anticlotting effect and is a vasodilator – so it can help to combat circulatory problems. It also promotes good digestion and is antispasmodic.

Ginger has a sedative effect and also reduces nausea and vomiting, including travel sickness. A study in 1990 at St Bartholomew's hospital, London, found that ginger reduced the incidence of nausea for post-operative patients. Its efficacy was comparable with metoclopramide, a widely used antiemetic drug.

Research published in the *Journal of Nutrition* in 2000 showed that an extract of ginger reduced blood cholesterol levels as well as inhibiting low-density lipoprotein (LDL) oxidation. This suggests that ginger could help to protect against the development of atherosclerosis and heart disease. Ginger can help to sweat out a cold. It is an antiseptic expectorant and thus helpful for treating catarrhal coughs. It is also reputed to lower fever.

Australian studies in 2000 revealed that several constituents of ginger had an anti-inflammatory effect. It may, therefore, be helpful for chronic inflammatory conditions such as arthritis. The essential oil is prescribed for external use in a rub for rheumatism and muscular pain.

Its antispasmodic effects make ginger a helpful remedy for period pains and digestive cramps. It can also cure flatulence and diarrhoea.

Cultivation

Ginger is a tropical plant, so must be grown indoors or in a heated greenhouse. Plant rhizomes in a sunny or slightly shady position in a neutral to alkaline soil, and keep well watered.

PREPARATION AND DOSAGE

For internal use

TO TREAT nausea and vomiting, poor digestion, period pains, flatulence, diarrhoea
POWDER Take 0.5-1.5g a day in water, or mixed with food.
LIQUID EXTRACT Take up to 1ml a day in a glass of water.
TINCTURE (1:5 in 60% alcohol) Take up to 30 drops a day in a glass of water.

For external use

TO TREAT painful muscles or joints
CREAM (containing rhyzome powder or essential oil) Apply to the affected parts two or three times a day (but not for acute joint inflammation).

IF SYMPTOMS PERSIST, CONSULT A DOCTOR

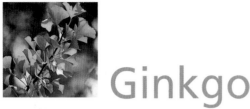

Ginkgo

Ginkgo biloba Ginkgoaceae **Also called** Maidenhair tree

Described by Charles Darwin as a living fossil, ginkgo is the world's oldest surviving tree species. It has grown in China for more than two hundred million years – and individual trees live for a thousand years or more. The ginkgo was brought to Europe in the 18th century as an ornamental tree.

Parts used

Leaves

● Ginkgo is cultivated for the pharmaceutical industry, particularly in the Bordeaux region of France and South Carolina in the USA.
● The crop is gathered by machines that cut branches from young trees.
● Ginkgo leaf is used for tinctures, dry extracts and a range of pharmaceutical products.

Constituents

Ginkgo's active elements are ginkgolide terpenes and polyphenols – mainly flavonoids: antioxidants that strengthen blood vessels and improve the circulation.

Medicinal use

Ginkgo has been used in Chinese herbal medicine for more than 4000 years to treat memory loss in the elderly. Pharmacological research has now begun in earnest. Research in 1999 showed that taking ginkgo extract counteracts declining mental faculties. A daily dose of 120-160mg, given to elderly people for 12 weeks, helped to improve concentration and memory as well as reducing mood swings and apathy.

The extract's effectiveness may be due to its effect on the circulation. Research has shown that ginkgo combats age-related deterioration of blood vessels in the brain. It also strengthens the veins and reduces bleeding in the capillaries and can be used to remedy another age-related condition called acrocyanosis – what appears to be permanent bruising, especially on the hands and feet.

In 1997 Chinese scientists found that ginkgolides had physiological effects that may one day benefit asthma sufferers and help to prevent conditions such as atherosclerosis.

Herbalists prescribe ginkgo to enhance mental alertness in people of any age, and to treat impotence.

Cultivation

Place this very hardy plant in a rich, well-drained soil in a sunny location.

CAUTIONS

● No adverse side effects have been reported to date.
● Overdose can cause stomach upsets and dizziness.
● Do not give to children.
● Avoid if taking anticoagulant or blood-thinning drugs.
● Do not take if pregnant or breastfeeding.
● Before surgery, tell your surgeon if you are taking ginko supplements.

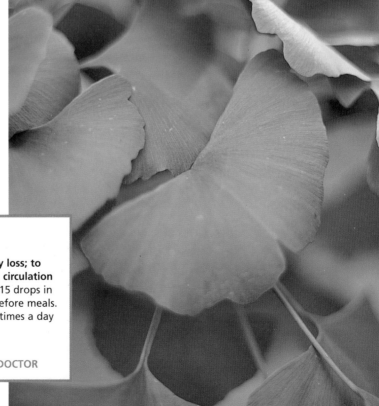

PREPARATION AND DOSAGE

For internal use

TO TREAT mood swings and memory loss; to improve mental alertness and blood circulation
TINCTURE (1:4 in 25% alcohol) Take 15 drops in a glass of water, three times a day before meals.
DRY EXTRACT Take 50-100mg three times a day before meals.

IF SYMPTOMS PERSIST, CONSULT A DOCTOR

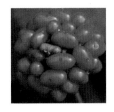

Ginseng (American)

Panax quinquefolius Araliaceae

The Chinese discovered the tonic effects of ginseng thousands of years ago. The perennial's tuber-like root resembles a human body – and in Chinese, ginseng means 'root man'. The species P. quinquefolius is cultivated in the American Midwest and exported all over the world.

Parts used

Roots

● Roots are gathered in autumn from plants that are 6 or 7 years old.
● Dried ginseng is white; scalded ginseng is red.
● Ginseng comes in different grades: the price is based on how rich in active components the root is.
● Ginseng is often mixed with – and sometimes tainted by – unrelated chemical components.

Constituents

The source of the root's tonic properties are terpenes called ginsenosides; in American ginseng the major ginsenoside present is R_{b1}.

Medicinal uses

Ginseng's botanical name *Panax* comes from panacea, a Greek word meaning all-healing, and the root has long been used as a cure all. Ginseng is renowned for its energy giving properties. It is thought to combat fatigue and is often used as a stimulant. Research is promising: ginseng appears to have several beneficial effects. It is an anabolic substance and stimulates protein synthesis. And Italian clinical trials conducted in 1986 found that ginseng improved mental performance on several levels.

Many alternative practitioners regard ginseng as a valuable way of relieving both physical and mental stress. It is prescribed for nervous exhaustion and to help recovery during convalescence. It may be taken on its own or combined with other stimulant plants such as tea and cola, and with vitamins.

Ginseng may be beneficial in the treatment of diabetes. In 1987 Chinese studies found that ginseng stimulates insulin release, and a 1988 study published in the *Journal of Traditional Chinese Medicine* found that ginseng increases the number of insulin receptors in bone marrow.

Cultivation

Sow seeds in spring. Ginseng likes a cool climate, a shady position and a warm, damp, rich, well-drained soil.

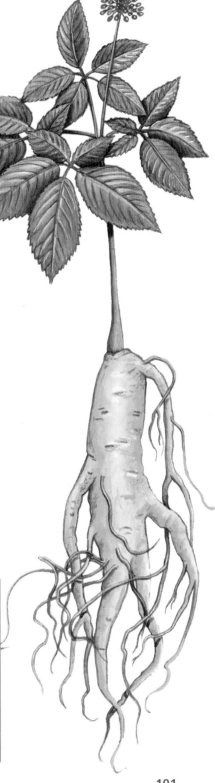

CAUTIONS

● No toxicity recorded to date.
● Prolonged use may cause unwanted hormonal effects such as period problems and hypertension.
● Do not exceed 2g of powder a day, and limit treatment periods to one month on, then two months off.
● Avoid during pregnancy and if breastfeeding.
● Do not give to pre-pubescents.
● Avoid if suffering from obesity, insomnia or high blood pressure.
● If you are diabetic, consult your doctor before taking ginseng.
● Tell your surgeon you are taking ginseng supplements before surgery.

PREPARATION AND DOSAGE
For internal use
TO TREAT stress, nervous exhaustion
CAPSULES (500mg) Take 2 capsules with breakfast and 2 with a midday meal.
INFUSION Add 1 dessertspoon dried root to a cup of boiling water. Steep for 3-5 minutes. Drink 2-4 cups a day.

IF SYMPTOMS PERSIST,
CONSULT A DOCTOR

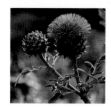

Globe artichoke

Cynara scolymus Compositae/Asteraceae

Native to the Mediterranean, the globe artichoke is now cultivated all over western Europe. Although widely enjoyed as a vegetable since the 15th century, its medicinal powers were not recognised until the 20th century. The herbaceous perennial grows up to 1.5m tall, with a thick, upright, ridged stem. The large, jagged leaves are grey-green, with a whitish down on their underside. Thistle-like, purple-green flowers surrounded by thick leaf-like bracts appear in summer.

Parts used

Leaves and flowers

• The leaves are picked, then dried and used in extracts, capsules, decoctions and tinctures.
• The unopened flowerheads and fleshy bases are eaten as vegetables.

Constituents

The leaves are rich in organic and phenolic acids, including the bitter, aromatic cynarin. They also contain sesquiterpene lactones, flavonoids, potassium salts, provitamin A and numerous enzymes.

Medicinal uses

Globe artichoke preparations are mainly used to treat digestive problems, especially those concerned with the liver and gall bladder.

In 2001 German scientists noted that the flavonoids in the plant's leaves could stimulate bile flow and encourage regeneration of liver cells. Earlier, the same team had also shown that the leaf extract can help to lower blood cholesterol levels. In 2002 Japanese researchers recorded the same effect and identified the sesquiterpene lactones as the active components.

The flavonoids, assisted by the acids and potassium salts, also act as diuretics, easing kidney problems.

Cultivation

Sow globe artichoke seeds in early spring in rich, well-drained soil in a sunny spot. Protect plants from frost during a harsh winter.

CAUTIONS

• Do not use any globe artichoke preparation to treat gallstones.
• Taking globe artichoke is not recommended when breastfeeding, as it reduces the flow of milk.
• The sesquiterpene lactones can cause allergic reactions, in which case, all globe artichoke preparations should be avoided.

PREPARATION AND DOSAGE

For internal use

TO TREAT liver and kidney problems, high blood cholesterol and indigestion

DECOCTION Put 30-40g of dried leaves into 1 litre of boiling water. Infuse for 10 minutes. Strain and drink 3 cups a day, 15-20 minutes before meals.
CAPSULES (50-100mg dry extract) Take 1-2 capsules, two or three times a day before meals.
CAPSULES (300mg dried leaf extract) Take 1 capsule a day.
TINCTURE Put 500g of dried leaves into 1 litre of alcohol and leave for 15 days. Take 1-4 teaspoons in half a glass of water, three times a day.

IF SYMPTOMS PERSIST, CONSULT A DOCTOR

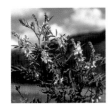

Goat's rue

Galega officinalis Fabaceae **Also called** Galega, French lilac

Growing wild in southern Europe and parts of Asia, goat's rue is a bushy perrenial that can reach a height of 1-1.5m. If bruised, the leaves emit a goaty smell, possibly accounting for its name. The leaves consist of six to eight bright green leaflets, and blue, pink or white, butterfly-shaped flowers appear all summer. When ripe, its long seedpod twists and bursts open to scatter the seeds.

Parts used
Flowers
• The flowers are collected when they are in full bloom between July and September.
• Once dried, they are used in infusions, powders and tinctures.

Constituents
The alkaloid galegine and its derivatives, are found throughout the plant. Goat's rue also contains chromium, flavonoids and tannins, which effect the clotting of blood.

Medicinal uses
Goat's rue can be useful as a supplementary treatment for Type 2 (non-insulin dependent) diabetes as it is rich in chromium which helps to combat the body's inability to absorb glucose. Also, animal studies in Scotland have shown that its galegine can lower blood sugar levels. While the herb is helpful, it is important that a diabetic patient also adheres to any prescribed regular courses of medication.

In addition, the Scottish research noted the ability of galegine to reduce appetite suggesting its potential for use in weight control. Goat's rue is also recommended for digestive problems and is known to relieve chronic constipation. It is a diuretic, helping to prevent swelling resulting from fluid retention, and

---

PREPARATION AND DOSAGE
Preparations containing goat's rue should only be taken in consultation with a doctor or medical herbalist. As high doses are potentially toxic, it is very important to observe the exact dosages prescribed.

---

can increase perspiration as well. Galegine is also responsible for the plant's antibacterial powers as shown by scientists in India in 2001. This, combined with the known anti-inflammatory effect of its flavonoids, may explain why goat's rue is sometimes used to treat fever.

Cultivation
Goat's rue can be grown from seed, planted in autumn. It is suited to deep, moist, well-drained soil, and should be positioned in the sun or a lightly shaded spot.

CAUTIONS
• As goat's rue can react adversely, especially with other drugs, it is essential to seek medical advice before using the plant.
• Prescribed doses of goat's rue must be closely adhered to since excessive consumption can lead to dangerous reductions in blood sugar.
• Although goat's rue preparations are sometimes prescribed to increase breast milk production, it is best to avoid them, until toxicity studies have been undertaken. Toxicity in the milk of lactating sheep has been reported.

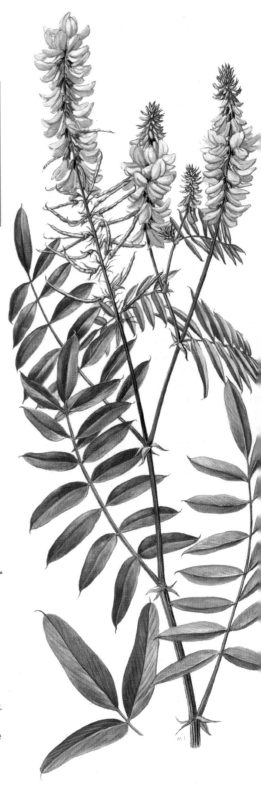

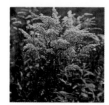

Goldenrod

Solidago virgaurea Asteraceae/Compositae

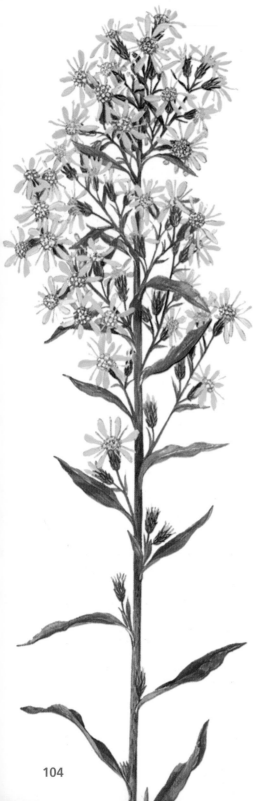

A common garden perennial, goldenrod bears feathery yellow plumes that brighten up the autumn border. The plant grows widely in Europe. Its use in traditional medicine to promote wound-healing gave rise to the plant's nickname 'woundwort'.

Parts used

Aerial parts

- Plants are gathered in autumn.
- They are dried and broken up into small fragments.
- Goldenrod is used for infusions, decoctions, tinctures and syrups.

Constituents

The plant contains an essential oil, tannins that have astringent qualities, flavonoids such as quercitin and rutin, triterpenoid saponins and phenolic acids – antiseptic substances that reduce inflammation.

Medicinal uses

Goldenrod is a diuretic and an expectorant. It also heals wounds ulcers and other skin ailments. The astringent tannins in goldenrod contribute to its healing qualities and combat diarrhoea. Its flavonoids reduce the permeability of blood vessels and increase their strength, thus improving circulation.

Goldenrod is a remedy for inflammation and infection of the urinary tract – cystitis and urethritis, for example. The plant's analgesic and anti-inflammatory properties have been attributed to a phenolic acid called leiocarposide.

CAUTIONS

- To date, no side effects or toxicity have been recorded.
- People with chronic kidney disease should consult a doctor before using goldenrod.

The herb has long been used to prevent and eliminate bladder stones and to stimulate urination. Its efficacy was proved by Polish studies in 1986 and 1988 that showed the diuretic effects of leiocarposide, and its value in treating bladder stones.

Gargling with an infusion of goldenrod can soothe a sore throat and coughs, while drinking the infusion will help chronic nasal catarrh and hayfever.

The herb may be prescribed for vaginal and oral thrush: German research in 1987 backed this application by showing one of the plant's saponins – virgaureasaponin – to be an effective antifungal.

Cultivation

Grow from seed - it will spread by self-sowing once established. It likes well-drained soil in a sunny border.

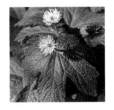

Golden seal

Hydrastis canadensis Ranunculaceae **Also called** Indian turmeric, Yellow puccoon

Originating in North America, golden seal was used as a healing herb by the Cherokee Indians. The plant belongs to the buttercup family, though it looks more like a miniature raspberry. Its dark yellow rhizome spreads horizontally. This is short and thick and has many slender roots.

Parts used
Rhizome
• The rhizome is harvested in autumn after three years or more.
• It is dried and cut up.
• The dried rhizome is ground for capsules or made into liquid extracts.
• Golden seal is usually used as a tincture and may be combined with other plants such as witch hazel.

Constituents
The main active rhizome components are alkaloids, including hydrastine and berberine. Hydrastine constricts blood vessels and raises blood pressure; berberine attacks bacteria and stimulates the immune system.

Medicinal uses
Golden seal has long been used in traditional medicine for stopping bleeding, and is prescribed for blood loss between menstrual periods. The rhizome is good for blood circulation making it useful for treating piles,

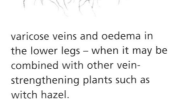

varicose veins and oedema in the lower legs – when it may be combined with other vein-strengthening plants such as witch hazel.

Golden seal is prescribed for catarrh, tinnitus, eczema, and eye and ear infections.

In 1999 American scientists found that golden seal increased immunoglobulin production, indicating that it strengthens the immune system.

Studies published in *Planta Medica* in 2001 reported on the antibacterial activity of berberine, while Chinese scientists found that berberine restored a regular heartbeat, suggesting that golden seal might be useful for arrhythmia.

Cultivation
Very hard to cultivate, golden seal needs a humus-rich, well-drained moist soil, preferably in woodland.

CAUTIONS
• The alkaloids in golden seal are toxic at high doses.
• Never take more than 2g a day.
• Do not use for more than three weeks at a time and take a break of two weeks between courses.
• Golden seal is not recommended for people with high blood pressure.
• Do not take in pregnancy or when breastfeeding.
• Do not give to children.

PREPARATION AND DOSAGE

For internal use

TO TREAT period problems, chest infections, poor circulation
CAPSULES (540mg) Take 1 capsule three times a day. (See Cautions, left.)
TINCTURE Take 20 drops in water three times a day.

IF SYMPTOMS PERSIST, CONSULT A DOCTOR

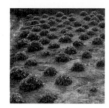

Gotu kola

Centella asiatica Apiaceae **Also called** Indian pennywort.

A tropical perennial, gotu kola grows mainly in Madagascar, China and Indonesia, thriving in damp habitats beside ponds and lakes or in paddy fields. It is a small, herbaceous plant, recognisable by its clusters of frilly, fan-shaped leaves and bears white flowers beneath the foliage in summer.

Parts used
Whole plant, leaves
- The whole plant or leaves are collected at any time and used fresh or dried in infusions, decoctions and powders.
- The plant extract is used for tablets, capsules and preparations for external use such as ointments.

Constituents
Its active compounds are triterpenoid saponins, including asiaticoside and brahmoside, which have wound-healing properties. It also contains flavonoids, which help to strengthen the veins, and traces of essential oil.

Medicinal uses
Taken by mouth, gotu kola has a positive effect on vein and lymph disorders. It has reputed vasodilatory effects and the whole plant is useful for strengthening veins and treating the symptoms of weak veins such as capillary bleeding, varicose veins and haemorrhoids.

A review published in *Angiology* in 2001 documents the effectiveness of gotu kola in treating chronic vein problems.

CAUTIONS
- A few cases of allergic reactions have been reported. Otherwise, the plant has, to date, caused no adverse side effects when used in prescribed doses.
- Do not take internally if pregnant.

Used externally, gotu kola can help to treat skin disorders, including superficial wounds and minor burns. In 1988, Italian researchers showed that its triterpenoids can stimulate the synthesis of connective tissue in human skin, which is likely to contribute to its wound-healing ability. Also, a study in Cumbria in the UK in 2000 found that the use of gotu kola externally when pregnant helped to reduce stretch marks.

The plant is also believed to have anti-inflammatory properties and has been used to ease rheumatic complaints, and to treat eczema.

As a tonic, it is used to strengthen the nervous and immune systems.

Cultivation
Gotu kola can be grown from seed, planted in spring, in a moist, sunny or lightly shaded plot. Because it needs temperatures above 10°C, it is normally grown indoors in the UK.

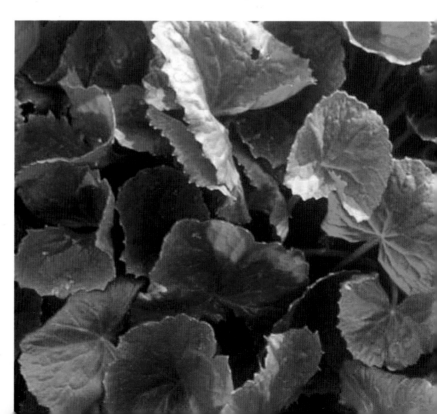

PREPARATION AND DOSAGE
For internal use
**TO TREAT poor circulation, vein problems and skin problems, immune system, nervous system
CAPSULES (300mg dried leaf)**
Take 2 capsules with food, twice a day.

For external use
**TO TREAT skin damage
OINTMENT** Massage in thoroughly once or twice a day, as directed, after the damaged area has been disinfected.

IF SYMPTOMS PERSIST, CONSULT A DOCTOR

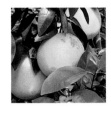

Grapefruit seed

Citrus paradisi Rutaceae **Also called** Fruit of paradise

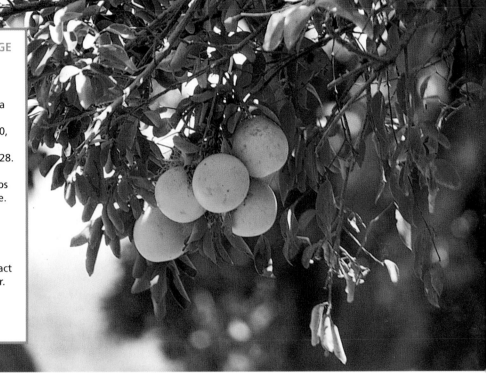

*First described in the 18th century,
the grapefruit tree, which grows up
to 8m high, is thought to have
developed as an accidental hybrid
in the West Indies. It is derived by
crossing the sweet orange and
pomelo trees and has been
cultivated since 1823, when the
first seeds were taken to Florida.*

Parts used

Seeds and pulp
- The fruit is harvested from
September until spring.
- It is commercially processed to
obtain grapefruit seed extract.

Constituents

Grapefruit seed extract contains
flavonoids and other phenolic
compounds, amino acids, fatty acids
and vitamins E and C.

Medicinal uses

Grapefuit is believed to possess antimicrobial properties and is indicated
in the treatment of bacterial, fungal,
viral and parasitic infections.

It can be used to combat colds,
influenza and sore throats, as well as
intestinal infections and diarrhoea.

In vitro studies on commercial
grapefruit seed extract performed in
Texas in 2002 demonstrated
powerful antibacterial activity. But
other studies that have confirmed
the antimicrobial efficacy of
commercial extracts have also
detected the presence of synthetic
preservatives, causing some scientists
to doubt the natural plant's efficacy.

Although it is likely that the
flavonoids and triterpenoids of
natural grapefruit seed will be
shown to display antibacterial

effects, further research is necessary
to clarify this issue. In the meantime,
organically produced grapefruit seed
extract is recommended.

Cultivation

Grapefruit is grown commercially in
subtropical climates in a range of
soils, using rootstocks best suited to
the soil type.

CAUTIONS

- If you are taking medication,
consult your doctor before using
grapefruit seed, as it can increase
the effects of several drugs.
- Preparations made from grapefruit
seed extract may irritate the
digestive system.

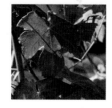

Grape vine

Vitis vinifera Vitaceae

For thousands of years the grape vine has provided fruit, wine and herbal medication. It bears clusters of sweet-smelling pale green flowers followed by bunches of grapes, fruits which contain four seeds. Its leaves turn fiery red in autumn.

Parts used

Leaves and grape seed

• The leaves and seeds are collected when the grapes ripen in autumn.
• The precise moment for harvesting the leaves is determined chemically in order to maximise the amount of active constituents.
• The leaves are air-dried away from sunlight and used to make infusions, powders (for capsules), tinctures and extracts.
• The seeds are separated from the grape and used to make extracts.

CAUTIONS

• No toxicity or side effects have been recorded to date, even after prolonged use.

Constituents

The leaves are rich in anthocyanins – pigments that give them their autumn colour and their capacity to strengthen blood vessels. They also contain organic acids, sugars and vitamins A, B_1, B_2 and C as well as tannins that have anti-inflammatory properties. Both leaves and seeds contain antioxidants that may offer protection against certain cancers and heart disease.

Medicinal uses

Studies have confirmed that vine constituents benefit the circulatory system. In 1994, Italian researchers showed that vine anthocyanins prevented free radical damage to tiny blood capillaries. Grape seed extract is one of the richest sources of antioxidant proanthocyanidins. Vine may help to erase marks and spots beneath the skin caused by capillary bleeding – a condition known medically as purpura.

Clinical trials in Milan in 1999 also confirmed that anthocyanins are good for treating chronic (long-term) vein weakness. Vine is thus an appropriate treatment for oedema – heaviness and swelling in the lower legs. It is also prescribed for piles.

Other therapeutic uses include the treatment of high blood pressure and high blood cholesterol levels. Herbalists may also recommend grape vine for heavy periods, some liver and urinary complaints, diarrhoea and as a digestive aid.

Grape seed is used externally to treat eye inflammation. It is also an expectorant and can soothe coughs.

Cultivation

Vines can be grown on a warm, south-facing wall or in a greenhouse or conservatory. They do best on shaly clay soils.

PREPARATION AND DOSAGE

For internal use

TO TREAT vascular disorders, haemorrhoids, blood marks under the skin
INFUSION Add 2g dried leaves to a cup of boiling water. Leave to infuse for 10 minutes. Take 1-3 cups a day.
GRAPE SEED CAPSULES Take 30-100mg a day.
LIQUID EXTRACT Take 30ml liquid extract a day (providing 50mg grape seed extract).

IF SYMPTOMS PERSIST, CONSULT A DOCTOR

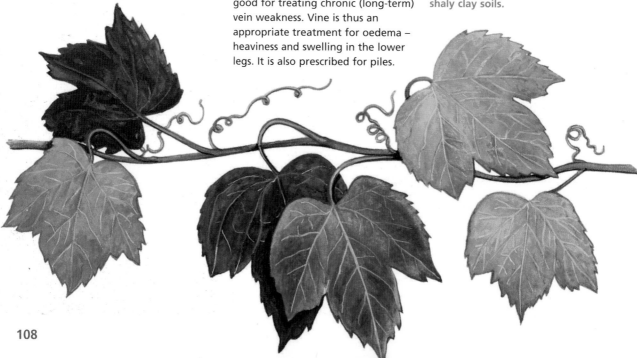

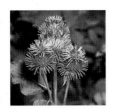

Great burdock

Arctium lappa (A. majus) Asteraceae

Common throughout the northern hemisphere, great burdock is generally regarded as a weed. The plant thrives on roadsides and building sites and grows to almost 1m tall. Its flowerheads, covered in spiny hooks that stick to fur and clothing, inspired the inventors of the Velcro fastening system.

Parts used

Roots and leaves

- The wrinkled greyish brown root is whitish and hard inside.
- The plant is harvested in July just before flowering.
- The root is used mainly for extracts and powders; the bitter-tasting leaves are used in infusions.
- In herbal medicine, great burdock is often combined with other plants.

Constituents

Burdock root stores plant sugars known as inulin: the sweetness can be tasted when the root is chewed. It also contains antibacterial and antifungal compounds. The leaves contain arctiopicrin, a bitter substance responsible for the plant's characteristic taste.

Medicinal uses

In traditional medicine, burdock root was used mainly to cleanse the blood and to treat eczema and psoriasis. Leaf poultices were applied to painful rheumatic joints.

Today, the plant is still used for skin disorders: the leaf is prescribed topically in creams or lotions for cracked weeping skin, grazes and insect bites, while the root is taken internally for ailments associated with oily skin such as acne, boils and other spots.

The root has diuretic and purging effects, aiding the removal of the body's waste products and making it a useful detoxifier.

Experiments have shown that the root has antibacterial and antifungal properties. It also lowers blood sugar levels and may have potential in the treatment of diabetes.

Root extracts have oestrogenic effects and could prove useful in treating menstrual disorders.

Cultivation

Sow seeds in spring in a wild part of the garden. Burdock does well on rough ground in a sunny location.

CAUTIONS

- No toxicity or side effects have been recorded to date.
- Do not give to children under 15.
- Do not take in pregnancy.
- Do not use burdock if you are suffering from diarrhoea.

PREPARATION AND DOSAGE

For internal use

TO TREAT skin complaints – acne, spots, boils, whitlows
INFUSION Put 5g dried leaves into 1 litre of boiling water. Leave to infuse for 10 minutes. Drink 2 cups a day.
CAPSULES (350g root powder) Take 1 capsule three times a day before meals with a glass of water. The dose may be increased to 5 capsules a day.

For external use

TO TREAT eczema, itching, cracked skin, grazes, insect bites
CREAMS, OINTMENTS, LOTIONS Apply as directed by the manufacturer.

IF SYMPTOMS PERSIST, CONSULT A DOCTOR

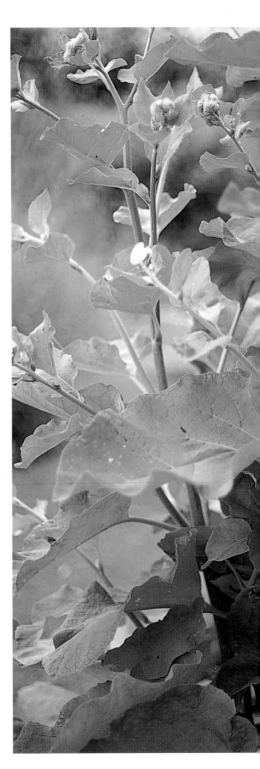

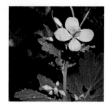

Greater celandine

Chelidonium majus Papaveraceae

Colonising hedgerows, waste ground and damp areas such as ditches, the greater celandine bears small yellow flowers from April to July. The whole plant is covered in fine bristly hairs. If you snap the stalk or root it exudes dark orange sap.

Parts used

Whole plant including root

• The plant is dug up and dried when in flower.

• Greater celandine is rarely used as an infusion on its own, but is blended with other plants such as dandelion or turmeric.

• Dry extract of greater celandine is made into capsules.

• The orange sap is used fresh.

Constituents

This plant's active compounds are alkaloids. The main one in the plant as a whole is protopine, an antispasmodic. The root also contains chelidonine, another antispasmodic alkaloid that also lowers blood pressure. In addition, greater celandine contains organic acids and carotenoids.

Medicinal uses

In traditional Asian medicine, greater celandine is used to calm the nervous system. The sap has long been a country remedy for wart removal. Today, the herb tends to be prescribed for liver problems.

The herb's antispasmodic action can ease spasms in the upper digestive tract and other digestive disorders, and is also helpful in the treatment of coughs and asthma.

Greater celandine acts against bacteria and viruses. And in 2002 Korean scientists reported that it may also be an anticancer agent.

In vitro studies in Germany in 1996 suggest that greater celandine could have a role to play in treating illnesses of the nervous system. The plant has mild analgesic and sedative qualities and can be used to ease rheumatic pain.

Cultivation

Greater celandine likes moist soil and tolerates sun and shade. Do not plant in gardens used by children or cultivate for home use.

CAUTIONS

• Greater celandine is poisonous in large amounts and can cause nausea and dysentery: only take this herb under professional supervision.

• Pregnant or breastfeeding women should avoid this herb.

• Avoid if you have low blood pressure.

• Do not give to children.

• Limit use to two weeks at a time.

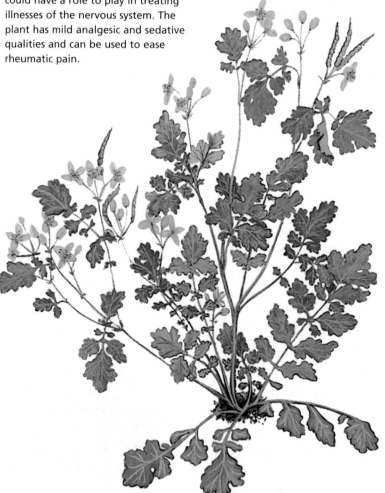

PREPARATION AND DOSAGE

For internal use

Greater celandine preparations should only be taken internally in consultation with a qualified medical herbalist

For external use

TO TREAT skins conditions such as warts, ringworm and eczema
FRESH SAP Apply to the affected area one to three times a day.

IF SYMPTOMS PERSIST, CONSULT A DOCTOR

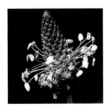

Greater plantain

Plantago major, P. lanceolata Plantaginaceae **Also called** Common plantain, Ribwort plantain

The flat rosette of leaves at the base of the greater plantain, Plantago major, blights many lawns. The leaves of the ribwort plantain, P. lanceolata, are spear shaped and upright. Both plants bear tiny flowers in cylindrical or egg-shaped spikes. Plantain is common in Europe and grows freely on embankments and waste ground.

Parts used

Leaves

● Leaves are collected from June to September, preferably before the plant flowers, and dried.
● Both species are used in soothing remedies, usually applied externally.
● They are also used in infusions, liquid extracts and capsules.

Constituents

The leaves of both plantains contain an iridoid called aucubin, and flavonoids – antioxidants that strengthen blood vessels and are often anti-inflammatory. Plantain also contains soothing mucilages.

Medicinal uses

Both forms of plantain have long been used in country lotions and potions to treat external complaints from itchy, chapped skin, cuts and grazes to insect bites or sore eyes.

Taken internally, the plant has a gentle expectorant action and the mucilage it contains soothes sore and inflamed mucous membranes, making it ideal for coughs and mild bronchitis. Bulgarian research in 1982 showed plantain extract to be an effective way of treating chronic bronchitis, and in 1983 it was shown that plantain relieved constriction of the airways. Taken internally, it can ease asthma, catarrh, laryngitis, pharyngitis, and various allergic reactions that affect breathing.

The iridoids in plantain are anti-inflammatory: Spanish scientists looking at plant iridoids in 2000 found aucubin to have demonstrable anti-inflammatory effects.

Plantain appears to contain antibacterial properties. Norwegian studies in 2000 showed that a polysaccharide extract from greater plantain fought pneumococcal infection. And a recent Swedish study suggested that injections of these polysaccharides could protect against streptococcus infection.

Cultivation

Plantain is an invasive plant. Grow in a wild part of the garden in a sunny or lightly shaded position.

CAUTION

● No adverse side effects or toxicity have been reported to date.
● Do not use plantain in pregnancy.

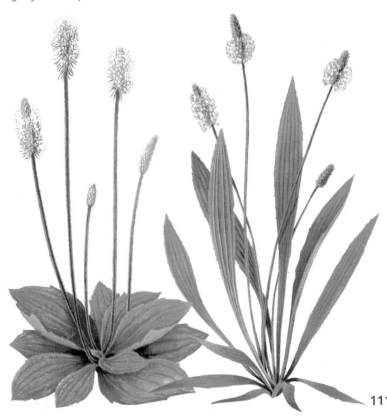

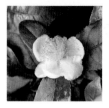

Green tea, black tea

Camellia sinensis Theaceae **Also called** Tea plant

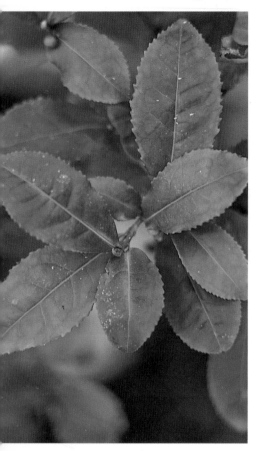

Originating in China and India, tea is still a vitally important crop in both countries. Black and green tea are both prepared from the same plant – the leaves are simply cured in different ways. The shrub can reach a height of 10m but it is normally clipped to just 1m. Tea flowers are white and sweet smelling; fruits are round capsules.

Parts used
Leaves
- The leaves, gathered all year round, usually by hand, are used to make green or black tea.
- The topmost leaves are more aromatic; just the leaf bud and two adjacent young leaves are picked.

- Black tea is fermented; green tea is gently steamed – and its active constituents are stronger.
- Tea is drunk as an infusion, either on its own or blended with other plants such as mint or lemon.
- Tea leaf is used in pharmaceutical preparations including powders and extracts.

Constituents
The main active constituent of both green and black teas is caffeine, which has a stimulating effect on the central nervous system. Tea contains phenolic acids, flavonoids and tannins. However, the fermentation process alters the polyphenols in black tea, and green tea appears to be the more medicinally powerful.

Medicinal uses
Tea leaves have been used for thousands of years to make a thirst-quenching infusion and a medicinal beverage. In traditional Chinese medicine, green tea is prescribed for a wide range of ailments including headaches, depression and fatigue. It is also reputed to prolong life.

Recent research has focused on the cancer-fighting potential of green tea. Several animal studies have found that antioxidant polyphenols in green tea inhibit various cancers – particularly those of the prostate, pancreas, colon and rectum. These antioxidant compounds work by blocking the formation of cancer-causing compounds such as nitrosamines, suppressing the activation of carcinogens and neutralising cancer-causing agents.

The stimulant and diuretic effects of both green and black teas are largely due their caffeine content. The stimulant action makes tea a good remedy for nervous exhaustion; its diuretic effect is a useful complement for people

following weight loss programmes. Tea is also antibacterial, and its tannins make it an effective remedy for treating diarrhoea.

A cooled infusion of tea can be applied externally to soothe tired eyes and skin inflammation; in 2002 American research confirmed that tea pigments have anti-inflammatory properties.

Cultivation
This tropical plant grows best in warm humid climates and in Britain would need to be cultivated in a heated greenhouse.

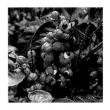

Guarana

Paullinia cupana Sapindaceae

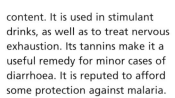

Native to the Amazon region of South America, guarana is a climbing woody vine with a fluted stem. Clusters of yellow flowers are followed by bright red fruits. Each fruit contains one bulky black seed surrounded by red, fleshy skin, and looks like a somewhat sinister eye.

Parts used

Seeds

• Seeds are collected when ripe. They are grilled, and their outer coating is removed.

• They are ground in water to make a paste, rolled into bars and cured.

• The seeds can also be dried and roasted or powdered for capsules.

Constituents

Guarana has a high caffeine content – more than twice as much as coffee. Caffeine stimulates the central nervous system, increases the metabolic rate and is a mild diuretic. Guarana also contains small amounts of theobromine (a stimulant present in chocolate) and theophylline, and larger quantities of starch. Its bitter taste comes from astringent tannins.

Medicinal uses

Guarana is a traditional South American preparation, valued for the energising effect of its high caffeine

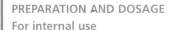

content. It is used in stimulant drinks, as well as to treat nervous exhaustion. Its tannins make it a useful remedy for minor cases of diarrhoea. It is reputed to afford some protection against malaria.

Guarana is believed to increase the breakdown of fats and is used to complement slimming diets. In 2001, a US clinical trial found that people taking a herbal preparation containing guarana lost significantly more weight than a group taking a placebo. Guarana was also found to reduce fats present in the blood.

In guarana's native Brazil, studies performed in 1988 found that it inhibited blood clotting. This suggests that guarana has potential in the treatment of thrombosis. And in 1997, Brazilian researchers found that guarana increased the stamina of mice during exercise. They also observed that guarana enhanced the animals' memories – they performed better in a maze – and appeared to reverse induced amnesia. However, these effects have not, so far, been replicated in human subjects.

Cultivation

Guarana is a native of the Amazon rainforest and requires a hot, humid, but shaded environment. It will not grow at temperatures below 18°C.

CAUTIONS

• Guarana can cause rapid heart rate, upset stomach, headache, agitation and insomnia. Discontinue if these symptoms appear.

• Do not take if pregnant or breastfeeding.

• Avoid if you have cardiovascular disease or high blood pressure.

• Avoid excessive or prolonged use.

• If taking prescribed drugs, especially anticoagulants, consult a doctor before using guarana.

PREPARATION AND DOSAGE

For internal use

TO TREAT nervous exhaustion CAPSULES (200mg) Take 2-3 capsules a day. (See Cautions).

TO TREAT excess weight (as a complement to slimming programmes) CAPSULES (200mg) Take 2-4 capsules a day. (See Cautions)

TO TREAT mild diarrhoea POWDER Put 2 level teaspoons into 250ml boiling water. Leave to infuse for 15 minutes. Drink 2-3 cups a day.

IF SYMPTOMS PERSIST, CONSULT A DOCTOR

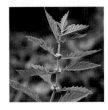

Gypsy wort

Lycopus europaeus Lamiaceae

At one time gypsies used to darken their skins with the dye yielded by gypsy wort, hence its name. The plant likes damp places and is commonly found on the banks of streams. Gypsy wort bears clusters of tiny white flowers, spotted with purple, from July to September.

Parts used

Aerial parts

● The plant may be used fresh or dried.

● It is made into infusions, powders, tinctures or extracts.

Constituents

The main active compounds in gypsy wort are flavonoids, tannins and phenolic acid derivatives including caffeic acid and rosmarinic acid. The plant also contains a bitter essential oil and the minerals fluoride and manganese. Gypsy wort owes its medicinal properties to its combination of active constituents and not to one single substance. For example, if manganese is removed from the plant's extract, there is a marked reduction in its effect on the thyroid gland. The same effect occurs when the tannins are removed.

Medicinal uses

Gypsy wort's main use is in the treatment of an overactive thyroid gland – medically known as hyperthyroidism. The plant extract affects iodine metabolism and the release of the hormone thyroxine. These effects were demonstrated in studies published in the *Journal of Endocrinology* in 1984. Gypsy wort is also recommended for treating hormonal disturbances, period problems and breast pain related to hyperthyroidism.

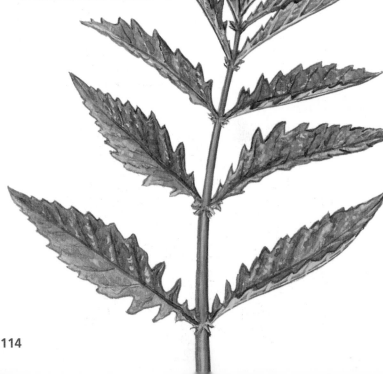

The plant has other hormonal actions: it can inhibit the production of sex and milk-producing hormones and glucagon, the hormone that increases blood sugar. The tannins in gypsy wort contract the tissues of the body, so helping to suppress dry coughs and stem bleeding.

In 2000 Chinese scientists found that a leaf extract inhibits an enzyme required for uric acid production. An excess of uric acid can lead to gout – so there may be potential for using gypsy wort in its treatment.

CULTIVATION

Plant in damp soil in a sunny or lightly shaded position. The seeds can be sown in autumn or spring.

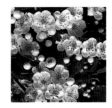

Hawthorn

Crataegus laevigata (*C. oxyacantha*) Rosaceae **Also called** May tree, Midland hawthorn

Widely used as hedging throughout Europe, the bushy hawthorn, or May tree, can reach 10m in height. According to country folklore the flowers' sweet but putrid scent was bequeathed by the Great Plague of London, which was raging at May blossom time in 1665.

Parts used
Flowers and berries
- The flowers quickly spoil and must be picked while in bud or just before they open.
- The flowers must not be allowed to lose their scent.
- They are spread out in thin layers on cloth and dried away from sunlight in a well-aired place.
- Both berries and flowers are used in infusions, capsules and tinctures.

Constituents
The hawthorn flower contains aromatic amines such as tyramine, which are known to be good for the heart. It also contains flavonoids – antioxidants that dilate and protect blood vessels and help to prevent cardiovascular disease. The berries contain anthocyanins – pigments that are thought to be helpful in maintaining healthy blood vessels.

Medicinal uses
The use of hawthorn for medicinal purposes dates back to the Middle Ages. At first, only the fruits were used but today both fruits and flowers are known to have beneficial properties. Traditionally, hawthorn

CAUTIONS
- Hawthorn is a long-term preventative remedy. Do not attempt to treat any form of heart disease without consulting a doctor.
- Large amounts may cause drowsiness: avoid driving.

was recommended for angina, hardening of the arteries, high blood pressure and heart palpitations.

Hawthorn's effects on the heart and circulatory system have been the subject of extensive research – and scientists have proved its usefulness in the treatment of cardiovascular illnesses. It strengthens the heart and encourages a regular heartbeat. It improves the flow of blood to the heart and, by relaxing the involuntary muscles, helps to lower blood pressure. It dilates the blood cells and reduces the capillaries' resistance to blood flow: this effect was demonstrated in animal trials conducted in France in 1985. And finally, by reducing heart palpitations, hawthorn has a calming effect on the central nervous system.

Herbalists prescribe hawthorn for rapid or irregular heartbeat. It is also recommended as a tonic for a weak heart – such as the tired heart of a very old person. Hawthorn may also be prescribed, in combination with valerian, for minor sleeping disorders in both adults and children.

Cultivation
Hawthorn can be grown from cuttings. It is very hardy and tolerates most soils, but prefers an alkaline, rich, moist loam.

PREPARATION AND DOSAGE
For internal use
TO TREAT rapid and irregular heartbeat, weak heart (as a tonic), minor sleeping problems
INFUSION Put 1-2 teaspoons of dried flowerheads into a cup of boiling water. Cover, infuse for 10 minutes, then strain. Drink 2-3 cups a day for three weeks out of every four.
TINCTURE 1:4 in 25% alcohol Take 20 drops with water after meals three times a day.

IF SYMPTOMS PERSIST, CONSULT A DOCTOR

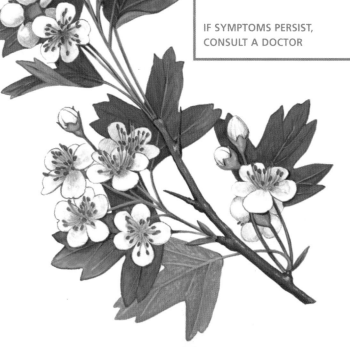

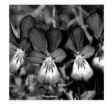

Heartsease

Viola tricolor Violaceae **Also called** Wild pansy

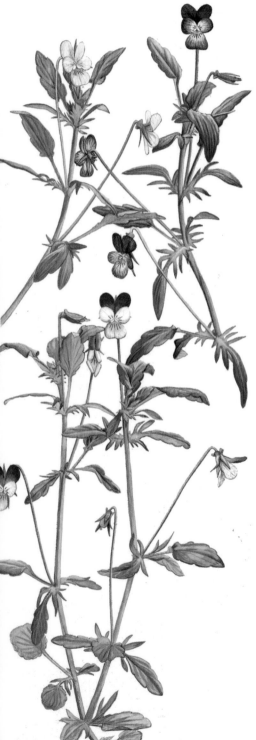

A common sight in hedgerows and on wasteground in summer, the wild pansy or heartsease grows to a height of around 40cm. This herbaceous annual has angular, branching stems with spear-shaped, deeply indented leaves. A single, delicate flower — usually purple, yellow or white, but often a mix of all three colours — sits elegantly at the end of each long stalk.

Parts used

Flower, leaves and stems

• The aerial parts are gathered from heartease from June to late August, in the early morning before the flowers have opened.

• After drying quickly but gently, out of direct sunlight, the leaves, stems and flowers are all used to make infusions, powders, tinctures, extracts, capsules and syrups.

Constituents

Salicylic acid and its derivatives have been identified in the aerial parts of heartsease. There are also mucilages, anthocyanosides, tannins, flavonoids and peptides.

Medicinal uses

The anti-inflammatory action of the salicylic acid in heartsease makes the plant highly effective when applied on a compress to ease skin problems such as acne, eczema, impetigo and seborrhoea (a scalp ailment caused by excessive secretions of sebum). Also, heartsease may be used to treat inflammation caused by

---

CAUTIONS

• Raw or untreated heartsease can be slightly toxic, so avoid it.
• Never use heartsease internally for young children.
• Excessive use of heartsease can cause adverse skin reactions.

rheumatism. Taken internally it can treat respiratory tract infections and its mucilage also has an expectorant effect which can be beneficial.

The plant's anthocyanosides and flavonoids help to keep blood vessels healthy and improve the circulation. This is why it is often prescribed for arteriosclerosis (hardening of the arteries) and heart conditions, which could account for the plant's name.

In addition, heartsease is known as a laxative and diuretic, helping to eliminate toxins and treat urinary tract infection. The tannins can boost immunity, and research in Norway has recently shown that the plant's peptides can help to fight infection.

Cultivation

Suited to any well-drained soil. Plant seeds in spring in a sunny or lightly shaded location. It grows as a short-lived perennial in mild areas.

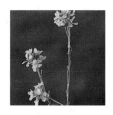

Hedge mustard

Sisymbrium officinale, formerly *Erysimon officinale* Brassicaceae

A roadside plant that grows vigorously in the wild to a height of around 60cm, hedge mustard has hairy, blackish green stems and serrated leaves varying greatly in size. Tiny yellow flowers, just 3mm across, appear from April to as late as November, the petals forming a cross shape. Its fruit consists of elongated pods, which hang in thin clusters and contain acrid, yellow seeds. The whole plant tastes and smells similar to mustard, and its leaves are sometimes used to flavour sauces and soups, as well as in salads and omelettes.

Parts used

Whole plant, leaves, flowering tops
- The leaves are picked in spring, and in summer with the flowers.
- Both leaves and flowers are usually dried before being used for infusions and tinctures. However, fresh leaves and flowers are also used.

Constituents

Hedge mustard contains an essential oil, rich in sweet-smelling sulphur compounds, consisting mainly of glucosinolates. It has also been found that the seeds contain small quantities of cardenolides.

Medicinal uses

The sulphur compounds in the essential oil of hedge mustard act as an expectorant, helping to loosen phlegm and dissolve mucus. This means that the plant can help to soothe coughs and treat throat and respiratory problems, such as catarrh,

bronchitis, hoarseness, voice loss and weakness in the lungs, caused by inflammation in the airways. Hedge mustard is therefore a common ingredient in cough syrups, and is known in France as 'singer's plant' because of its ability to restore the voice to full power.

Hedge mustard is also known to stimulate the gastric juices and can act as a diuretic. This makes the plant useful for cleansing the system and easing a number of digestive ailments, including bloating and stomach problems in general.

Testing several natural substances for their ability to protect the immune system from damage by bacterial infection, Japanese researchers recently showed that the sulphur compounds in hedge mustard were the most effective.

Cultivation

Hedge mustard can be grown from seeds, planted in either spring or autumn. It is suited to moist or dry, acid to alkaline soil, and prefers a sunny or lightly shaded spot.

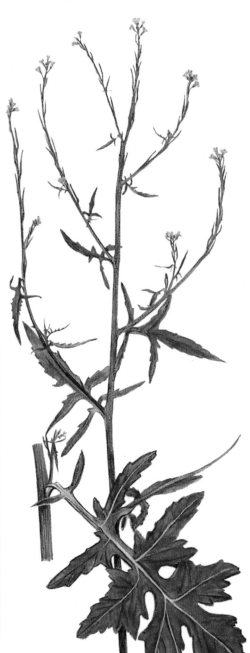

CAUTIONS

- Excessive use of hedge mustard can induce unwanted side effects, including slowing of the heartbeat.
- Hedge mustard should never be given to young children.

PREPARATION AND DOSAGE

For internal use

TO TREAT hoarseness, laryngitis, pharyngitis and inflammation of the airways
INFUSION Add 5g of dried plant to 1 cup of boiling water. Cover. Leave to infuse for 10 minutes. Strain. Drink 2-4 cups a day.
TINCTURE Take 30 drops in a glass of water, three to four times a day.

For external use

TO TREAT voice loss
GARGLE Make the infusion as described above, and use three or four times a day.

IF SYMPTOMS PERSIST, CONSULT A DOCTOR

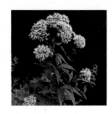

Hemp agrimony

Eupatorium cannabinum Compositae/Asteraceae

A native of damp woodlands, marshes and riverbanks throughout Europe and in many parts of Asia and North Africa, hemp agrimony, a herbaceous perennial, can grow to a height of about 1.5m. It has downy leaves on its distinctive red stems, which are crowned in late summer by a mass of tiny bright pink to mauve flowers. Its fruits mature into seedpods, topped with a tuft of soft, white hairs.

Parts used
Whole plant
- The leaves are usually collected in spring before the plant flowers.
- The roots are collected in spring or autumn.
- Its flowers are picked at the end of the flowering season in early autumn.
- The parts are dried and used to prepare infusions and tinctures.

Constituents
An essential oil in the leaves gives the plant its characteristic smell. The leaves also contain bitter elements, alkaloids, flavonoids, saponins, tannins, pyrrolizidine and a resin. The roots contain some essential oil, as well as some bitter compounds and pyrrolizidine alkaloids.

Medicinal uses
Hemp agrimony is well known for its ability to help to eliminate toxins from the body by stimulating the action of the kidneys and liver. It is widely prescribed for skin ailments, linked to toxin build-up due to bile and liver disorders, and for treating rosacea and acne. Animal studies have, in fact, observed that because of the bitter elements, an aqueous extract of the plant can stimulate the flow of bile in rats and exert a protective action on the liver.

Research has also established that a constituent of the essential oil, p-cymene, can help to boost the immune system, increasing resistance to the viral infections that can cause influenza, colds and sore throats.

One of the bitters found in the leaves and roots, eupatoriopicrine, has recently been shown to have anticancer properties. This exciting new development is currently being investigated further.

Cultivation
Hemp agrimony grows best in moist soil in a sunny or partially shaded spot. Grow from seed in spring but do not use in home preparations taken internally.

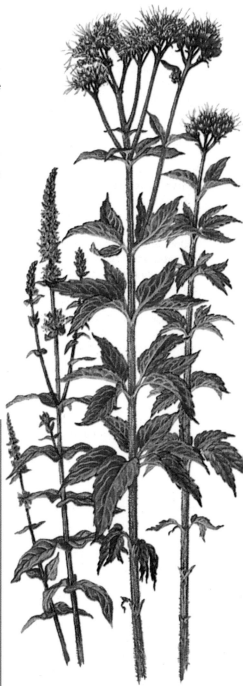

CAUTIONS
- Consult a medical herbalist before taking the plant internally.
- Only use the dose prescribed.
- When taken in large amounts the pyrrolizidine alkaloids in hemp agrimony can have a toxic effect.
- Avoid hemp agrimony if pregnant or breastfeeding.

PREPARATION AND DOSAGE
Hemp agrimony infusions and tinctures are sometimes used to treat liver and kidney problems. However, any preparations for internal use are best taken only as prescribed by a qualified medical herbalist.

For external use
TO TREAT skin irritations, blotches, rosacea, acne
TINCTURE, DECOCTION Add 2-4 teaspoons to 1 litre of boiling water. Cool and apply on a compress to affected areas.

IF SYMPTOMS PERSIST, CONSULT A DOCTOR

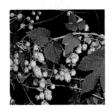

Hop

Humulus lupulus Cannabaceae

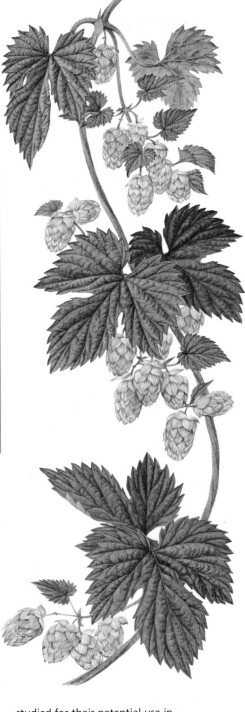

Growing at altitudes of up to 1500m in the hedgerows and forests of Europe, the hop is a climbing perennial. The tough, twisting stem bears heart-shaped leaves, divided into sharply indented lobes. Flowers of different sexes grow on separate plants. It is the female flowers that produce the decorative cone-like 'hops' that have been used since ancient times in medicines and in brewing.

Parts used

Female flowers (cones)

● The female flowers, or cones, are picked when they are yellowish green in colour in autumn.
● Once dried, the cones have an aromatic, bitter taste. They are mainly used in brewing, but are also made into infusions, powders and extracts for medicinal use. In balneotherapy (therapeutic use of baths), they are employed for their calming properties.

Constituents

The aromatic taste of the plant is due to an essential oil composed of mono and sesquiterpenoid hydrocarbons and oxygenated compounds. The compounds that cause its bitter taste include humulone and lupulone. Oestrogenic substances are also present.

CAUTIONS

● Two of the bitters found in hops, humulone and lupulone, may have toxic side effects.
● Hops are not recommended for people who have a tendency to suffer from depression.
● Hops can cause contractions of the uterus, and are therefore not recommended during pregnancy.
● Women who are breastfeeding are advised to take only small amounts of any hop preparation.
● Some people have an adverse allergic reaction to preparations that contain hops.

PREPARATION AND DOSAGE

For internal use

TO TREAT insomnia
INFUSION Put 10g of hop cones into 1 litre of boiling water. Infuse for 10 minutes. Drink 1 cup, just before going to bed.
TINCTURE, LIQUID EXTRACT Take 20 drops in water, three times a day.

For external use

TO TREAT nervous problems
INFUSION Prepare as above and add 1 litre to a warm bath. Soak for 20 minutes.

IF SYMPTOMS PERSIST, CONSULT A DOCTOR

Medicinal uses

The sedative and sleep inducing properties of the hop, particularly of the essential oil and its oxygenated compounds, have been confirmed by various studies. Indeed, clinical trials in Germany showed a preparation of hops and valerian to be as effective as benzodiazepines in remedying sleep disorders. This combination was also shown to be effective as a treatment for nervous problems in adults and children.

The bitter compounds are known to help the digestive system to work more efficiently, and research has also revealed that the humulone and lupulone bitters can destroy bacteria and are antispasmodic.

The hop, along with several other plants that contain compounds with similar properties to the female hormone oestrogen, are being studied for their potential use in treating problems relating to the menstrual cycle and menopause.

Cultivation

Cuttings taken in autumn can be planted out in spring in rich, well-drained soil, in sun or light shade. Or buy ready-grown young plants.

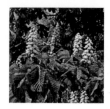

Horse chestnut

Aesculus hippocastanum Hippocastanaceae **Also called** Conker tree

A native of Anatolia, the horse chestnut is an elegant tree that can reach a height of 30m. It is thought that the tree gets its name from the tiny horseshoe-shaped marks – complete with what look like nail holes – that cover its branches. These are leaf scars, left behind when the leaves fall. The fruit, a prickly capsule, contains the large seed, known as a conker.

Parts used

Conkers (seeds) and bark

• Conkers are collected in September and October when ripe.
• Conkers are used raw or stabilised by being soaked in alcohol.
• The bark is stripped from the branches in spring.
• Conkers and bark are used in infusions, powders and dry or soluble extracts. They may be combined with other herbs, such as butcher's broom.
• Horse chestnut is also made into ointments, creams and gels.

Constituents

Conkers contain a saponin known as aescin, which constricts blood vessels, counteracting oedema (swelling) and inflammation. They also contain flavonoids and tannins. The bark is rich in coumarins, notably aesculetin, which has vitamin P properties.

CAUTIONS

• Do not give to children.
• Do not take if pregnant or breastfeeding.
• Avoid if suffering from kidney disease or damage.
• Individuals taking anticoagulant drugs should seek advice from a doctor before taking horse chestnut.
• Horse chestnut can be toxic in large amounts.
• Used externally the plant may, in rare cases, cause an allergic reaction.

Vitamin P is a term used for bioflavonoids – pain-relieving substances that have an antibacterial effect and promote circulation.

Medicinal uses

Horse chestnut is an effective treatment for vein disorders and fragile capillaries. In 1994 French scientists showed that aescin increases blood flow, decreases capillary permeability, has an anti-inflammatory action and protects against free radical damage. Horse chestnut is therefore a good remedy for haemorrhoids, varicose veins and chronic (long-term) venous insufficiency, which can cause oedema (swelling) in the lower legs.

Topical aescin gels are prescribed for haemorrhoids, ulcers, varicose veins, sports injuries and bruising.

Cultivation

This hardy tree can be grown from seed – a conker. Plant in a rich, well-drained soil in sun or light shade.

PREPARATION AND DOSAGE

For internal use

TO TREAT vein and capillary disorders including oedema, piles and varicose veins

INFUSION Put 1 sachet into 200ml of boiling water. Drink one to three times a day after meals.

CAPSULES (75mg) Take 2-3 capsules a day, at mealtimes.

LIQUID EXTRACT Put 20 drops in a glass of water and take three times a day.

TABLETS (300mg) Take 1 tablet a day.

For external use

TO TREAT haemorrhoids (piles), sports injuries

CREAM, GEL, OINTMENT Apply three or four times a day.

IF SYMPTOMS PERSIST, CONSULT A DOCTOR

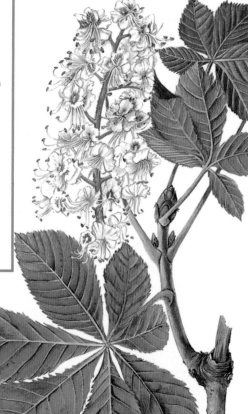

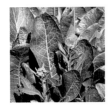

Horseradish

Armoracia rusticana Brassicaceae

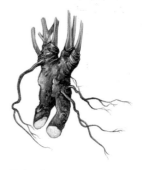

More familiar as a piquant condiment to accompany beef, horseradish has been used in Europe as a medicine for centuries. It has large leaves and a thick root with brown skin and white flesh. The root is rich in vitamin C, and sailors used to take it with them on long voyages to prevent scurvy.

CAUTIONS
- Do not use pure, untreated juice or extract of horseradish as its caustic effects can irritate the digestive tract.
- Do not give to children.
- Not recommended for individuals with gastric ulcers or those suffering with thyroid disorders.
- Externally, the essential oil may cause skin irritation and burning.
- Keep away from the eyes.

Parts used
Roots
- The root – similar to a large parsnip – is collected in autumn.
- It may be used in tinctures but this is rare: it is best used fresh and can be kept for months in a refrigerator.
- Horseradish is used in some pharmaceutical products.

Constituents
Horseradish contains an essential oil rich in sweet-smelling sulphur compounds known as glucosilinates. These compounds are found only in plants belonging to the mustard family. They can irritate the skin, causing blistering and burning. Horseradish contains twice as much vitamin C as lemon, and also contains B group vitamins and minerals, including potassium, calcium, iron and phosphorus.

Medicinal uses
Horseradish stimulates the appetite and digestive juices, making animal and vegetable fats more easily digested. This makes it a good accompaniment for oily fish and rich meat. Traditional herbalists prescribed it for its strong diuretic properties to treat kidney stones and urine retention.

Horseradish is still used for urinary infections and fluid retention. The fact that it increases perspiration means it can be used to lower fevers. Its high vitamin C content, antibacterial action and expectorant qualities make it a good remedy for coughs and bronchitis.

It is a rubefacient, that is, it heats the skin temporarily, and can be useful for treating painful ailments such as arthritis and gout.

Cultivation
Easily grown from root cuttings in well-drained, rich soil, in sun or partial shade. But beware – once established it is hard to control.

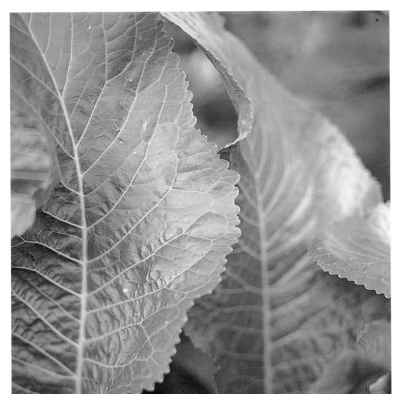

PREPARATION AND DOSAGE
For internal use
Horseradish should only be used medicinally in consultation with a medical herbalist

For external use
TO TREAT rheumatic pain, arthritis
POULTICE Spread fresh, grated root on a linen cloth. Lay on the affected area, with cloth against the skin, until a glowing sensation is felt.

IF SYMPTOMS PERSIST, CONSULT A DOCTOR

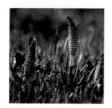

Horsetail

Equisetum arvense Equisetaceae **Also called** Bottle brush

Thriving in swamps and marshes, horsetail is found widely in Europe and the USA. Its fertile stem dies away and is replaced by a tall sterile stem bearing several rings of leaves. The plant, which looks much like a baby's bottle brush, was once employed as an abrasive to scour pots or to smooth rough wood.

Parts used

Sterile stem

• Stems are gathered in summer.

• Stems with brown marks are rejected, as these indicate the presence of parasites.

• Once dried, stems are only suitable for use if they remain green.

• Horsetail is mainly used as a powder, but it can be used fresh or as a liquid extract or tincture.

Constituents

Horsetail is rich in minerals. The main one is silica, believed to have a connective tissue-strengthening and antiarthritic effect. The stem also contains flavonoids – which have antioxidant and diuretic actions – organic acids and nicotine.

Medicinal uses

Traditionally, extracts of horsetail have been used to treat a wide range of ailments including genitourinary infections, kidney problems, prostate problems, obesity, arthritis, bleeding ulcers and tuberculosis. The silica in horsetail is thought to strengthen connective tissue – in tendons, ligaments, cartilage and bone – which helps to explain its use in treating rheumatic complaints.

Horsetail is also prescribed to combat cellulite, a fatty deposit that collects around the thighs and buttocks. It provides a source of minerals for people prone to bone fractures and is used to treat tetany – involuntary jerking and trembling.

Horsetail is prescribed for internal and external bleeding, and vaginal discharge. In 2002 Russian scientists demonstrated its protective effects against hepatitis.

Cultivation

Horsetail prefers swampy or marshy ground in the sun or light shade. It is an invasive weed in the garden.

CAUTIONS

• Do not use horsetail for more than six weeks at a time.

• Do not take it if pregnant or breastfeeding.

• Horsetail may irritate the digestive tract.

• Do not take if you have heart or kidney disease.

• Be careful not to confuse horsetail with the poisonous marsh horsetail (*Equisetum palustre*).

PREPARATION AND DOSAGE

For internal use

TO TREAT kidney problems, rheumatism, cellulite, brittle bones, involuntary shaking

INFUSION Put 2-4g dry stem into 200ml boiling water. Leave to infuse for 10-15 minutes. Or use one horsetail teabag to a cup of boiling water and allow to infuse for 5-10 minutes. Drink 1 cup a day.

COLD MACERATION Put 2-4g dry stem into 200ml of cold water. Leave to macerate (soak) for 12 hours and strain. Drink half of this, twice a day.

POWDER Take 2g three times a day.

LIQUID EXTRACT Take 25 drops in a glass of water four times a day.

IF SYMPTOMS PERSIST, CONSULT A DOCTOR

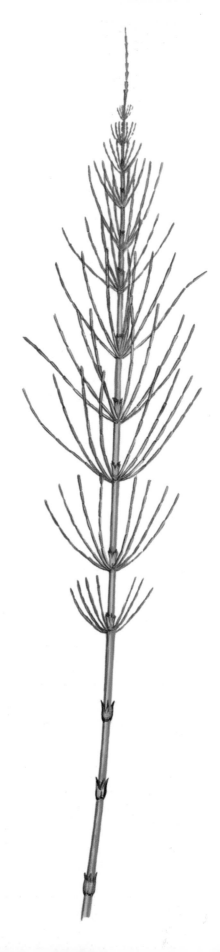

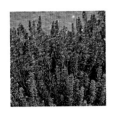

Hyssop

Hyssopus officinalis Lamiaceae

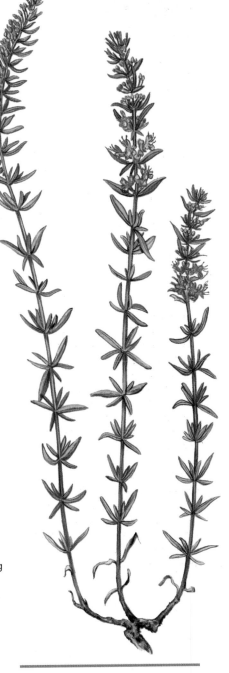

Used as a cleansing herb from Biblical times, the aromatic hyssop, a bushy evergreen shrub up to 60cm in height, grows widely in the Mediterranean region. It is a constituent of scented liqueurs such as Chartreuse and imparts a fine flavour to honey when bees have access to its flowers.

Parts used

Aerial parts

- Hyssop is picked at the beginning of the flowering period.
- It is dried for use in infusions.
- The flowers may be distilled and yield a pungent, spicy essential oil.
- The essential oil is made into creams and lotions for external use.

Constituents

Hyssop flowers contain a strongly aromatic essential oil composed of many compounds including camphor and terpenes. The plant also contains tannins and flavonoids, as well as caffeic and rosmarinic acids.

Medicinal uses

Hyssop's antispasmodic action makes it useful for treating coughs, asthma and bronchitis. It can also soothe stomach cramps. This effect was demonstrated by Italian researchers in 2002, who found that the essential oil inhibited contraction of animal intestines.

Hyssop is an expectorant and is recommended as a treatment for catarrhal coughs and bronchitis. It also raises blood pressure and stimulates perspiration – energising, tonic effects that can help to fight chronic fatigue.

The herb is antiseptic, antifungal and antiviral. A paper published in *Antiviral Research* in 1990 reports that leaf extracts demonstrate strong activity against HIV, the virus responsible for AIDS. Scientists think that caffeic acid may contribute to hyssop's antiviral effect.

Externally, an infusion of the leaves may be used to treat bruises and aching muscles. The oil is also used in various rubs for bruises.

Cultivation

Sow seeds in spring in well-drained, neutral to alkaline soil. Hyssop does best in a sunny border.

PREPARATION AND DOSAGE

For internal use

TO TREAT asthma, bronchitis, sore throat

INFUSION Put 1-2 teaspoons dried flowers into a cup of boiling water. Cover, infuse for 5-10 minutes and strain. Drink 3 cups a day.

GARGLE Use the infusion as a gargle three times a day for sore throat.

For external use

TO TREAT bruises

PREPARATIONS OF ESSENTIAL OIL IN A CREAM OR LOTION Apply to the bruise twice or three times a day as directed.

IF SYMPTOMS PERSIST, CONSULT A DOCTOR

CAUTIONS

- No adverse side effects or toxicity reported to date.
- Do not take the essential oil internally.
- Do not take if pregnant or breastfeeding or have high blood pressure.
- Do not give to children.
- Seek medical advice if using for more than three consecutive days.
- People allergic to oregano and thyme (members of the same plant family) may be allergic to hyssop.

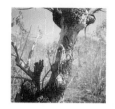

Indian frankincense

Boswellia serrata Burseraceae **Also called** Frankincense

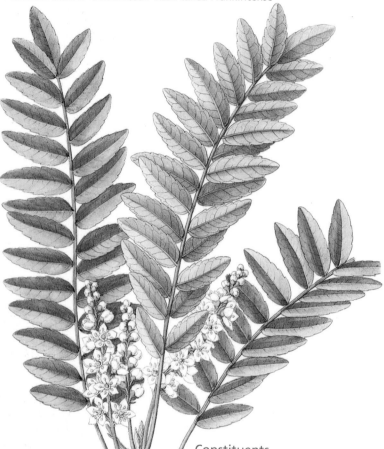

This deciduous tree from India has ash-coloured bark that peels away in flakes. The oval leaves are long and grow opposite one another, while white flowers grow in clusters. The resins (gum) of Boswellia species have long been used for incense, most famously the frankincense mentioned in the Bible. However, B. serrata is also known for its medicinal properties.

Parts used

Gum

• The gum is collected all year round and can be used fresh or dried to make powders and decoctions.

• The essential oil is also extracted.

Constituents

The gum contains several triterpenoid acids known as boswellic acids, which are thought to impart the therapeutic actions of Indian frankincense. Various sugars are also present in the gum. Ingredients of the essential oil, which is obtained from the gum, include pinene, phellandrene and sesquiterpene alcohols.

Medicinal uses

Indian frankincense is traditionally used as an anti-inflammatory agent and this action was verified in a British study in 2000. This, coupled with its antiseptic and expectorant properties, explains its use in treating infections of the respiratory system. It is also used to help skin problems and vaginal infections. It is

believed to aid the digestive system and treat diarrhoea and intestinal infections. Indian frankincense also stimulates blood circulation and has been used in the treatment of piles. The aroma of the essential oil is reputed to have sedative effects and can relieve anxiety.

A German review published in 2002 documents the effectiveness of boswellic acids in treating arthritis, chronic colitis, ulcerative colitis, Crohn's disease, bronchial asthma and reactive swelling around a brain tumour, as shown by clinical trials.

In 2002 Swiss research suggested that extracts of Indian frankincense may have the potential to destroy certain types of cancer cells.

Cultivation

Plant in moist but well-drained soil. It requires full sun and temperatures of 15°C and above.

CAUTIONS

• Pregnant women should not use Indian frankincense.

• Some individuals may experience heartburn or hot hands and feet.

• Indian frankincense is usually used for 8-12 weeks at a time.

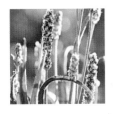

Ispaghula

Plantago ovata Plantaginaceae **Also called** Blond psyllium

Native to western Asia and India, ispaghula is a small annual herb with many erect stems. Its leaves are narrow, lance-shaped, indented and hairy and have vertical, parallel veins. Its white flowers grow in cylindrical spikes. Its seeds are pink or greyish brown, shaped like small oval boats and measure around 2mm in length.

Parts used

Seed and its outer coating

- When ripe, the seed is harvested, threshed and dried in the sun.
- The seed is then used to make bulk-forming laxatives in the form of powders, drinkable solutions and granules.

Constituents

Up to 30 per cent of the seed is composed of mucilage, which is responsible for its laxative effects. In addition to this, the seed contains proteins, lipids and sterols.

Medicinal uses

The mucilage present in ispaghula is not absorbed by the digestive tract and so helps to bulk out the stools. The result is a marked improvement in both the movement and the softness of the stools. Because of this gentle action, ispaghula is a popular remedy for constipation, as well as remedying diarrhoea.

Ispaghula should be used on its own and not combined with stimulant laxatives such as senna. A clinical trial performed in Germany in 1994 documents the efficacy of ispaghula husk in treating irritable bowel syndrome. Ispaghula is also reputed to soothe gastric inflammations, as well as urinary tract infections.

It has also been suggested that ispaghula mucilage may reduce both blood sugar and cholesterol levels. A Spanish study performed in 2001 demonstrated the ability of ispaghula husk to lower blood glucose levels after eating.

Cultivation

Plant in well-drained soil and locate in light shade. The seeds are obtained at the beginning of autumn, and can be saved for sowing the following spring.

CAUTIONS

- Laxatives, including ispaghula, should not be used for prolonged periods without the consent of a doctor.
- Ispaghula should never be used by anyone suffering from undiagnosed abdominal pains, intestinal blockage; or a diagnosed intestinal illness.
- While taking the laxative, you should also eat a healthy, high-fibre diet, drink plenty of fluids (important for older people), and take some physical exercise.

PREPARATION AND DOSAGE

For internal use

TO TREAT constipation, high cholesterol

CAPSULES (430mg) Take 2 capsules before each meal with a large glass of water.

POWDER SACHET (3-6g) Take 1 or 2 with a main meal diluted in a large glass of water.

GRANULES Take 3 teaspoons during main meals with a large glass of water.

IF SYMPTOMS PERSIST, CONSULT A DOCTOR

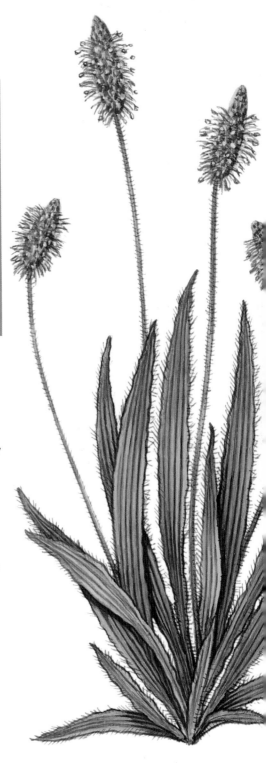

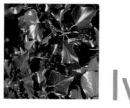

Ivy

Hedera helix Araliaceae

This evergreen shrub grows wild throughout Europe and Asia, creeping or climbing in woods, in hedgerows and on walls. Little roots on its branches act as crampons and allow it to climb. Ivy's shiny dark green leaves are of two kinds: unlobed on flower-bearing branches and sharply divided into three to five lobes on non-flowering branches. The small greenish yellow flowers are followed by spherical, usually black fruits.

Parts used

Wood and leaves
• The wood is taken from mature branches and the bark is stripped off. The wood is then cut into small pieces for use in infusions or syrups.
• The leaves, which are picked when young and fresh, are for external use only in ointments and creams.

Constituents

Ivy wood contains saponins which have antispasmodic and expectorant actions. The leaves contain the same saponins, as well as sterols, phenols and flavonoids. There are also mucilages, which soothe coughs, tannins and anthocyanins. The alkaloid emetine is also present.

Medicinal uses

When taken internally, ivy wood is recommended as a treatment for coughs during attacks of bronchitis. This is due to its ability to ease spasms, release phlegm and soothe a sore throat. German research performed in 1997 has demonstrated ivy wood's ability to ease spasms, while extracts from ivy leaves have been shown to release phlegm.

The leaf extract has also been found to attack fungal infections and other germs and may act against tumours.

Extracts of ivy wood and leaves are used in cellulite-reducing cosmetic products that are applied topically as a complement to slimming regimes. Creams containing extracts of ivy are also used externally to treat itching skin, burns, warts, scabies and rheumatism.

Cultivation

Ivy can be grown in a variety of soils and in heavily shaded locations. Grow from semi-ripe cuttings in summer.

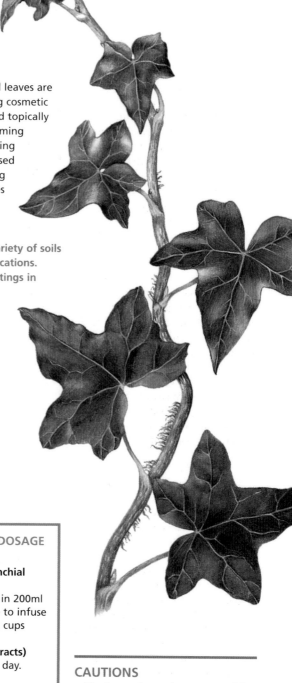

PREPARATION AND DOSAGE

For internal use

TO TREAT coughs, bronchial attacks
INFUSION Put 1 sachet in 200ml of boiling water. Leave to infuse for 5 minutes. Take 1-2 cups a day at mealtimes.
SYRUP (made from extracts) Take 1-3 tablespoons a day.

For external use

TO TREAT itching skin and cellulite
CREAM, GEL Apply to affected area two or three times a day.

IF SYMPTOMS PERSIST, CONSULT A DOCTOR

CAUTIONS

• The leaves have shown no toxicity but there is a risk of contact dermatitis when they are handled during harvesting or preparation.
• The berries are poisonous.
• Excessive use can lead to diarrhoea, an upset stomach and vomiting, as well as slowing the heartbeat.

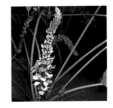

Japanese arrowroot

Pueraria lobata Fabaceae **Also called** Kudzu.

Native to semi-tropical regions of Asia, Japanese arrowroot is a climber that can reach 30m. Its dark green leaves are composed of three lobes and are held on long leafstalks. Japanese arrowroot has been a feature of Chinese medicine since 200 BC, but it is more often grown as a cooking ingredient. Its yellowish, light brown roots are cylindrical. Its fruits are seedpods containing black seeds.

Parts used

Roots and leaves

• The leaves are gathered in the autumn and the roots are harvested in spring or autumn.
• The leaves and roots are dried for use in decoctions, powders and liquid or dry extracts.
• The plant's primary use is as a thickening agent in cooking. The cooked roots and leaves are used as setting agents in jellies.

Constituents

The plant contains numerous active elements including isoflavonoids (daidzein, daidzin, puerarin), coumarins and saponins.

Medicinal uses

Japanese arrowroot protects the liver and helps the body to metabolise alcohol. Japanese research published in 1998 verified this, suggesting that the protective action on the liver was due to several saponins.

Japanese arrowroot is also reputed to suppress the craving for alcohol. American research published in

CAUTION

• The plant has to date caused no adverse side effects.
• However, medical consultation is usually advisable when treating serious ailments.

PREPARATION AND DOSAGE
For internal use
TO TREAT liver ailments, hormonal disorders during the menopause and alcohol dependency
DECOCTION Put 10g of crushed roots into 500ml of boiling water. Gently reduce the amount of water by half under a low flame and strain. Drink half a cup, four times a day.
POWDER Take 500mg, three to six times a day.
DRY EXTRACT Take 300mg, three to six times a day.
LIQUID EXTRACT Put 60 drops into a glass of water. Take three to six times a day.

IF SYMPTOMS PERSIST, CONSULT A DOCTOR

1998 showed that puerarin, daidzin, and daidzein decreased alcohol consumption in alcohol-preferring rats.

It has been demonstrated that the plant affects the hormonal system in a similar way to oestrogen and it is recommended for balancing the hormones during the menopause.

It is also reputed to ease muscular aches and pains, and is beneficial in the treatment of digestive disorders, as well as colds and flu. It increases blood flow to the heart and brain and is indicated in the treatment of angina and high blood pressure.

Cultivation

Plant in well-drained soil, preferably in the sun. Sow seeds in spring at 13-18°C – soaked seeds are best.

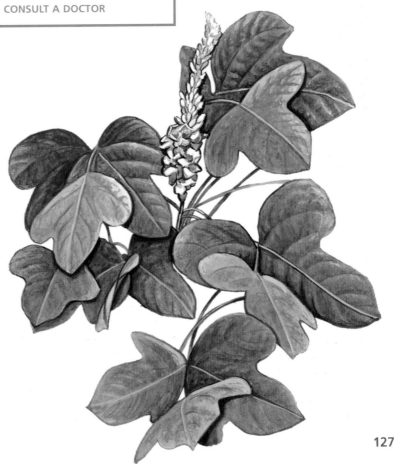

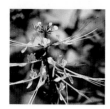

Java tea

Orthosiphon stamineus (O. aristata) Lamiaceae/Labiatae

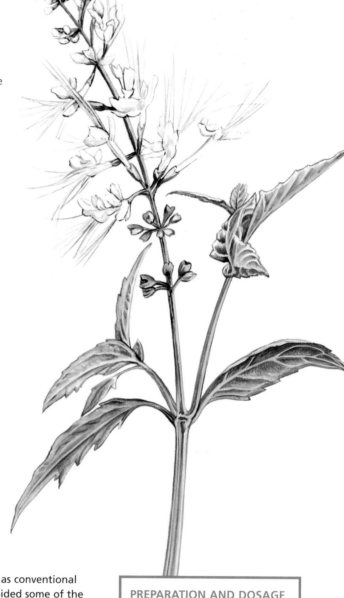

This attractive shrub from Southeast Asia can grow to a height of almost 1m. It has irregular, indented leaves, which grow in pairs opposite one another. A distinctive feature of the plant is the white or lilac flowers with wispy stamens that extend 2cm beyond the petals. They are known as cats' whiskers.

Parts used

Leaves and flowers

● The leaves and the flowers are harvested at the beginning of the flowering period, then dried and broken into fragments.
● The plant is used to make infusions, powder capsules and extracts.
● Indonesia is the principal exporter of Java tea.

Constituents

The most significant compounds in Java tea are polyphenols and, in particular, flavonoids, among which is sinensetin. Very small quantities of essential oil have been detected and Java tea also contains a large amount of potassium.

Medicinal uses

Java tea is believed to be beneficial in the treatment of gout, rheumatism, and renal and urinary infections. Human experiments in 1998 showed that Java tea has a mild diuretic effect and can increase the excretion of urea and uric acid. A Thai study in 2001, involving patients suffering from kidney stones, found that a daily dose of Java tea infusion was as effective as conventional drugs and it avoided some of the side effects. An increase in excretion of calcium and uric acid in the urine was observed.

Another study showed that certain terpenic compounds extracted from the leaves of Java tea inhibited the proliferation of cancer cells.

Java tea's diuretic and bile-stimulating effects mean that it is often used to complement slimming diets. Another traditional use is in the treatment of diabetes.

Cultivation

Plant in well-drained soil in a sunny or lightly shaded location.

CAUTIONS

● No adverse side effects have been recorded when the plant is used in therapeutic doses.
● It is not recommended for pregnant or breastfeeding women.

PREPARATION AND DOSAGE

For internal use

TO TREAT bile disorders, kidney stones and gallstones
INFUSION Put 5g into 1 litre of boiling water. Leave to infuse for 5 minutes. Drink 1-3 cups a day, the last one several hours before going to bed.
CAPSULES (150mg dried aqueous extract or 325mg powder) Take 2 capsules with a large glass of water three times a day at mealtimes.

IF SYMPTOMS PERSIST, CONSULT A DOCTOR

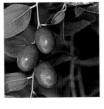

Jujube

Zizyphus jujuba (Z. vulgaris) Rhamnaceae **Also called** Chinese date

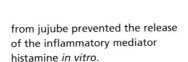

This small tree grows to a height of 6-8m and is common throughout the Mediterranean region. The bark on its trunk is brown and covered in small cracks and its branches are thorny. Jujube leaves are oval and fluted and its flowers are yellowish green and grow in small clusters. Its fruit, the jujube, is a berry that contains a single seed.

Parts used

Fruit

● Jujube berries are harvested in September and October, as soon as they turn brown.

● They are then dried and their seeds are removed. The dried flesh is used to make decoctions and a flour that is mixed to a paste.

● Jujube can be combined with other plants with soothing qualities, such as carob and marshmallow.

Constituents

The flesh of the berry is rich in mucilages, which have soothing properties. It also contains flavonoids, saponins (such as zizyphus saponins I, II and III), and vitamins A, B and C.

Medicinal uses

Jujube is one of the four 'pectoral' fruits that are especially good for chest ailments (the other three being dates, figs and raisins). In traditional Chinese medicine jujube is used to rebuild strength and stamina when the body is in a weakened state such as during convalescence or chronic fatigue syndrome. It has been shown to possess several pharmacological properties: it acts against bacteria, inflammation, fevers and diabetes.

Jujube is believed to modify the immune response and reduce allergic reactions. In 1997, for example, Japanese scientists showed that triterpene oligoglycosides isolated from jujube prevented the release of the inflammatory mediator histamine *in vitro*.

Jujuba also has a sedative effect and can help with insomnia. In 2002 Chinese scientists found that the glycoside jujuboside inhibited the stimulation of the hippocampus in the brain, which may account for jujube's sedative effects.

Taken orally, the jujube fruit is used to relieve hoarseness, voice loss, inflammatory throat infections, coughs and bronchitis.

Its astringent, binding action makes it an effective remedy for diarrhoea, taken on its own or with other soothing plants such as carob and marshmallow. It can also reduce perspiration including night sweats.

Cultivation

Plant in well-drained, moist or dry soil in a sunny spot. Protect from hard frosts. Jujube can be grown from seed, suckers or cuttings.

PREPARATION AND DOSAGE

For internal use

TO TREAT voice loss, sore throat, cough, bronchitis, diarrhoea

DECOCTION Put 30-50g of ground fruit into 1 litre of water. Boil for 30 minutes and strain. Drink as required.

PASTILLES Take as directed for chest ailments or to soothe a sore throat.

IF SYMPTOMS PERSIST, CONSULT A DOCTOR

CAUTIONS

● No harmful side effects have been associated with the consumption of jujube berries.

● However, pregnant or breast-feeding women should not take jujube as a herbal medicine.

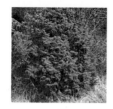

Juniper

Juniperus communis Cupressaceae

This evergreen shrub is found throughout Europe and its blue-black berries have long been used for medicinal purposes. They were believed to protect against the plague and cure snake bites. Juniper grows slowly but can reach a height of 15m. Whorls of evergreen leaves, like short, sharp needles, cover its erect stems. In April and May yellow or blue flowers appear on the male or female plants respectively.

Parts used

Fruit

• Harvesting of juniper berries should not take place before the autumn of the third year of growth.

PREPARATION AND DOSAGE

For internal use

TO TREAT urinary problems
DECOCTION Put 10g of berries into 750ml of boiling water. Leave to boil for 20 minutes, then filter. Drink 2-3 cups a day.

TO TREAT digestive problems
INFUSION Put 0.5-2g of crushed berries into a cup of boiling water. Cover and infuse for 10 minutes, then strain. Drink 15 minutes before meals.
TINCTURE Put 10-20 drops of tincture (1:5 in 45% alcohol) into a small glass of sweetened water. Take three times a day.

For external use

TO TREAT muscle pains, rheumatism, neuralgia, tendinitis
INFUSION (as above) Put 100-200ml into the bath water.
ESSENTIAL OIL Dilute, allowing 3 drops to 10ml of carrier oil. Massage affected area two or three times a day.

IF SYMPTOMS PERSIST, CONSULT A DOCTOR

• The whole of the berry is used: crushed for infusions and decoctions or ground to a powder for capsules.
• Juniper is also available in the form of tinctures and an essential oil.
• Juniper berries are often combined with other diuretic plants such as spiny restharrow and goldenrod.

Constituents

About 0.5 to 2 per cent of the berry is made up of an essential oil that is rich in monoterpenes. It also contains some bitter elements, which promote digestion. Flavonoids and tannins are also present.

Medicinal uses

Juniper berries are used to stimulate the appetite and to treat flatulence and other digestive disorders. The berries are also antiseptic and diuretic and are therefore used to treat minor urinary problems. In 1987 Italian research showed that juniper is anti-inflammatory.

The essential oil is used to treat neuralgia and rheumatism, while an infusion added to bath water has a gentle, relaxing effect which relieves tendonitis and muscle pains.

Juniper has also been shown to be active against viruses and research in 1994 suggested its potential for treating diabetes.

Cultivation

Juniper will grow in most soil types. Plant in sun or light shade from ripe seeds or cuttings taken in autumn.

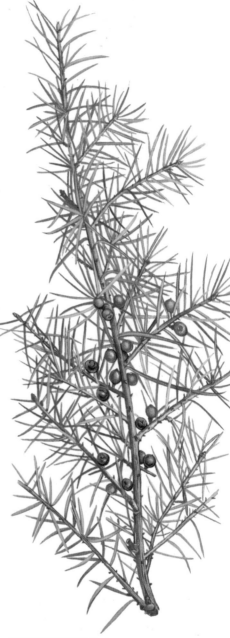

CAUTIONS

• Juniper must not be taken if you suffer from kidney disorders.
• Prolonged use (more than six consecutive weeks) or an overdose can lead to albumin or blood in the urine, kidney pains or cardiovascular complications.
• Sensitive individuals may experience an allergic skin reaction.
• Juniper must not be taken by pregnant or breastfeeding women.
• Diabetics should consult their doctor before taking juniper.

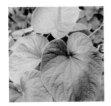

Kava kava

Piper methysticum Piperaceae **Also called** Kava pepper.

An evergreen shrub that grows on the islands of western Polynesia, kava has, in the past, been very popular as a treatment for stress. This pepper plant does not produce fruit but propagates itself by putting out runners and shoots underground. It can reach 10m in height and has fleshy stems and heart-shaped leaves.

Parts used
Roots
● The roots are processed into extracts but this use is now banned in Europe.
● The Polynesians soak the roots in water to obtain a drink once used in rituals and reputed to create feelings of calm and well being.

Constituents
The plant's resin contains unsaturated a-pyrones such as kawain and yangonin, which have several derivatives (kavalactones). The amount of resin varies from 5 to 20 per cent according to the variety and whether it has come from the main root or lateral roots.

Medicinal uses
Numerous experiments have clearly revealed the sedative effects of kava kava and its extracts. A paper published in *CNS Drugs* in 2002 documents the ability of kava and kavalactones to treat anxiety.

In 1990 Australian scientists showed that kava exerted analgesic effects in two animal models of pain. The plant also induces mild euphoria.

Kava kava is used in the treatment of urinary tract infections because of its reputed antiseptic and anti-inflammatory qualities. American research published in *Phytomedicine* in 2002 revealed that an extract of kava inhibited cyclooxgenase, an enzyme required for the synthesis of certain inflammatory mediators.

CAUTIONS
● The UK Government banned kava kava after 70 cases of liver damage were associated with it. Studies are being conducted to establish if the herb is safe for future use.
● Kava-containing products have been associated with liver-related injuries including hepatitis, cirrhosis and liver failure.
● Kava products are still available on the Internet but, in view of the above, cannot be recommended.

Cultivation
As a tropical plant, kava kava needs the warmth of a well-heated greenhouse. The plant can be grown in rich, well-drained soil in partial shade for ornamental purposes but cultivation for the purposes of preparing home preparations is not recommended. See CAUTIONS.

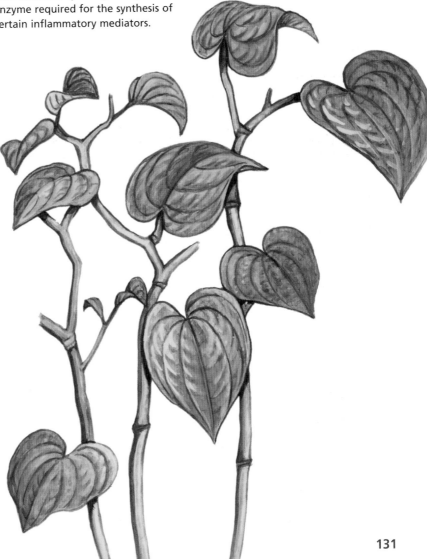

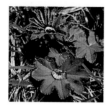

Lady's mantle

Alchemilla vulgaris Rosaceae **Also called** Alchemilla

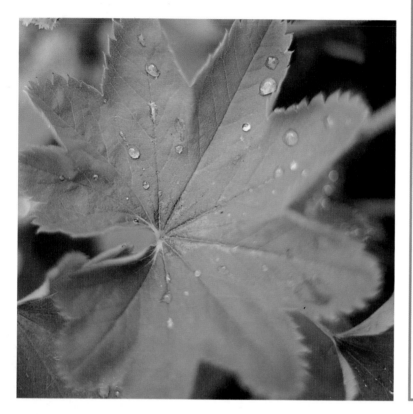

This perennial plant occurs throughout Europe and is easily recognised by its large, fan-shaped leaves made up of 8-10 serrated lobes. Its Latin name Alchemilla means alchemy, and stems from the medieval alchemists' fascination with the plant. They collected the dew from the slightly concave leaves, calling it 'heavenly water' and believed it to have magical powers. Lady's mantle bears clusters of little green flowers and its yellow, rounded fruit contains one seed.

Parts used

Flowers, leaves and roots
• The flowers, leaves and roots are picked from May to September, and then dried in a shady place.
• The plant is used in infusions, tinctures and liquid extracts.

Constituents

Lady's mantle contains large amounts of tannins (6 to 8 per cent). It also contains flavonoids (2 per cent) and some salicylic acid.

Medicinal uses

Due to its tannin content, lady's mantle has astringent and coagulant properties, and is therefore able to tighten the tissues and stop bleeding. Traditionally it has been used in a compress for placing over wounds to speed healing.

Taken internally lady's mantle is a valuable herb for treating irregular or excessive menstrual bleeding. A strong infusion taken frequently also treats mild diarrhoea.

When applied externally, the plant helps to relieve itching and inflammation and is used to treat cellulitis (a skin infection), gingivitis,

insect bites and (in a sitz bath) ailments affecting the vulva such as itching and vaginal discharge.

A 1986 French study showed that lady's mantle inhibits the breakdown of the skin's elastic and connective tissues, supporting its use to treat stretch marks and ageing skin.

Cultivation

Sow seeds in moist, well-drained soil in a sunny or slightly shady position in early spring.

CAUTIONS

• Pregnant and breastfeeding women should avoid lady's mantle.
• Seek medical advice if also taking aspirin or anticoagulant medication.

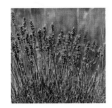

Lavender

Lavandula officinalis Lamiaceae

This small, bush-like shrub, a native of the Mediterranean region, grows to a height of 30-60cm. Its stems are erect and its leaves are narrow and silvery green. All parts of the plant are aromatic, but its flowers particularly so. The Romans used lavender to perfume their washing water and it remains one of the most popular and well-known herbs. The tiny purple flowers appear on spikes above the foliage in summer.

Parts used
Flowers
● After being gathered between May and June the flowers are dried for use in infusions and capsules or they may be processed to extract the essential oil (essence of lavender).
● Ointments, creams and gels are made with a base of the essential oil.
● Lavender oil is mainly produced in southern France.

Constituents
Lavender contains an essential oil (fresh flower, 0.1 to 1 per cent; dry flower, 1 to 3 per cent). There are over 40 constituents including linalyl acetate, linalool and terpinene-4-ol.

Medicinal uses
Lavender is well known for its sedative and calming effects. In 2001 Japanese researchers found that the scent of lavender reduced mental stress, indicating its use in the treatment of depression, anxiety and tension headaches. It has other valuable properties, such as easing spasms, helping digestion, relieving flatulence and improving the passage of bile. It is believed to help some types of asthma.

Lavender is antiseptic and antibacterial and soothes minor skin infections, insect bites and burns.

Lavender is used in therapeutic baths to treat blood circulation problems and it can ease rheumatic pains as well as lowering fevers.

Cultivation
Plant seeds in spring in well-drained, neutral to alkaline soil in full sun.

CAUTIONS
● Pregnant or breastfeeding women should avoid using lavender, although many midwives advocate its use during labour.
● The essential oil must not be ingested, although small amounts may be applied to the skin for the almost instantaneous relief of minor burns.

PREPARATION AND DOSAGE

For internal use

TO TREAT nervous agitation
INFUSION Put 2-3g of the flowers into a cup of boiling water. Leave to infuse for 5-10 minutes, then strain. Drink 3-4 cups a day between meals.

TO TREAT: minor sleep difficulties
INFUSION (see above) Drink 1 cup just before going to bed.
CAPSULES (300mg powder) Take 1 or 2 before going to bed.

TO TREAT digestive problems
INFUSION (see above) Drink ½ cup twice a day.

For external use

TO TREAT period pains
ESSENTIAL OIL Dilute, allowing 3 drops per 10ml of carrier oil, and massage enough of this mixture to cover the lower abdomen and lower back. Apply twice a day.

IF SYMPTOMS PERSIST, CONSULT A DOCTOR

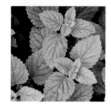

Lemon balm

Melissa officinalis Lamiaceae **Also called** Bee balm

This perennial herb is native to the eastern Mediterranean but now grows wild all over Europe. Its stems are erect and form dense clumps about 70cm high. All parts of lemon balm are hairy and have a strong lemon scent. Its pointed oval leaves have rounded indentations and prominent veins. Lemon balm's white or pinkish flowers grow at the point where the leaves join the stem and its fruits are small and brown.

Parts used

Leaves
- After collection in July to September (when flowering begins) the leaves are dried in the open air.
- Lemon balm is used mainly for infusions or powder capsules. The plant may also be processed to release its essential oil.
- The plant has a traditional use in liqueurs such as Benedictine.

Constituents

Lemon balm contains flavonoids, tannins and phenol acids, including rosmarinic acid. A small amount of essential oil consisting mainly of citrals is also present and due to the low yield, this is one of the most expensive essential oils sold.

Medicinal uses

Lemon balm is most often prescribed to treat intestinal problems such as sluggish digestion, bloating, belching and flatulence. Experiments have clearly shown the plant's capacity to relieve stomach spasms and aid digestion. In 2001, a German trial found that a herbal preparation containing lemon balm improved the symptoms of dyspepsia.

The plant is also used to treat minor sleep problems as well as nervousness and mild depression. For these purposes it is combined with other plants, such as lime flower, hawthorn and passionflower. A Spanish review published in 2001 also documents the use of lemon balm for treating attention deficit disorder and hyperactivity in infants.

In 2003, a trial in Iran found that taking lemon balm reduced agitation and impaired symptoms of mild to moderate Alzheimer's disease.

Earlier research has demonstrated the antiviral properties of lemon balm, which is used to treat herpes. The plant also appears to have an effect on the thyroid gland and has been used to treat hyperthyroidism.

Cultivation

Planted in moist soil in a sunny or lightly shaded location. Sow seeds and cuttings in autumn or spring.

CAUTION
- Avoid long-term usage (1-3 months) as lemon balm may reduce hormonal activity in the sex glands.

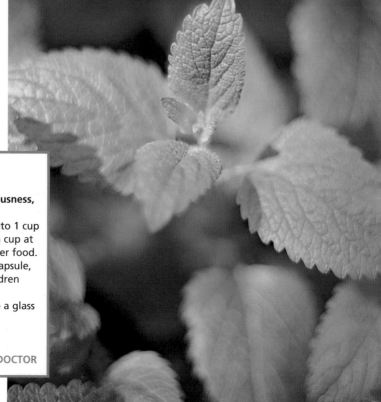

PREPARATION AND DOSAGE
For internal use
TO TREAT digestive problems, nervousness, depression, minor sleep problems
INFUSION Put 2-3g of dried leaves into 1 cup of boiling water, then strain. Drink a cup at midday and a cup in the evening after food.
CAPSULES (200mg powder) Take 1 capsule, three times a day before meals. Children should take 2 a day.
SOLUBLE EXTRACT Put 50 drops into a glass of water. Take three times a day.

IF SYMPTOMS PERSIST, CONSULT A DOCTOR

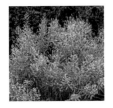

Lemon verbena

Aloysia triphylla (*Lippia citriodora*) Verbenaceae

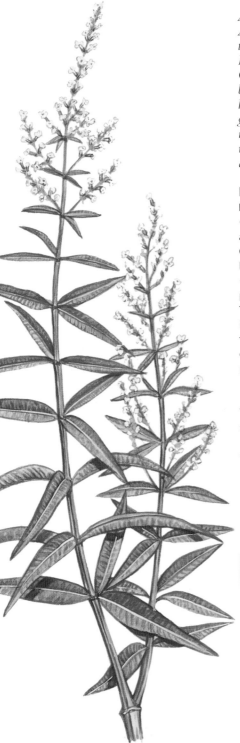

A native of North and South America, lemon verbena is a shrub that can grow to a height of 1.5m. It was introduced into Europe from Chile in 1794. The dried leaves became popular in pot pourri. It has long, thin leaves that grow in groups of three (thus the Latin name triphylla) or four. Its small, whitish flowers have four petals and are followed by fleshy fruits.

Parts used

Leaves

● The leaves are collected twice a year, once in July and again in October, and then spread in a thin layer to dry.
● Once dry, the leaves give off a pleasant lemony scent if crushed. They are used to make delicious infusions or are processed to release the essential oil, which is often combined with other plants to produce a natural sedative.

Constituents

The plant contains flavonoids and a small quantity of essential oil, whose main component is citral, responsible for the plant's characteristic scent.

Medicinal uses

Although research carried out on lemon verbena has concentrated mainly on its sedative properties,

no absolute conclusion has yet been reached. The opposite has, in fact, been the case, since a recent study showed that an infusion of the plant had no sedative and calming effects.

Lemon verbena is reputed to possess antispasmodic properties and is indicated in the treatment of indigestion, flatulence, diarrhoea and colic. The plant is also used to relieve asthma, lower fevers; it also possesses antibacterial and insecticidal properties. In 2002, a Portuguese study demonstrated the antioxidant properties of an infusion of lemon verbena.

The leaves are used in herbal medicine – like the aerial parts of peppermint and lime – as stimulants to help digestion. They can be found in pharmacies and food shops.

Cultivation

Plant in light, well-drained soil in a sunny location. Cuttings should be planted in summer.

PREPARATION AND DOSAGE

For internal use
TO TREAT digestive problems
INFUSION Put 1 sachet into a cup of boiling water. Leave to infuse for 5 minutes, then strain. Drink 2 cups a day after the main meals.

IF SYMPTOMS PERSIST, CONSULT A DOCTOR

CAUTIONS

● To date, no toxicity has been associated with lemon verbena, although excessive use should be avoided, as it has been associated with hormonal changes.
● The herb is not recommended for people with kidney disorders.
● Pregnant or breastfeeding women should not take lemon verbena.
● While using lemon verbena exposure of the skin to sunlight should be kept to a minimum.

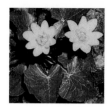

Lesser celandine

Ranunculus ficaria or *Ranunculus bulbosus* Ranunculaceae **Also called** Pilewort

This perennial plant carpets woodland floors, grassy banks and meadows throughout Europe. Its gleaming green leaves are heart-shaped and held on long stalks, which encase the main stem. The roots are long and swollen and the plant's brilliant yellow flowers bloom in spring. The plant has long been a remedy for haemorrhoids, which has given rise to its alternative name of pilewort.

Parts used
Whole plant
● Lesser celandine is uprooted in spring when in full bloom and then dried in a shady place.
● The dried herb is used in pharmaceutical creams, ointments and suppositories.

Constituents
The lesser celandine is rich in heterosides belonging to the saponin group, which are known to constrict blood vessels. The main saponin is protoanemonin, an irritant but thought to be the active ingredient. The plant also contains essential oil, tannins and vitamin C.

Medicinal uses
The astringent and soothing properties of lesser celandine indicate its use, externally, as a treatment for piles in which bleeding may be present. A paper published in *Phytochemistry* in 1984 attributed the anti-haemorrhoidal properties of lesser celandine to its saponin constituents. The plant has also been used externally to treat itching, inflamed skin and warts.

No part of the plant should be taken internally; this is due to the protoanemonin it contains, which is a severe irritant.

Cultivation
Plant in moist, neutral to alkaline soil in sun or shade in a wild part of the garden, as it is invasive.

CAUTIONS
● Like many members of its family, lesser celandine can irritate the skin and mere contact with the fresh plant can cause blisters. It is rendered less toxic when dried, but medical herbalists now restrict its use to external applications only.
● Excessive use is not recommended.
● Pregnant and breastfeeding women should avoid lesser celandine.

PREPARATION AND DOSAGE
For external use
TO TREAT haemorrhoids
CREAMS, OINTMENTS OR SUPPOSITORIES (containing 3% extract) Apply twice a day.

IF SYMPTOMS PERSIST, CONSULT A DOCTOR

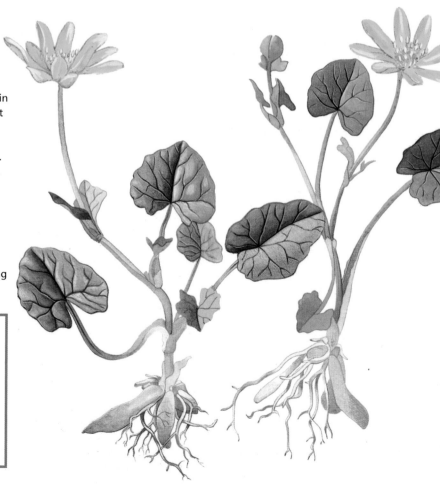

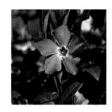

Lesser periwinkle

Vinca minor Apocynaceae

A native of the Mediterranean, lesser periwinkle is favoured by gardeners as a groundcover plant. Its crawling stems root at intervals to produce erect flower-bearing stems. It is a perennial evergreen whose leaves are shiny, leathery and unlobed. Vinca comes from the Latin word vincio (meaning 'I bind') and alludes to the plant's long stems, which were used for tying and binding. Violet-blue, five-petalled flowers appear in spring. Its fruit consists of pairs of seedpods, which split to release their seeds.

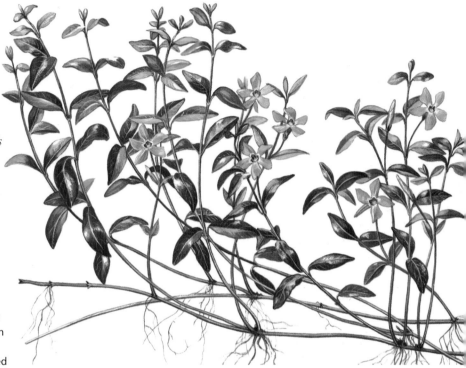

Parts used

Leaves

● Harvesting of the leaves takes place before the flowers bloom, when their alkaloid content is at its highest. The leaves are then dried in the open air.

● Despite their bitter taste, the dried leaves are used for infusions. In powder and extract forms they are used in pharmaceutical products.

Constituents

The active compounds are indole alkaloids, the most important being vincamine, which is much used by the pharmaceutical industry for its ability to stimulate blood circulation in the brain.

Medicinal uses

In the past lesser periwinkle was used as a treatment for skin ailments. However, recent research has shown that its alkaloids, mainly vincamine, dilate blood vessels in the brain thus improving cerebral circulation. A review published in 1999 documents these vasodilator properties, as well as the plant's ability to enhance brain activity and its usefulness in treating brain disorders relating to poor blood circulation.

Lesser periwinkle is prescribed to combat the mental effects of ageing, such as loss of concentration and loss of memory. An Austrian study performed in 1996 found the plant to be more effective than a placebo in improving symptoms of dementia. The plant is also used to stop both internal and external bleeding.

Lesser periwinkle can also help to ease stomach-related problems and soothe sore throats and other types of oral inflammation.

CAUTIONS

● Extracts of lesser periwinkle can only be obtained on medical herbalist prescription. Do not harvest garden plants.

● Pregnant women should not use lesser periwinkle.

Cultivation

Plant in moist soil in a sunny or lightly shaded position. It is possible to grow from cuttings in summer. Once established lesser periwinkle can become invasive.

PREPARATION AND DOSAGE

For internal use

TO TREAT effects of ageing, inadequate blood circulation
CAPSULES (290mg powder) Take 1 capsule three times a day at mealtimes.
TINCTURE Take 15 drops two or three times a day.

IF SYMPTOMS PERSIST, CONSULT A DOCTOR

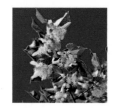

Lime tree

Tilia cordata, T. platyphyllos (and their hybrids) Tiliaceae **Also called** Linden tree

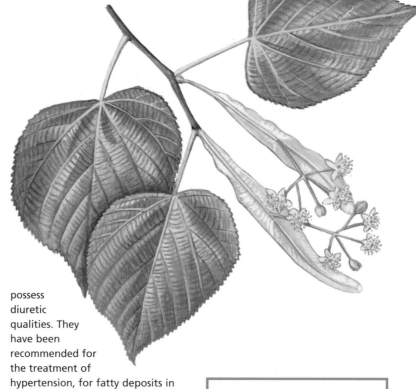

This tree, which grows as high as 20-40m, has grey bark that is smooth but cracks with age. Its leaves, whose size vary according to species, are an asymmetric heart-shape with serrated edges. The sweetly scented light yellow flowers grow in clusters and have long, greenish yellow bracts that are joined to the flower stalk.

Parts used

Flowers, bracts and sapwood

• The flowers are collected from both wild and cultivated trees when two-thirds of the flowers have bloomed, and then dried in thin layers away from sunlight.

• The sapwood (the inner layer of bark and the wood immediately under it) is collected from wild trees in sustainable environments and dried in large well-aired sheds.

• The flowers are used for infusions and the sapwood for powders and extracts.

Constituents

The flowers contain phenolic acids, proanthocyanadins, tannins, flavonoids, mucilages and a small quantity of essential oil that has a sedative effect. The sapwood also contains phenolic compounds and phloroglucinol.

Medicinal uses

Taken internally, the flowers are prescribed for minor sleep problems and nervous conditions. A hybrid of *Tilia cordata* and *T. platyphyllos* was shown by Portuguese scientists in 2001 to possess sedative effects.

In 1985 the antispasmodic effect of lime flowers was demonstrated, which has been attributed to the plant's phenolic compounds and phloroglucinol. The ability to relax smooth muscle is also attributed to the sapwood. Lime-tree flowers also possess diuretic qualities. They have been recommended for the treatment of hypertension, for fatty deposits in blood vessels (as they dilate the vessels), and to relieve migraines.

The sapwood is a purgative and also stimulates the secretion and elimination of bile. It is taken by mouth to treat gallstones, bloating and digestive problems.

Used externally, lime-tree flowers can soothe cracked and chapped skin, insect bites and skin irritations.

Cultivation

Plant in moist, well-drained soil in a sunny location. Trees can be grown from seed planted when ripe.

CAUTIONS

• Do not exceed the stated dose as this may affect heart function.

• Lime tree should not be taken by anyone with a heart disorder, except as directed by a medical herbalist.

• Pregnant or breastfeeding women should not take lime tree.

PREPARATION AND DOSAGE

For internal use

TO TREAT minor sleeping problems

INFUSION Put 5g of dried flowers into 1 litre of boiling water. Leave to infuse for 5 minutes, then strain. Drink 1 cup in the evening before bed.

TO TREAT digestive problems caused by the liver, gallstones, bloating

TINCTURE (1:5 in 25% alcohol) Take 5ml in water three times a day before meals.

For external use

TO TREAT cracked or chapped skin, insect bites

SOLUTION (with a base of lime flowers) Apply to the affected area several times a day.

IF SYMPTOMS PERSIST, CONSULT A DOCTOR

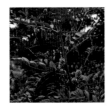

Liquorice

Glycyrrhiza glabra Fabaceae

This perennial shrub is native to southern Europe. It has upright branched stems to about 1m high, bearing alternate leaves made up of 7-17 bright green leaflets. Its small pale blue to lilac flowers grow in spikes. It has thick, woody rhizomatous roots and creeping stems that can reach 2m in length. The fruit is a reddish brown pod.

Parts used

Roots

• The roots are collected in autumn from plants that are at least three years old.
• Once washed, the roots are dried in the sunshine.
• The roots are used in segments, in powders (for infusions and macerations) or as a juice.

Constituents

A large proportion of the root is composed of polysaccharides. Other components include coumarins, a small amount of phytosterols (mainly oestriol), flavonoids, saponins (in particular glycyrrhizin and glycyrrhizinic acid) and some traces of essential oil that give the plant its aroma and sweet taste. The pharmacological activity is due to the flavonoids and saponins.

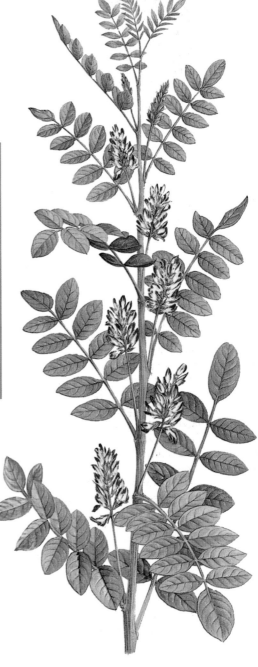

Medicinal uses

The glycyrrhizin and glycyrrhizinic acid in liquorice impart several medicinal properties: it can be used to treat gastric ulcers and inflammation, it releases phlegm and soothes coughs, eases asthma, stimulates the immune system and helps to fight dental plaque and tooth decay, as well as mouth and throat infections.

Liquorice root is also used to treat digestive problems such as bloating, spasms, sluggish digestion, belching and flatulence. The plant has a slight oestrogenic effect and its flavonoids, can help to protect liver cells and combat free radicals.

Liquorice can also be used to treat skin inflammation and infections. Research published in 1980 demonstrated the anti-inflammatory effects of glycyrrhizinic acid against erythema (reddening of the skin) caused by exposure to ultraviolet light. Liquorice also stimulates the secretion of aldosterone, a hormone that causes water and sodium retention, but prevents the retention of potassium. As a result, it has adverse side effects if taken in large doses, particularly in people with heart or liver problems.

Cultivation

Plant in rich, well-drained soil in a sunny location. The seeds should be sown in spring.

CAUTIONS

• Any treatment using liquorice must be accompanied by a low-salt diet and should never last longer than 4-6 weeks.
• The maximum daily dose of glycyrrhizin is 100mg. Care should be taken not to consume too many drinks or sweets containing liquorice during the treatment.
• The plant should not be taken during pregnancy or if suffering from high blood pressure, heart problems, or any illnesses that hinders the elimination of salts from the body, such as liver disorders.
• Liquorice is not recommended for individuals with kidney disorders.

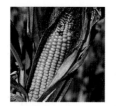

Maize

Zea mays Poaceae **Also called** Sweetcorn, Corn

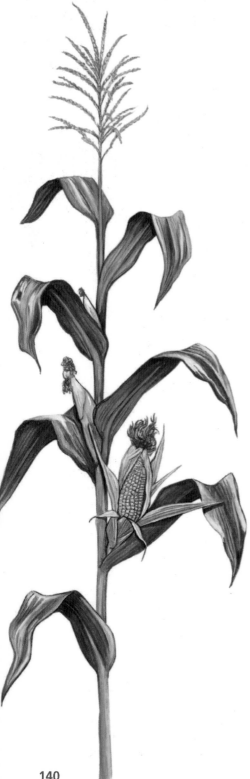

A robust annual, maize is native to the Andes and Central America. Its stalk can grow as high as 3m, with long, ribbon-like leaves curling downwards from it at regular intervals. The female flowers, found halfway up the stalks, produce the cobs, which are long, cylindrical ears of corn, surrounded by a mass of silky stamens then large bracts, and topped with a tuft of feathery styles. Delicate strands of tiny male flowers grow in loose clusters from the top of the stalk.

Parts used

Stamens and seeds of female flowers (corn cobs)

• The corn cobs are picked during summer, before pollination, and the stamens, also known as 'cornsilk', are carefully removed.

• These must be dried quickly, but can also be used fresh. Preparations made from cornsilk include infusions and extracts.

• Corn oil is extracted from the seeds. It is used for cooking, and in medicines and cosmetics.

Constituents

Maize stamens contain saponins, tannins, phytosterols, mucilage, potassium and an essential oil. The oil that is found in the seeds, or corn kernels, makes up to about 20 per cent of their content and is rich in healthy, unsaturated fatty acids.

CAUTIONS

• Cosmetics containing maize oil have been known to induce contact dermatitis in people who have particularly sensitive skin.

• Women who are pregnant or breastfeeding should not consume large amounts of maize (corn) oil.

PREPARATION AND DOSAGE

For internal use

TO TREAT cystitis, inflammation of the urinary tract, water retention caused by kidney problems, kidney stones
INFUSION Put 1 teaspoon (2g) of dried cornsilk into 1 cup of water. Bring rapidly to the boil, then infuse for 5 minutes. Drink 1 cup three times a day.
CAPSULES (150mg dry extract) Take 2-4 capsules a day.

IF SYMPTOMS PERSIST, CONSULT A DOCTOR

Medicinal uses

Maize stamens are mainly used for their anti-inflammatory and general healing powers, which have been confirmed by a number of scientific studies. It is because of these powers, coupled with cornsilk's ability to act as a diuretic, that its preparations are most often used to treat urinary tract problems such as cystitis, water retention caused by kidney problems and kidney stones. Sometimes the plant's ability to ease inflammation is employed in treating gout.

Cornsilk preparations are also reputed to stimulate the secretion of bile, which is why they are often prescribed for liver and gall-bladder disorders. It is also believed that cornsilk can help to lower blood pressure and blood sugar levels.

Maize oil from the seeds, or kernels, is an ingredient in cosmetics used to soften and moisturise the skin, and to combat wrinkles.

Cultivation

Maize can be grown from seeds. Plant them in late spring in any rich, well-drained soil. The plant grows best in a sunny location.

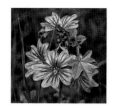

Mallow

Malva sylvestris Malvaceae

Common throughout Europe, the mallow is a robust plant with a thick stem and downy, lobed leaves. It grows wild by the roadside, on embankments and on waste ground. The showy, mauvish flowers are attractively streaked with crimson veins. The fruit of the mallow is a circle of small nuts, each containing a single seed.

Parts used

Leaves and flowers

- The leaves are collected in spring, before the plant is in bloom. Flowers are gathered from to June to September.
- Both flowers and leaves are arranged in thin layers and left to dry in a dark place, so as not to destroy their anthocyanic pigments.
- Once dried, the leaves and flowers are used to prepare infusions, decoctions and powders.

Constituents

Both the leaves and flowers are rich in soothing mucilages. Anthocyanin pigments, responsible for the colour of mallow flowers, also contain polysaccharides and flavonoids.

Medicinal uses

Mallow is well known for its soothing effect on the bronchial tubes and is most frequently used to ease bronchial ailments and coughs.

The plant can also be taken to calm inflammation in the digestive tract and to treat symptoms of constipation and colitis.

Externally, mallow soothes skin irritations and, as a gargle, is good for oral problems; the decoction can also be applied to babies' gums to soothe teething pain.

Japanese studies published in 1989 have shown that mallow's anti-inflammatory action is due to its mucilage content.

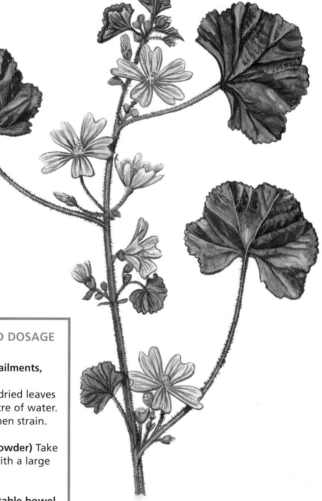

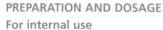

PREPARATION AND DOSAGE

For internal use

TO TREAT bronchial ailments, coughs

INFUSION Put 5g of dried leaves and flowers into 1 litre of water. Boil for 5 minutes, then strain. Drink 1-3 cups a day.

CAPSULES (250mg powder) Take 3-5 capsules a day, with a large glass of water.

TO TREAT colitis, irritable bowel syndrome (IBS), constipation

INFUSION Put 10-15g of dried flowers into 1 litre of boiling water. Infuse for 10 minutes, then strain. Drink 3-4 cups a day.

For external use

TO TREAT skin and mouth problems

DECOCTION Put 30g dried flowers and/or leaves into 1 litre of boiling water. Infuse for 10 minutes, then strain. For itching and dry skin, apply to the affected area several times a day. For inflammation of the mouth and voice loss, gargle or use as a mouthwash several times a day.

IF SYMPTOMS PERSIST, CONSULT A DOCTOR

Scientists are now exploring new uses for the plant as recent research has revealed that the polysaccharides contained in mallow and the related marshmallow root (see p.143) can help to strengthen the immune system.

Cultivation

Mallow is grown from seeds. Plant them in late spring, in a sunny or lightly shaded spot. Mallow grows in any well-drained soil and thrives in poor soils.

CAUTION

- Very high doses of preparations that contain mallow have been known to have a laxative effect.

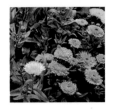

Marigold

Calendula officinalis Asteraceae/Compositae **Also called** Calendula.

Originally from the Mediterranean region, marigold has been cultivated for its ornamental, culinary and medicinal qualities for many centuries. The ancient Romans used it in a broth that was said to uplift the spirits. Soft, green leaves spring from its robust, angular stems, and the vivid, orangey gold flowers appear from early June right up to the time of the first winter frosts.

Parts used

Flowers

● The flowers are gathered from June onwards, just as they begin to bloom, and are left to dry on racks in a dark, well-ventilated place.
● Dried marigold flowers are used in ointments, gargles and compresses.
● Occasionally, marigold is used internally as an infusion or tincture.

Constituents

Marigold flowers contain flavonoids, carotenoid pigments, which give them their orange colour, and an essential oil, rich in triterpenoids – thought to be responsible for its anti-inflammatory properties.

Medicinal uses

Applied externally marigold has long been an effective treatment for skin problems such as cuts, itching, cracked skin, sunburn and insect bites, and is used in many skin cosmetics. It is also recommended as a treatment for mouth infections.

A number of investigations into the healing powers of marigold flowers have highlighted not only their anti-inflammatory and

antibacterial properties, but also their ability to fight off infection caused by viruses and parasites. Research in Italy in 1994 found that triterpenoids in the plant are responsible for its anti-inflammatory powers, and trials have shown that these compounds can help to ease swelling caused by fluid retention.

Marigold is also reputed to be capable of staunching bleeding and calming muscular spasms.

Cultivation

Marigold grows easily from seeds. Plant in spring in well-drained, neutral to alkaline soil, preferably in a sunny or lightly shaded location.

CAUTION

● Marigold preparations should only be taken internally under the supervision of a medical herbalist.
● Do not take in pregnancy.

PREPARATION AND DOSAGE

For external use

TO TREAT cracked skin, cuts, insect bites, sunburn
COMPRESS Put 5g dried flowerheads into 1 litre of boiling water. Infuse for 5 minutes, then strain. Apply to the affected area as a compress three or four times a day.

TO TREAT mouth infections
GARGLE Prepare the infusion as described above for a compress. Leave until just warm; use as a gargle two or three times a day.

IF SYMPTOMS PERSIST, CONSULT A DOCTOR

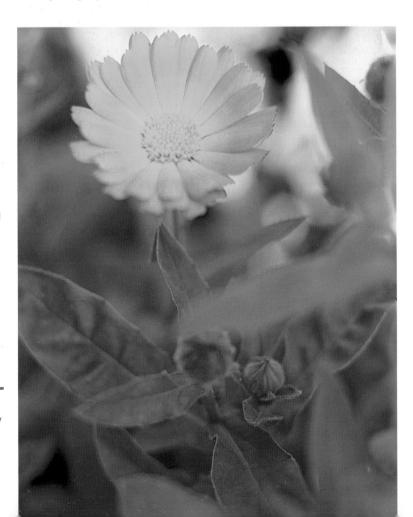

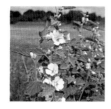

Marshmallow

Althaea officinalis Malvaceae

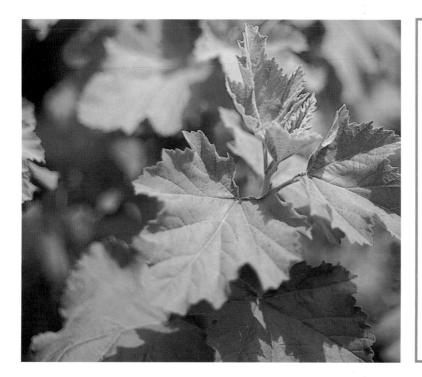

Found on damp ground all over Europe, the marshmallow can reach a height of 1m. The down on its stems and large leaves give the plant a velvety look, and in late summer delicate pinky white flowers appear briefly, followed by flat, round fruits. But the marshmallow is mainly valued for its thick, white, fibrous roots, which the Romans considered a delicacy.

Parts used

Roots and leaves

• The roots are dug up in autumn, two years after planting. They are dried, then used to make infusions, powders, extracts, and syrups.
• The leaves are sometimes picked in summer and used for infusions.

Constituents

A large proportion of the root consists of mucilage. Some phenolic acids and flavonoids are also present.

Medicinal uses

Marshmallow is well known for its soothing and anti-inflammatory properties, and it is widely prescribed to calm dry coughs and treat other respiratory ailments, including sore throats and bronchitis. It is also very effective in soothing mouth ulcers, dental abscesses, boils, acne and burns, when applied directly to the affected area on a compress.

Tests have shown that the high level of mucilage in marshmallow root is responsible for its power to reduce inflammation. Other research has confirmed the antiseptic powers of marshmallow, as well as its ability to fight infection by stimulating the immune system.

Perhaps of less importance than its medicinal powers is the recent discovery in Japan that marshmallow may have a whitening effect on the skin. This action may be of interest to the cosmetics industry, which has long incorporated the plant into moisturising creams, because of its softening and soothing properties.

Cultivation

Marshmallow can be cultivated from seeds. Plant them in spring in any type of moist soil, in a plot where they will receive plently of sunshine.

CAUTIONS

• Marshmallow can become toxic if combined with substances such as alcohol, tannins and iron.
• If you are taking other medicines, check with your doctor before using a marshmallow extract, as it can affect their absorption.
• Marshmallow has been shown to lower blood sugar levels. Therefore, It may interfere with the action of other therapies or medications being used to control blood sugar levels, such as insulin for diabetes.

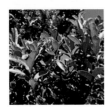

Maté

Ilex paraguariensis Aquifoliaceae **Also called** Paraguay tea

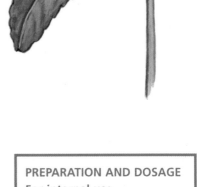

A South American evergreen, the maté tree grows wild near streams, but is cultivated on a large scale in Brazil, Paraguay and Argentina. Maté tea, made by infusing the leaves, is regarded as the national drink throughout much of South America. The tree can reach a height of 10m, and bears oval, leathery leaves, similar to those of holly – but without thorns.

Parts used

Leaves

- Where grown commercially, the maté tree is pruned low to make harvesting easier.
- Leaves are picked from trees at least four years old, from December to August.
- They are dried rapidly over a fire and chopped into small pieces.
- The dried leaf, known as green maté, is used in drinks and infusions.

Constituents

The chemical composition of maté is complex. Once dried, up to 10 per cent of the leaf is composed of phenol acids, and there are also saponins, flavonoids, a little resin and some traces of essential oil.

CAUTIONS

- Excessive use of maté tea can overstimulate the nervous system.
- Do not take if you have sleep problems.
- Do not take maté if you suffer from heart or circulatory problems.
- Use of maté should be avoided when pregnant or breastfeeding.
- Maté is on the list of banned stimulants for sports participants.
- Recent South American studies suggest a possible link between drinking large amounts of maté tea and an increased risk of developing cancer of the lungs or oesophagus.

The main active compounds, however, are caffeine and theobromine, a diuretic and cardiac stimulant.

Medicinal uses

Because maté contains high levels of caffeine, a potent stimulant, it is used to combat fatigue. Maté is also a diuretic and is widely used for kidney problems.

All the research conducted on caffeine shows that it increases alertness and intellectual capacity and generally stimulates the central nervous system. It has been shown that caffeine can raise the base metabolic rate by about 10 per cent. Together with the caffeine in maté, the theobromine, phenol acids, flavonoids and saponins all contribute to this energising effect.

Research published in *Planta Medica* in 1988 showed that maté can also suppress the appetite. That finding, and a 1995 study demonstrating the ability of maté infusions to break down fats in the blood, suggest that the herb may be useful for weight loss regimes. A further British trial in 2001 found that maté taken in combination with guarana and damiana could cause weight loss.

Recent French research has indicated that maté may help to protect against hardening of the arteries, a cause of many major heart and circulatory disorders. It is also prescribed to alleviate the pain of tension headaches and rheumatism.

Cultivation

Maté is a tropical tree and needs to be grown indoors or in a heated greenhouse, as it will not survive temperatures below 7°C.

PREPARATION AND DOSAGE

For internal use

TO TREAT lethargy, nervous exhaustion, kidney problems
INFUSION Put 2-3g of dried leaves into 1 cup of boiling water. Leave to infuse for 5 minutes, then strain. Drink 1-3 cups a day, preferably before 5pm to avoid any difficulty in falling asleep at night.

IF SYMPTOMS PERSIST, CONSULT A DOCTOR

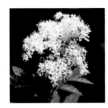

Meadowsweet

Filipendula ulmaria (Spirea ulmaria) Rosaceae **Also called** Queen of the meadow

Growing in abundance in the temperate parts of Europe and Asia, meadowsweet loves damp places, where it grows up to around 2m tall. The fern-like leaves, made up of three to nine pairs of indented leaflets, grow alternately along the hollow, red-veined stem. Clusters of sweet-smelling, creamy white flowers blossom from June to September. Their fragrance made them a popular flavouring for beers and wines in the Middle Ages.

Parts used
Stems, leaves and flowers
● The aerial parts are picked in June and July, as the first flowers appear.
● They are dried in a shady, well-aired place, until they turn slightly yellow, then used for infusions and tinctures.

Constituents
Meadowsweet is rich in tannins, hence its sharp astringent taste. It also contains flavonoids and a fragrant essential oil, largely made up of salicylates, which have an anti-inflammatory effect.

Medicinal uses
Meadowsweet is highly effective in treating flu symptoms, headaches, toothache, and joint pain caused by rheumatism and gout. It can also stimulate sweating. Its salicylates confer its anti-inflammatory and pain-relieving powers and the flavonoids also contribute to this effect, as well as helping to soothe muscle spasms and digestive tract problems, including gastric ulcers. Studies in the Ukraine have confirmed the plant's benefits in ulcer treatment.

Meadowsweet has antibacterial and healing powers, in which its tannins and flavonoids play a major role. For centuries, it has been prescribed for urinary tract infections and as a diuretic – often being recommended for overweight and bloating due to water retention.

Cultivation
Meadowsweet can be grown from seeds. They should be planted in spring in moist, water-retentive, rich alkaline soil, in a sunny or lightly shaded plot.

CAUTIONS
● Avoid if allergic to aspirin.
● Do not use meadowsweet in combination with standard 300mg aspirin tablets, to avoid overdose. It can, however, be taken by those on low-dose aspirin (75mg a day).
● Meadowsweet may constrict the airways: it should never be taken by people with asthma.
● Do not take when pregnant or breastfeeding.

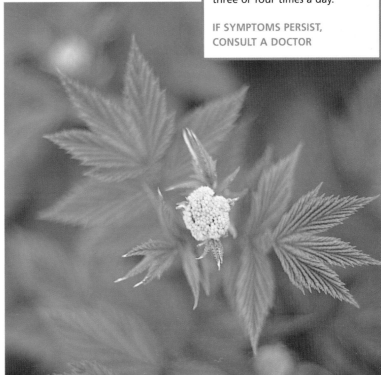

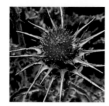

Milk thistle

Silybum marianum (Carduus marianus) Asteraceae/Compositae **Also called** Our lady's thistle

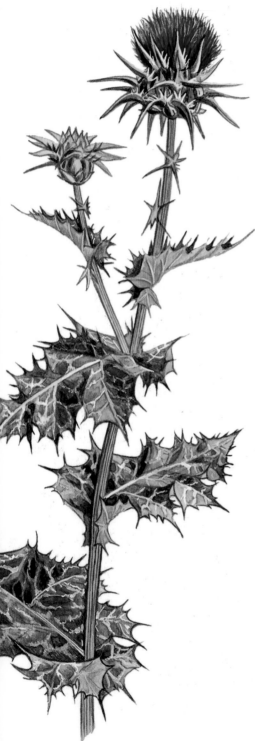

A tough herbaceous plant that thrives on dry wasteground, the milk thistle is common in many parts of Europe and Asia. Its shiny, indented leaves are fringed with spines and have milky white veins, the result, according to myth, of milk from the Virgin's breast falling onto the plant. Crimson-mauve flowers made up of hundreds of florets crown the tops of the stems in summer. These are followed by tufted seeds.

Parts used

Leaves and seeds

• Leaves and seeds may be used fresh or dried.

• The leaves are picked at the end of summer. They are dried, cut into small pieces or crushed into powder, and used in infusions.

• The seeds are collected in autumn, dried and used in powders, dry extracts and tinctures.

• Milk thistle is often combined with other plants used to treat bile problems, such as globe artichoke.

Constituents

The seeds contain silymarin, a mixture of several compounds that are known to protect the liver. The leaves contain flavonoids – antioxidants that are good for the circulation – and b-sitosterol, a substance that emulsifies fats and breaks down cholesterol deposits.

CAUTIONS

• Milk thistle can be allergenic: stop using if you have a reaction.

• Do not use to treat problems caused by an obstruction to the flow of bile, such as gallstones.

• It is not advisable to use the plant when pregnant or breastfeeding.

• An overdose of any milk thistle preparation can cause vomiting.

Medicinal uses

In a number of studies, the silymarin in milk thistle has been shown to have antioxidant properties which help to protect the liver and other parts of the body from damage by free radicals. This is why milk thistle is recommended as a supplementary treatment for chronic hepatitis and cirrhosis. Spanish studies have also noted silymarin's anti-inflammatory action, and its soothing powers are sometimes employed to treat piles.

In addition, milk thistle infusions and tinctures are known to calm muscular spasms and stimulate the flow of bile from the gall bladder. They are therefore recommended as a treatment for bile-flow and minor digestive problems. The plant is also reputed to stimulate menstruation.

Cultivation

Milk thistle grows readily from seed. Plant in a wild part of the garden in a sunny, well-drained spot.

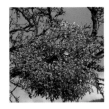

Mistletoe

Viscum album Viscaceae

Common throughout Europe, mistletoe is a parasitic shrub that sinks its roots into the branches of trees with a soft bark, such as ash, poplar and old apple trees. Its smooth, many-branched stems bear leathery, evergreen leaves. In May, it bears clusters of tiny, yellowish flowers. The fruit, a sticky white berry, ripens in early winter.

Parts used

Leaves and fruits (berries)

● The leaves are gathered in spring and autumn and dried rapidly until they turn a yellowy green.

● Despite their unpleasant bitter taste, the leaves are used in preparations that are taken internally. These include infusions, extracts, capsules and other pharmaceutical products.

● Sometimes the berries are also picked and used medicinally.

Constituents

The significant active compounds in mistletoe are viscotoxins and lectins, poisonous substances, but which, in tiny doses, are believed to boost the immune system.

Medicinal uses

The capacity of mistletoe to lower blood pressure has been verified by experimental data, and seems to be due to the combined effects of a group of compounds rather than to one specific active agent.

Research in Germany has shown that mistletoe has a stimulating effect on the immune system and inhibits the growth of tumours – an effect attributed to its viscotoxins and lectins. This could make mistletoe useful in fighting cancer, if the toxicity of these components can be controlled.

It has also been claimed that the plant can treat hardening of the arteries, but results of human clinical trials have proved disappointing.

Cultivation

Mistletoe is a parasitic plant, only found in the wild on trees at least 15 years old. Rubbing its berries into crevices in the underside of the bark of a suitable soft-barked tree, such as apple, willow or rowan, can encourage mistletoe to grow there.

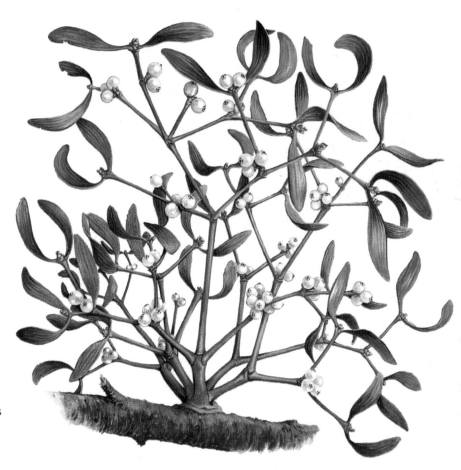

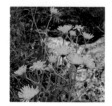

Mouse-ear hawkweed

Hieracium pilosella (Pilosella officinarum) Asteraceae/Compositae

Common in Europe, North Africa and Asia, mouse-ear hawkweed is a tiny herbaceous plant with crawling shoots, or runners. Its elongated, oval leaves are coated in white hairs and form a rosette around the base of the plant. From May to September, when the plant is in bloom, dandelion-like flowers appear at the tips of the almost leafless stems.

Parts used

Whole plant

● The plants are collected in their wild state just after blooming. They are tied in bunches and left to dry in the open air.

● Mouse-ear hawkweed is used to make infusions, powders and dry or liquid extracts. It is also found in a number of pharmaceutical products.

Constituents

All parts of the plant contain umbelliferone, a coumarin, which has an antibiotic effect, flavonoids, which are diuretic, and phenols – substances with antiseptic and anti-inflammatory actions.

Medicinal uses

French studies in 1999 demonstrated the diuretic effects of the plant's flavonoids. Because it can help the body to eliminate excess fluid and waste, the plant is an effective treatment for swelling caused by water retention, especially in the legs and lower part of the body.

Mouse-ear hawkweed is also reputed to possess anti-inflammatory and antispasmodic properties. It is sometimes applied to wounds, and used to treat respiratory complaints such as asthma and bronchitis, as well as to ease inflammation in the kidneys and urinary tract.

Umbelliferone is known to help stimulate the flow of bile from the gall bladder, helping to keep the digestive system healthy, and research has shown that it also has an antibiotic effect. And in 1993, American scientists discovered that umbelliferone, as well as other coumarin derivatives, can help to fight off the HIV virus and it is thought that this ability might be harnessed for combating other types of viral infection.

Cultivation

Mouse-ear hawkweed can be grown from seed planted in spring. The plant thrives in any well-drained soil, in a sunny or lightly shaded spot. Confine to a wild or informal part of the garden.

CAUTIONS

● **No toxic side effects have been reported to date, even after prolonged use.**

● **Do not exceed the recommended dosage.**

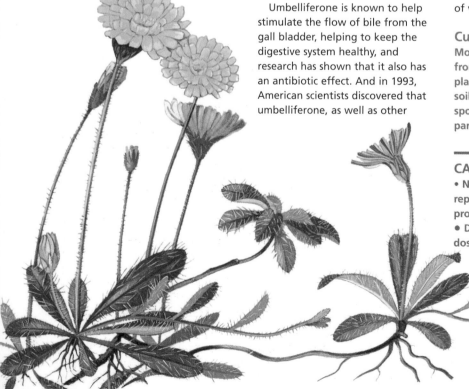

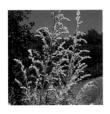

Mugwort

Artemisia vulgaris Asteraceae/Compositae

Throughout Europe and around the Mediterranean, tufts of mugwort grow wild beside woodland paths and streams. Its upright stems often have reddish marks and can reach a height of 1.5m. The deeply indented leaves are dark green on the top and white beneath. Tiny heads of small yellow or reddish brown flowers cluster around the stems in summer.

Parts used

Leaves and flowerheads
• Leaves and flowers are gathered in June or early July, just as the plant comes into bloom. Flowers taken from dry areas are said to have more beneficial properties than those that have grown in damp locations.
• After being cleaned and woven into garlands, the flowers and leaves are left to dry in a sheltered place.
• The dried plant is used to make infusions, powders, extracts, tinctures and a tonic wine.

Constituents

The presence of sesquiterpene lactones accounts for the bitter taste of mugwort. It also contains a little essential oil, flavonoids that have an antioxidant effect, coumarins, and some phytosterols, which appear to mimic the action of the female hormone, oestrogen.

CAUTIONS

• Mugwort should not be used when pregnant or breastfeeding.
• People who are taking blood-thinning drugs such as Warfarin should not use mugwort.
• Because of its sesquiterpenic lactones, contact with mugwort can cause allergic reactions such as dermatitis and conjunctivitis.
• Do not exceed the recommended or prescribed dose of mugwort.

Medicinal uses

Though few of its properties have been scientifically proven, mugwort is commonly prescribed to treat a whole range of digestive problems including slow digestion, indigestion and loss of appetite.

Mugwort is also known to be antispasmodic, so can help to ease intestinal cramps and is an effective remedy for period pains.

There are centuries-old references to the effectiveness of mugwort in warding off disease and in 1989, scientists in China demonstrated the plant's antibacterial powers.

The herb is still prescribed to fight bacterial and fungal infections, and can be of great benefit when treating fevers, skin inflammation and rheumatism. It is also used to eliminate worms, an ability attributed to its essential oil and sesquiterpene lactones.

Cultivation

Mugwort can be grown from seed, which should be planted in spring. It does best in well-drained, neutral to alkaline soil, preferably in a sunny position.

PREPARATION AND DOSAGE

For internal use
TO TREAT digestive problems, intestinal worms
INFUSION Put 1 dessertspoon of the dried plant into 150-200ml of boiling water. Leave to infuse for 5-10 minutes and strain. Drink 1-2 cups a day.
POWDER Take 2-4g a day.
TINCTURE Put 30 drops into a glass of water. Take three times a day.

TO TREAT menstrual pain
INFUSION Make as above and take 1-2 glasses a day for eight to ten days before a period.
TONIC WINE Add 20g dried herb to 1 litre of white wine and leave for ten days. Drink 2 glasses a day for eight days before a period.

IF SYMPTOMS PERSIST, CONSULT A DOCTOR

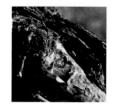

Myrrh

Commiphora myrrha Burseraceae

Found mainly in East Africa and Somalia, the commiphora, or myrrh tree has a thick, twisted trunk, that can grow to a height of around 5m. The tiny leaves are made up of two leaflets, each with a spine at its tip. Small yellow-red flowers grow on the spiny branches in summer. In the rainy season, the bark, which ranges in colour from orange to grey, if cut, releases a thick resin or gum.

Parts used

Resin

● During the rainy season, October to April, cuts are made in the bark of the tree, through which the resin oozes. This is white at first, then yellow and finally brownish red.

● The resin solidifies to form cracked translucent pieces of varying shapes and sizes. This is the precious myrrh, mentioned in the Bible. It has a strong aroma and a bitter taste – 'myrrh' is Hebrew for bitterness.

● The myrrh pieces break up easily, and are used to make tinctures.

Constituents

Myrrh's essential oil contains furanosesquiterpenes which have an anti-inflammatory effect and also give the wood a rich characteristic scent. The plant's resins are rich in alcohols and triterpenic acids.

Medicinal uses

Myrrh is one of the earliest plants to be put to medicinal use. Its healing powers were widely appreciated in the ancient world, and more recently studies have confirmed its antiseptic, anti-inflammatory, fever-reducing and analgesic actions. These are often employed in treating minor wounds as well as oral problems, such as inflammation, gum infections and damage caused by dentures.

Myrrh is also known to have the ability to relieve nasal congestion, and is reputed to help ease digestive problems due to trapped wind and muscle spasms.

Cultivation

Myrrh grows best in well-drained soil, preferably in the sun. It needs warmth of at least 10°C, so a heated greenhouse is best. Grow from seed in spring, or from a cutting taken at the end of the growing season.

CAUTIONS

● Myrrh is only suitable for external use. It should never be ingested.

● Prolonged use of myrrh is not recommended, because it can cause allergic reactions in some people.

● Individuals who suffer from any thyroid disorder should always seek the advice of a medical herbalist before using myrrh.

● Women who are pregnant or breastfeeding are advised to use myrrh sparingly.

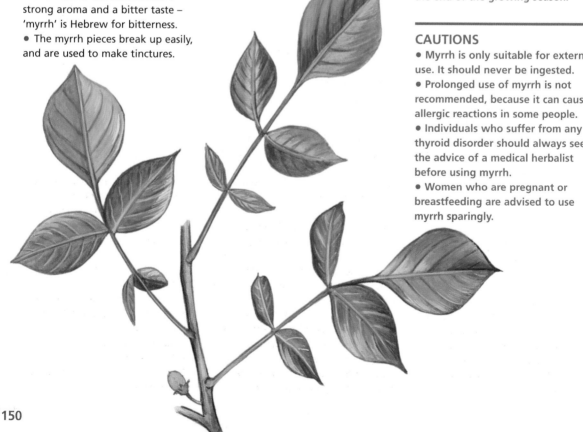

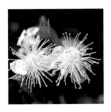

Myrtle

Myrtus communis Myrtaceae

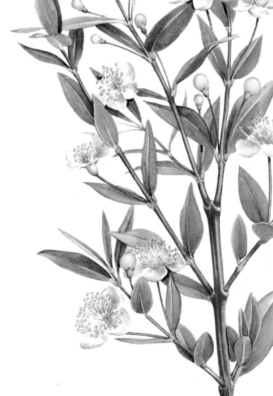

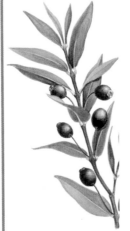

Native to scrubland around the Mediterranean, myrtle is an evergreen shrub with erect, hairy stems and shiny, pointed oval leaves, covered in tiny pits. White, sweet-smelling flowers, are followed by purple-black fruits, or berries, about the size of a pea.

Parts used

Leaves and berries
● The leaves are gathered in spring, then dried in the shade, so that they remain green.
● They are used in infusions and powders, and for their essential oil.
● The berries are picked in autumn. Fresh ones are sometimes chewed. In Corsica and Sardinia a popular drink is made by steeping the berries in alcohol.

Constituents

Myrtle leaves contain a small quantity of essential oil. The berries contain more and also tannins, and a number of organic acids.

Medicinal uses

Recent research has confirmed the antiseptic and decongestant powers of myrtle, which traditionally made it a valued treatment for respiratory and intestinal problems. It is also used occasionally to treat genital and the urinary tract infections. For its emollient and healing powers, it is recommended for treating skin infections, such as abcesses and boils, and the essential oil will kill infestations of lice.

The berries are chewed as an appetite stimulant because they are said to stimulate the gastric function.

Myrtle may have a new use, too, in treating diabetes. Tests show that it can reduce high blood sugar levels.

Cultivation

Grow myrtle from seeds in autumn, a young nursery plant or woody cuttings taken in summer, ideally in a sheltered spot. The neutral to alkaline soil should be well drained.

CAUTION

● As some essential oil components can irritate the digestive system, it is advisable to consult a doctor or medical herbalist before taking myrtle preparations internally.
● Do not take myrtle if pregnant or breastfeeding.

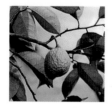

Nutmeg

Myristica fragrans Myristicaceae

Found in tropical countries, such as Brazil, Indonesia and the West Indies, the nutmeg tree can grow to a height of 20m. It has shiny evergreen foliage, but its clusters of delicate, yellow flowers do not appear until the tree is seven years old. The fleshy, pale yellow fruits each contain one large seed – the 'nut' – enclosed first in a hard, woody casing, then in a red or orangey membrane, known as mace.

Parts used

Seeds (nuts)
● The fruit is mostly picked in July and August, and the seeds removed.
● Using steam, about 8 to 15 per cent of the essential oil is extracted together with nutmeg butter (used in the pharmaceutical industry).

Constituents

Nutmeg's essential oil, which has a sharp taste and a peppery smell, is composed mainly of camphene and pinene, but also contains myristicin which is toxic.

Medicinal uses

Although nutmeg essential oil is reputed to be an aphrodisiac and tonic, it is seldom used for these purposes because of the toxicity of its myristicin content. Instead, it is reserved almost exclusively for use externally, as an anti-inflammatory remedy for joint pains, muscular injuries, rheumatism and tendinitis.

However, scientists in India have shown that the essential oil can help to lower blood cholesterol and to decrease fatty

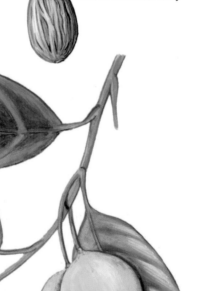

deposits around the liver, heart, and the aorta. In addition, Nigerian studies have shown that the essential oil can inhibit the formation of blood clots. All this evidence suggests that nutmeg could be useful in protecting against blockages and hardening of the arteries and associated heart and circulatory problems. Studies have also shown that it can lower harmful cholesterol.

One reason that nutmeg is used as a spice is because it aids digestion, and clinical studies have discovered that it can help to treat diarrhoea.

Cultivation

Grow from seeds when ripe, or woody cuttings at the end of the growing season. Use rich, well-drained sandy soil, preferably in a greenhouse heated to a minimum of 15-18°C and with high humidity.

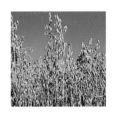

Oats

Avena sativa Poaceae

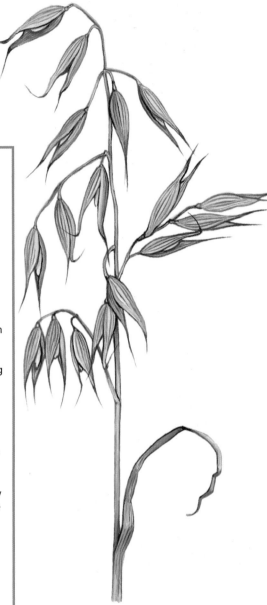

Grown in all temperate regions of the world, oats are an important cereal crop. Long, slender leaves grow along stalks, which can reach a height of around 1.5m. Clusters of flowers are followed by the tiny ears that enclose the seeds, or grain.

Parts used

Seeds (grain) and stems

● After harvesting, which takes place in late summer, the seeds and stems are dried.

● The grain is removed from the husk and pressed, then used along with the dried stalks in infusions, extracts and tinctures, as well as in skincare products and sun creams.

Constituents

Oat grains contain vitamins B_2, B_5 and E, the minerals calcium, iron, manganese and zinc, a soothing oil and a small quantity of alkaloids. The stems also contain flavonoids.

Medicinal uses

Herbalists have long used oats to help ease indigestion and to soothe the intestinal inflammation associated with diarrhoea. This anti-inflammatory action, probably due to the flavonoids, can also bring relief from rheumatism and gout.

In the ancient world oats were used to treat skin problems such as boils and impetigo; and recent

CAUTIONS

● Oats are not toxic and have no adverse side effects but they can cause flatulence and more frequent bowel movements. When eating them, it is advisable to drink plenty of water.

● Like many other cereals, oats are rich in gluten and therefore should be avoided by people suffering from coeliac disease.

PREPARATION AND DOSAGE

For internal use

TO TREAT stress, insomnia, minor nervous problems, rheumatism, gout

INFUSION Put 3g of dried plant into 250ml of boiling water. Infuse for 5 minutes. Strain. Drink 3-4 cups a day. For insomnia drink 1 cup before going to bed.

TINCTURE (1:5 in 45% alcohol) Take 20 drops in a glass of warm water, two or three times a day.

LIQUID EXTRACT Take 10-30 drops in hot water, before going to bed.

For external use

TO TREAT skin ailments

COMPRESS Make up the infusion described above, and soak a clean cloth with it. Apply this to the affected area.

DECOCTION Put 20g of dried plant into 1 litre of water. Allow to boil for 3 minutes, then leave for 10-20 minutes. Strain, then use added to bathwater. This is also effective when feeling weary and in need of a tonic.

IF SYMPTOMS PERSIST, CONSULT A DOCTOR

---

clinical trials in France have confirmed its efficacy for combating skin problems.

Oats are now widely used in cosmetics as its vitamin B_2 content can promote healthy skin and its vitamin E and oil are moisturisers.

Furthermore, oats have been shown to lower cholesterol. In a study in Mexico, men given oat-enriched cookies over an eight-week period showed around a 26 per cent drop in their cholesterol levels.

Vitamin B_5 is known for its ability to combat depression, stress, and fatigue, and alkaloids are said to

soothe the nerves. Their presence in oats may be why they are frequently prescribed for a whole range of minor nervous problems and as a general tonic. In controlled trials, athletes placed on an oat-based diet demonstrated an approximately 4 per cent increase in stamina.

Cultivation

Sow the seeds in spring in well-composted, well-drained soil in a sunny position.

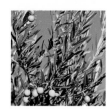

Olive

Olea europaea Oleaceae

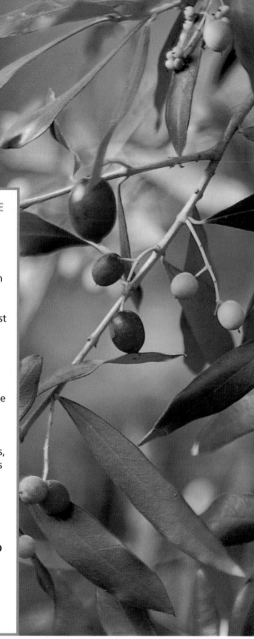

Widely cultivated throughout the Mediterranean region, the olive tree has a grey, twisted and grooved trunk and grows to a height of about 10m. Its tough, spear-shaped, evergreen leaves are greyish green on top and silvery white beneath. Its flowers are white and grow in little, erect clusters and its oval fruit, the olive, is green at first ripening to black, with a hard stone at its centre.

Parts used

Leaves and fruits

● Mature leaves are gathered in March and April, before the flowers come into bud.

● They are dried, broken into fragments and used for infusions, extracts and tinctures or combined with other plants in preparations that lower blood pressure.

● Olives are picked in November and December. Their oil is expressed cold from the ripe fruit for culinary use or for creams and liniments.

Constituents

The leaves contain secoiridoids, in particular oleuropein, which reduces blood pressure. They also contain triterpenes and flavonoids. Olive oil, obtained from the fruits, is rich in monounsaturated (oleic acid) and polyunsaturated fatty acids (linoleic and linolenic acids) as well as in vitamin E.

Medicinal uses

Due mainly to the oleuropeoside, olive leaves have several beneficial effects. They help to reduce blood pressure, dilate coronary blood vessels, regulate heart beat, lower blood sugar levels and are diuretic.

Olive leaves, often combined with hawthorn, are considered an effective treatment for mild cases of high blood pressure. Their ability to

lower blood pressure was shown by Egyptian researchers in animal studies in 2002.

The extract can also be used as a supplementary treatment for less serious forms of Type 2 (non-insulin dependent) diabetes. Spanish studies performed in 1992 showed that oleuropeoside lowered blood sugar levels in *in vitro* models of diabetes.

Olive oil is mildly laxative and, because it stimulates the secretion and elimination of bile, is used in the treatment of gallstones. It has also been used to treat stomach ulcers and to ease nervous tension.

Applied externally, olive oil softens and soothes the skin and is a component of protective sun creams and liniments to soothe burns.

Cultivation

Olive trees are grown from seeds or cuttings. They need well-drained soil and plenty of sunshine.

CAUTIONS

● To date, when used as directed or prescribed, neither olive leaf nor olive oil have any known adverse side effects.

PREPARATION AND DOSAGE

For internal use

TO TREAT mild cases of high blood pressure, mild forms of Type 2 diabetes

INFUSION Put 20 dried leaves in 300ml of water. Boil for 30 seconds and leave to infuse for 10 minutes. Strain. Drink at least 3 cups a day during meals.

CAPSULES (50mg dry extract) Take 1-2 capsules three times a day at mealtimes, with a large glass of water.

TABLETS (500mg olive leaf) Take 1 tablet a day with food.

TO TREAT gallstones.

OLIVE OIL To prevent gallstones, take 50ml in several small doses between meals. If suffering from gallstones, take 50 to 150ml to reduce pain.

For external use

TO TREAT sunburn, burns

OLIVE-OIL BASED CREAMS AND LINIMENTS Apply as directed several times a day.

IF SYMPTOMS PERSIST, CONSULT A DOCTOR

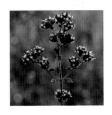

Oregano

Origanum vulgare Lamiaceae **Also called** Wild marjoram

A perennial that can reach a height of 30-80cm, oregano is common throughout Europe, particularly in dry places. Its pointed, oval leaves grow in pairs opposite each other along the woody, reddish stems. Between July and September, round clusters of pinkish crimson flowers appear at the top of the plant, offering passing bees an abundance of scented nectar. As well as having medicinal value, the aromatic plant is also a popular culinary herb.

Parts used

Aerial parts
- The best time for gathering oregano is in early July, just as the first flowers appear.
- Once picked, the aerial parts are dried and used for infusions or to extract the essential oil.

Constituents

Oregano is rich in flavonoids, and the essential oil contains thymol and carvacrol, which have both antiseptic and antispasmodic properties.

Medicinal uses

Researchers have demonstrated the ability of thymol and carvacrol in the essential oil to act against bacterial and fungal infections. For example, in 2001, American studies showed the power of the essential oil to act against the fungus *Candida albicans*, which can cause thrush. The essential oil is also beneficial in the treatment of urinary, lung and intestinal infections, and is known to have a stimulating, tonic effect.

Scientists have also demonstrated the antispasmodic powers of thymol and carvacrol, and oregano infusions are recommended for coughs and bronchitis, as well as for indigestion caused by stomach spasms.

Oregano can also be applied externally in ointments and massage oils to help ease rheumatic pain, period pain and headaches.

Cultivation

Oregano can be grown from seeds, sown in autumn. It thrives in dryish, neutral to alkaline soil with plenty of warmth and sunlight.

CAUTIONS

- In large doses oregano may cause excitability and irritability.
- Applied externally, the essential oil may cause skin irritations.
- Never ingest the essential oil, unless prescribed by a doctor or medical herbalist, as it can irritate the mucous membranes.
- Avoid oregano when pregnant, as it can stimulate the uterus.

PREPARATION AND DOSAGE

For internal use

TO TREAT abdominal wind, stomach upsets
INFUSION Put 20g of aerial parts into 1 litre of boiling water. Infuse for 10 minutes and strain. Drink 1 cup after every meal.

TO TREAT bronchitis
INFUSION (see above) Drink 3-4 cups a day.

For external use

TO TREAT rheumatic pain, headaches
MASSAGE OIL Soak 100g of aerial parts in 500ml of warmed olive oil for 30 minutes. Strain and apply three or four times a day to painful areas, including, if necessary, the forehead and temples. Otherwise apply a mix of 3 drops of essential oil to every 10ml of carrier oil.

IF SYMPTOMS PERSIST, CONSULT A DOCTOR

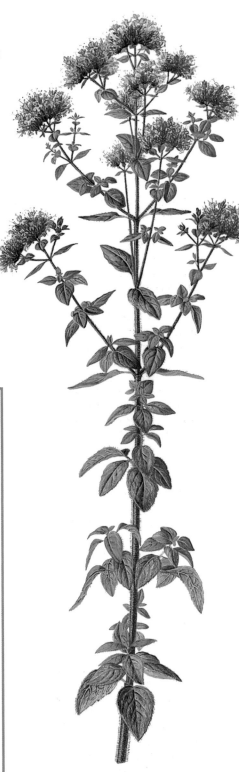

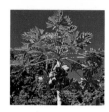

Papaya

Carica papaya Caricaceae **Also called** Pawpaw

Characterised by a tall, slender trunk crowned with a clump of leaves, the papaya tree grows in many tropical regions and can reach a height of 3-10m. The greenish male flowers are small and cluster under the leaves. The female flowers are bigger and grow singly or in groups of two or three towards the top of the trunk. The fruit, also called papaya, is a large berry, packed with orange flesh when ripe. It can have a diameter of 20-30cm and weigh as much as 5kg.

Parts used

Fruit sap

• Sap is collected from the unripe fruits when they are still on the trees by means of tap-holes.

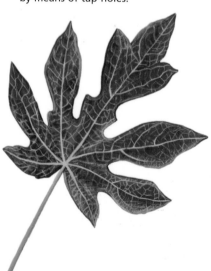

CAUTIONS

• Papaya is not recommended for pregnant or breastfeeding women.
• Papaya preparations may trigger allergies in susceptible individuals.
• Prolonged use should be avoided.
• Papainous injections may induce a fatal allergic reaction.
• Do not use papaya if you are taking anticoagulants.

• The sap, a white liquid or latex, has to be dried to preserve it and this is done outside in the sunshine.
• The dried sap is brown and smells like meat extract.
• Each fruit provides about 10g of fresh sap, which will produce up to 2g of raw dried papain in powder form. Papain is used for tablets, capsules and elixirs. It is also included in various pharmaceutical products.

Constituents

The sap contains a mixture of enzymes that are proteolytic (able to breakdown proteins). These include papain, chymopapain and papayaproteinases.

Medicinal uses

Papain kills stomach parasites as well as having a calming, soothing effect on the digestive system. Its proteolytic enzymes help stomach acids to break down proteins.

The plant is used to treat stomach and pancreatic disorders, abdominal bloating and nausea caused by migraine attacks. It is also used to treat various intestinal parasites, such as threadworms, ascaris (roundworms) and ancylostoma, as well as various blood vessel problems, such as varicose veins, ulcers and haemorrhoids. Italian studies performed in 1996 demonstrated that the sap exerted antifungal activity against *Candida albicans*, the microbe that is responsible for thrush.

Used externally, papaya acts against water retained in the tissues and is beneficial in the treatment of oedema, abscesses and wounds. Clinical studies performed in 1969

found that papaya may possess anti-inflammatory properties that would benefit patients recovering from operations or injuries.

The flowers can also be used in an infusion, which will ease coughs and soothe the throat and vocal cords.

Cultivation

Papaya can be grown from seed, planted in moist, rich soil in spring. It needs plenty of warmth and sunshine and will not tolerate frost, so must be grown under glass in a temperate climate.

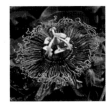

Passionflower

Passiflora incarnata Passifloracea **Also called** Maypo, Apricot vine

This climbing shrub is native to South America and can grow to 9m. It has three-lobed, indented leaves and grips on by means of tendrils. Its showy flowers grow singly and have white petals, surmounted by a crown of violet or pink filaments, and large stamens with orange-coloured sacs. This medicinal plant must not be confused with the cultivated variety that produces passion fruit.

Parts used

Leaves and stems
● The aerial parts of the plant are gathered at the end of summer.
● After drying, passionflower is used for infusions, tinctures, liquid extracts and powders.

CAUTION
● To date, no side effects have been recorded in therapeutic doses.
● Do not use if pregnant.

Constituents
In addition to a tiny percentage of maltol, passionflower contains traces of indole alkaloids and up to 2.5 per cent of various flavonoids.

Medicinal uses
Passionflower is used to treat insomnia, anxiety, muscle spasms, palpitations and digestive problems that have a nervous origin. It is a gentle remedy so is particularly suitable for use with children.
    Studies performed in 1974 suggest that maltol and ethyl maltol impart sedative effects. In addition, the flavonoids are likely to have a sedative action.

Cultivation
Plant seeds in spring, or semi-ripe cuttings in summer, in well-drained, sandy soil in a sunny location.

PREPARATION AND DOSAGE
For internal use
TO TREAT insomnia
INFUSION Put 1 teaspoon of dried plant into a cup of boiling water. Leave to infuse for 5-10 minutes and strain. Drink 1 cup at bedtime.
TINCTURE (1:8 in 25% alcohol) Take 25-75 drops a day in a glass of water.

TO TREAT vegetative dystonia, palpitations, nervous agitation
INFUSION (see above) Drink 1 cup, three times a day.
TINCTURE (1:8 in 25% alcohol) Take 25 drops in a glass of water three times a day.

IF SYMPTOMS PERSIST, CONSULT A DOCTOR

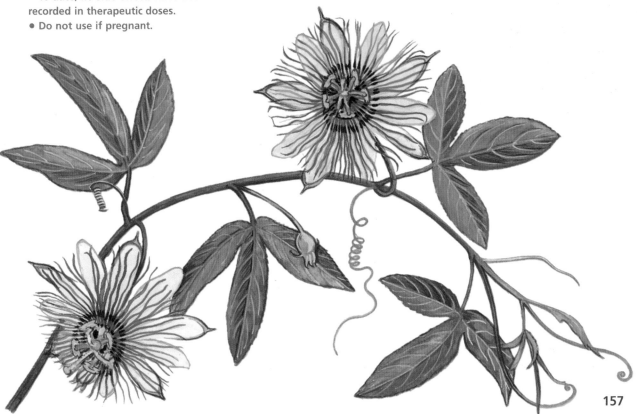

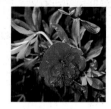

Peony

Paeonia officinalis, P. lactiflora (albiflora), P. suffruticosa Paeoniaceae

The large, showy flowers of this herbaceous perennial can be bright red, red-purple or white, and appear against the brilliant green leaves in early summer. Peony has a long history of medicinal use and takes its name from Paeon, the physician of the Greek gods. The source of the peony's medicinal properties lies in its swollen, tuberous roots. The peony has been used in Japanese and Chinese herbal medicine since ancient times, although it has long been cultivated for its ornamental qualities as well. Superstitions associated with the plant include the belief that its seeds can ward off evil spirits.

Parts used

Roots

- Harvesting of the roots takes place in October and November from plants that are four or five years old.
- The roots are dried, broken into fragments and used for infusions and decoctions.

Constituents

Chinese peony (*P. lactiflora*) contains paeoniflorin (a monoterpenic glycoside). The mountain peony (*P. suffruticosa*) contains paeonol and its glycosides, as well as suffruticosides. The common peony (*P. officinalis*) contains paeonine (an essential oil), tannins and resin.

Medicinal uses

The common peony has a sedative effect and is a remedy for nervous agitation and excitability. It acts on the sympathetic nervous system (which controls the body's involuntary activities) to relieve spasms in the smooth muscle of the gut.

By constricting the blood vessels peony has a beneficial effect on haemorrhoids and varicose veins. It can also be used to treat a lack of periods and period pains. In certain preparations, the plant can also be combined with other herbs such as Chinese anise and mugwort.

Like the common peony, the Chinese peony has a sedative, antispasmodic effect. In 2001 Chinese scientists demonstrated that paeniflorin found in Chinese peony prevented blood clot formation. The anti-inflammatory properties of this variety make it useful in treating rheumatism and other inflammatory conditions. Paeniflorin has also been used to treat eczema.

The paeonol compound found in the mountain peony kills bacteria and helps to prevent blood clots. A Taiwanese paper published in 2001 found that mountain peony exerted antiviral activity against the herpes simplex virus.

Cultivation

Plant in rich, well-drained soil in a sunny or lightly shaded location. Once established, do not move. Do not use in home preparations.

CAUTIONS

- This herb should only be taken under medical supervision.
- An overdose of the roots can cause gastroenteritis.
- Women who are pregnant or breastfeeding should avoid peony.

PREPARATION AND DOSAGE

Preparations such as decoctions, tinctures and infusions of peony can treat rheumatic, gastrointestinal and menstrual problems, and externally peony is used to soothe atopic eczema and rheumatic pains.

However, preparations should only ever be taken as prescribed by a qualified medical herbalist and with the consent of your doctor.

IF SYMPTOMS PERSIST, CONSULT A DOCTOR

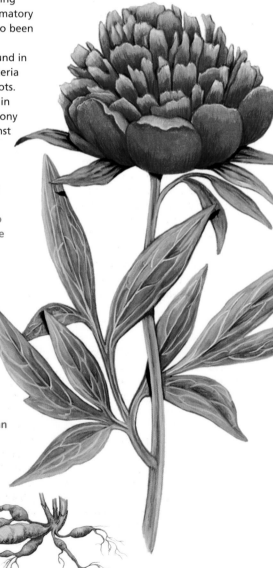

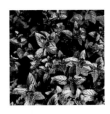

Peppermint

Mentha x. piperita Lamiaceae/Labiatae

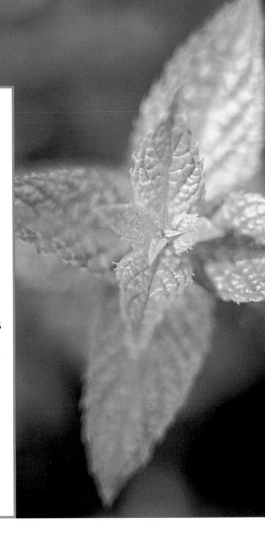

The peppermint we know today is a perennial cultivated as a cross between water mint and spearmint, it has square, purplish or crimson stems and its aromatic leaves are oval shaped but with pointed tips. The plant bears crimson whorls of flowers in late summer.

Parts used
Leaves
• The leaves are harvested when the plant is flowering in summer when they are at their most aromatic.
• Fresh or dried, the leaves are used for infusions. The essential oil is used externally.
• Peppermint has a wide variety of uses as a flavouring.

Constituents
Peppermint is rich in phenolic compounds (7 per cent), whose properties include antiviral, anti-inflammatory and antioxidant actions. It also contains generous amounts of flavonoids and tannins. The yield of essential oil is extremely high – 10-30ml a kg of the dried plant. The oil's composition varies according to the weather and when it is harvested. The oil's main constituents are menthol (30-50 per cent), menthone (15-35 per cent) and menthyl acetate (10 per cent).

Medicinal uses
Peppermint has antispasmodic, digestive properties due mainly to its essential oil and flavonoids. It is therefore taken internally to treat problems such as bloating, sluggish digestion, belching, flatulence and inadequate bile secretion.

A clinical trial performed in Taiwan in 1997 verified its carminative effect when peppermint oil was found to relieve the intestinal cramps suffered by individuals with irritable bowel syndrome (IBS). In 2001 American researchers also found it to be effective in children with IBS. In small doses it has a sedative effect and a tonic effect in large doses.

Externally the essential oil helps to soothe skin irritations and insect bites. Taken as an inhalation, it is useful in the treatment of colds and flu since the menthol component acts as a nasal decongestant. It can also be used as a mouthwash to treat oral infections and is believed to remedy headaches. Commercially, the largest use of peppermint oil is in the flavouring of chewing gum.

Cultivation
Suited to rich, moist soil. Place in a sunny or lightly shaded location.

PREPARATION AND DOSAGE
For internal use
TO TREAT bloating, sluggish digestion, belching, flatulence, inadequate bile secretion
INFUSION Put 1 dessertspoon of dried leaves into 150ml of boiling water. Leave to infuse for 10-15 minutes. Strain. Drink 1 cup after meals.
FOR A TONIC EFFECT Take 2 cups after meals.
FOR A SEDATIVE EFFECT Take 1 cup in the evening.

For external use
TO TREAT colds, oral infections
INHALATIONS, MOUTH WASHES Put a handful of leaves into a bowl of boiling hot water. Inhale the steam or cool and use as a mouthwash.

TO TREAT skin disorders
ESSENTIAL OIL Dilute, allowing 3 drops to 10ml of carrier oil. Apply to the affected area.

IF SYMPTOMS PERSIST, CONSULT A DOCTOR

CAUTIONS
• Use of the leaf, whether fresh or dried, poses no risk. However, the essential oil must be taken internally only under medical supervision.
• Do not give the essential oil to small children.
• The essential oil may exacerbate acid reflux problems.
• It is not recommended for pregnant or breastfeeding women.
• Prolonged use of the essential oil is not recommended and excessive use may cause an allergic reaction or irritate the stomach lining.

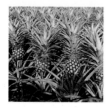

Pineapple

Ananas comosus (A. sativus) Bromeliaceae

Native to South America, the pineapple is a perennial with a large stem that can grow to 1m in height. Its fleshy, spiny leaves are shaped like spearheads. The flowers form a dense spike on the top of the stem. The fruit, topped by a crown of leaves, is made up of yellow or reddish yellow berries, which seem welded to one another.

Parts used

Ripe and unripe fruit and stem

• The best way of consuming pineapple is to eat the ripe raw fruit or to drink its juice.

• The stems are collected after the fruit is harvested.

• The fruit is also dried for use as a powder or extract in capsules.

Constituents

The fruit and the stem contain an enzyme called bromelain, which is proteolytic (it breaks down proteins). The fruit is also a source of vitamins A and C.

Medicinal uses

Bromelain is the key to pineapple medicinal uses. This enzyme breaks down proteins and also has anti-inflammatory and healing properties. It is prescribed for the treatment of swelling following injury or surgery. Research published in 1986 suggests that bromelain works by inhibiting the synthesis of inflammatory mediators as well as inhibiting platelet aggregation. Separate research performed in Germany in 1999 validates this antiplatelet activity, indicating its use in the treatment of thrombosis.

The unripe fruit stimulates the appetite and is an effective treatment for indigestion. The ripe fruit reduces stomach acidity and flatulence. The fibre content stimulates bowel movements, while the leaves are believed to be beneficial in the treatment of late or absent periods and period pain.

PREPARATION AND DOSAGE

For internal use

TO TREAT indigestion

CAPSULES (500mg powder) Take 2 capsules in the morning and 2 in the evening with water.

PURE JUICE Drink 1 glass a day.

IF SYMPTOMS PERSIST, CONSULT A DOCTOR

Cultivation

Pineapple is suited to tropical environments and grows well in heated, temperature-controlled greenhouses.

CAUTIONS

• Pineapple fruit and juice normally cause no side effects but should not be given to children under six years old, as bromelain can irritate the digestive mucous membranes.

• Excessive pineapple intake can cause stomach ache, diarrhoea and allergic reactions.

• Drinking large quantities of pineapple juice may induce uterine contractions in pregnant women.

• Pineapple should not be used while taking anticoagulants and may enhance the effects of some drugs. Check first with a medical herbalist.

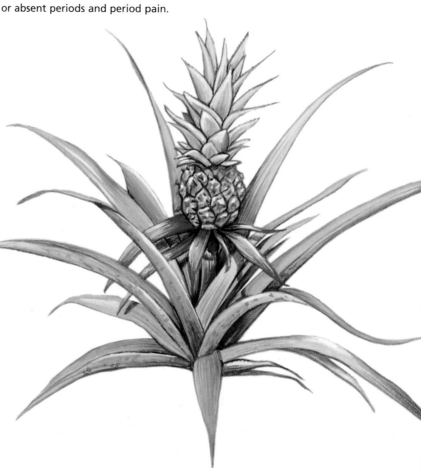

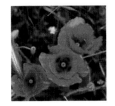

Poppy, common

Papaver rhoeas Papaveraceae **Also called** Corn poppy, Field poppy, Flanders poppy

Characterised by their blood-red, papery flowers and delicate hairy stems, poppies are annuals often seen growing wild on the edges of fields. The leaves are highly serrated and form large rosettes at the base of the flower stems. The fruit is an oval-shaped capsule enclosing hundreds of tiny black seeds.

Parts used

Petals

● After they have been carefully gathered and dried in May and June, the petals are used to make infusions and powder for capsules.
● Poppy flowers are a common ingredient in syrups.
● The flowers may be mixed with other plants that have similar qualities, such as lime, lavender and passionflower.

Constituents

Poppy petals contain mucilage, anthocyanins and a small amount of alkaloids, which constitute 0.07 per cent of the plant, the main one being rhoeadine. These exert similar but milder effects than those found in the opium poppy. The seed capsules of the plant are never used because they contain toxic alkaloids, but the seeds are used in cooking and are safe in small amounts.

Medicinal uses

The mucilage content of the petals has a soothing effect on the lining of the throat. Preparations with a base of poppy petals, often combined with blue mallow and marshmallow, provide an effective treatment for dry coughs and hoarseness.

Poppy possesses antispasmodic and sedative effects and is prescribed to treat the symptoms of nervous tension, particularly mild insomnia, in adults and children. It is also reputed to aid digestion and possesses mild analgesic qualities.

A French study performed in 2001 demonstrated the sedative effects of the plant. Analysis of the extract used showed the presence of anthocyanins but no alkaloids.

Traditionally, the common poppy has been used to treat cardiac rhythm abnormalities in adults whose hearts are otherwise healthy.

Cultivation

Suited to well-drained soil and a sunny location. Grow from seed.

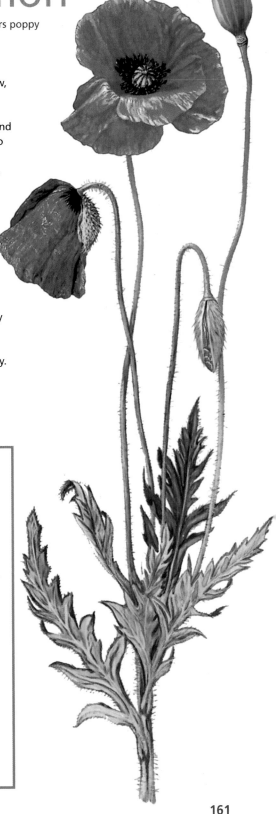

CAUTIONS

● It is best to consult a medical herbalist before taking the plant.
● Do not use in pregnancy.
● Keep out of reach of children. Cases of poisoning after ingesting poppy syrup have been recorded.

PREPARATION AND DOSAGE

For internal use

TO TREAT hoarseness, dry coughs
INFUSION Put 2 teaspoons (about 1.5g) of flowers into a cup of boiling water. Leave to infuse for 10 minutes and filter. Take 2 or 3 cups a day. Sweeten, if you wish, with honey.
TINCTURE Take 15 drops in water three times a day after meals.

TO TREAT mild insomnia
INFUSION Drink 1 cup at night before going to bed.
CAPSULES (375mg) Take 1 or 2 capsules before going to bed.
TINCTURE Dosage as above.

IF SYMPTOMS PERSIST, CONSULT A DOCTOR

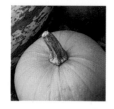

Pumpkin

Cucurbita pepo Cucurbitaceae

Grown in Central America for at least 9000 years, pumpkin is now cultivated all over the world for its enormous, globular fruit. The name pumpkin derives from 'pepon', a Greek word meaning mellow or sun ripened. A long prickly stem bears large downy leaves and deep yellow funnel-shaped flowers. These are followed by orange fruits containing numerous flat white seeds.

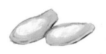

Parts used

Seeds and fruit flesh

● The flesh is eaten fresh, or dried for medicinal use.

● The seeds may be hulled and eaten whole, crushed for their oil or used in tinctures.

Constituents

The flesh is a good source of beta carotene and contains vitamin E – both cancer-fighting antioxidants. The seeds contain around 30 per cent unsaturated oil – mainly linoleic acid, and are rich in iron, phosphorus and zinc – known to benefit prostate problems and acne.

Medicinal uses

Pumpkin seed is prescribed to treat ailments of the prostate gland. In particular, the seeds' combination of high zinc content and diuretic effect makes it a good remedy for non-cancerous prostate enlargement. And a Swedish clinical trial found that a substance called curbicin, obtained from pumpkin seeds and dwarf palms, noticeably improved the symptoms of enlarged prostate.

Pumpkin seed oil is also reputed to be beneficial in ailments of the urinary system. A paper published in 1994 in the journal of Tongji Medical University describes the effectiveness of the seed oil in improving the function of the bladder and urethra.

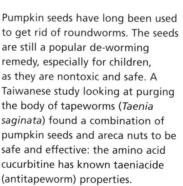

> ### PREPARATION AND DOSAGE
> **For internal use**
> **TO TREAT constipation, prostate problems, urinary problems**
> **CAPSULES** Take three 430mg pumpkin extract capsules a day.
> **TINCTURE (seed)** Take 150 drops a day in a glass of water.
>
> **TO TREAT worms**
> **SEEDS** Eat 60-100g hulled seeds a day to prevent or eliminate worms. Follow with a purgative such as castor oil.
>
> IF SYMPTOMS PERSIST, CONSULT A DOCTOR

Pumpkin seeds have long been used to get rid of roundworms. The seeds are still a popular de-worming remedy, especially for children, as they are nontoxic and safe. A Taiwanese study looking at purging the body of tapeworms (*Taenia saginata*) found a combination of pumpkin seeds and areca nuts to be safe and effective: the amino acid cucurbitine has known taeniacide (antitapeworm) properties.

Egyptian research published in 1995 found that pumpkin seed oil improved arthritic conditions, while a decoction of the seeds is used to remedy intestinal inflammation. Pumpkin flesh is high in fibre and acts as a gentle laxative. For external use, the flesh can be pulped and applied as a poultice to treat burns, while the oil is a soothing emollient.

Cultivation

Pumpkin thrives in warm and temperate climates. Grow from seed in a rich, well-drained soil and in a sunny position. Keep well watered once the fruit begins to swell.

CAUTIONS

● No adverse side effects or toxicity have been reported to date.

● Do not self-prescribe for prostate enlargement as this could be prostatic cancer: consult a doctor.

● Do not take if pregnant or breastfeeding.

● Excessive use of diuretics can lead to cramps and cardiovascular or renal problems.

● Do not exceed recommended doses of pumpkin seed: excessive intake may cause liver damage.

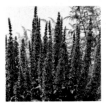

Purple loosestrife

Lythrum salicaria Lythraceae **Also called** Spiked loosestrife

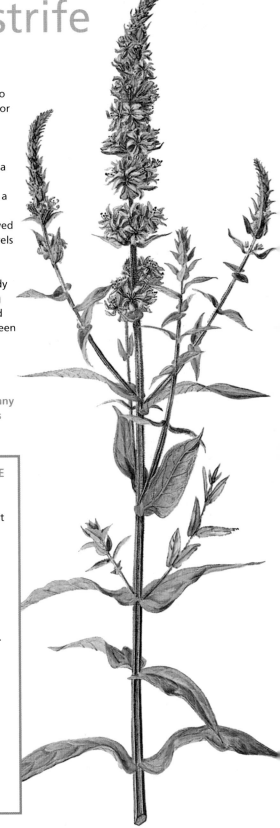

Thriving in marshy or swampy ground, purple loosestrife is a tall, handsome perennial. The plant can reach a height of 1.5m and bears striking purplish pink spikes of unscented flowers. It is popular as an ornamental border plant. It should not be confused with willow herb, which looks quite similar.

Parts used
Aerial parts
- Flowering stems are gathered in full bloom.
- Bunches are hung upside down in a well-ventilated room to dry.
- Dried stems are crumbled or powdered.
- Purple loosestrife is used for decoctions and liquid extracts.

Constituents
Purple loosestrife is rich in polyphenols, substances that are useful for treating vein disorders. These consist of flavonoids, which improve the circulation by strengthening blood vessels; anthocyanins, pigments that keep blood vessels healthy; and tannins, whose astringent qualities improve resistance to infection, are effective for treating diarrhoea.

Medicinal uses
Purple loosestrife has long been used in traditional medicine to treat diarrhoea, and externally to heal wounds, ulcers and to ease sore eyes. Today, its main use in herbal medicine is still as a treatment for diarrhoea, and it is considered suitable for infants. Experiments have demonstrated its efficacy, which has been attributed principally to its tannin content. As the plant is also antiviral, it is especially effective for viral forms of diarrhoea.

Finnish studies in 2000 found purple loosestrife to inhibit the growth of several types of bacteria as well as the *Candida albicans* fungus, which causes thrush. And a study published in the *Journal of Ethnopharmacology* in 1986 showed the herb to lower blood sugar levels in cases of hyperglycaemia.

The polyphenols in purple loosestrife make it a useful remedy for circulatory problems including haemorrhoids. It is also prescribed for heavy periods, bleeding between periods, vaginal discharge and vaginal irritation.

Cultivation
Plant in moist or wet soil in a sunny or slightly shaded location. Seeds can be sown in spring at 13-18˚C.

PREPARATION AND DOSAGE

For internal use
TO TREAT minor diarrhoea
DECOCTION Put 10g dried plant into 1 litre of water. Boil for 10 minutes and strain. Drink 2-3 cups a day.

TO TREAT loose motions in infants, minor diarrhoea in adults, circulatory problems
LIQUID EXTRACT Infants – 10-15 drops to a glass of water. Adults – 1 teaspoon in water three times a day for a maximum of two days.

For external use
TO TREAT wounds, eczema
TINCTURE & WOUND WASH Follow manufacturer's directions.

IF SYMPTOMS PERSIST, CONSULT A DOCTOR

CAUTION
- No adverse side effects or toxicity have been reported to date.

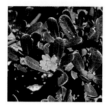

Purslane

Portulaca oleracea Portulacaceae

A small hairless, succulent with a fleshy stem and dark green, oval leaves, purslane is native to Asia but also grows in temperate regions of Africa and America. Its young shoots can be eaten raw in salads, steamed as a vegetable or cooked in soups. It was once believed that purslane spread around a bed could protect the sleeper from evil spirits.

Parts used

Aerial parts

- Purslane is harvested throughout summer.
- For medicinal use, the plant is dried and powdered or used fresh in decoctions and poultices.

Constituents

Purslane is rich in omega-3 fatty acids: 100g of fresh leaves contains 300-400mg fatty acids. The plant also contains mucilage (soothing to mucous membranes), and the antioxidant vitamins C, E and beta-carotene (the plant form of vitamin A) as well as glutathione, another antioxidant. Purslane is also rich in the minerals potassium and calcium.

Medicinal uses

Purslane is notable for its high levels of omega-3 fatty acids – substances more commonly found in fish oils. Omega-3s strengthen the immune and cardiovascular systems. Purslane is anti-inflammatory, improves blood circulation and prevents clotting in the arteries. The benefits of omega-3 fatty acids in the treatment of inflammation and autoimmune disease, including coronary heart disease, were outlined in a paper published in the *Journal of the American College of Nutrition* in 2002. The herb is prescribed for internal use to prevent cardio-vascular problems.

The plant's high concentrations of antioxidants means that it protects against cancer-causing and degenerative free radical damage – thus also slowing some of the effects of ageing. In addition, it may help to regulate blood cholesterol levels.

Purslane relaxes smooth muscle and has been shown to lower blood pressure: Scottish research published in 1993 found that the muscle relaxant properties were due to its high concentration of potassium.

The mucilage in purslane soothes gastrointestinal infections and inflammation and urinary infections. Researchers in the United Arab Emirates in 2000 found that an extract of the dried leaves and stems was both anti-inflammatory and analgesic, and further studies in 2001 confirmed these analgesic effects.

A Colombian paper in the *Journal of Ethnopharmacology* in 2002 reported purslane to be effective against worms. Purslane is also applied topically for muscle cramps.

Cultivation

Sow seeds in a sunny, well-drained position from May onwards. Purslane needs fertile soil and should not be allowed to dry out.

CAUTIONS

- Fresh, cooked purslane has caused no reported side effects.
- Overdoses of dry extract (capsules) can cause stomach upsets.

PREPARATION AND DOSAGE

For internal use

TO TREAT cardiovascular system, helping to prevent heart problems
CAPSULES (200mg) Take 2-3 capsules a day with a large glass of water.

For external use

TO TREAT muscle cramps
COMPRESSES, POULTICES Put 100g of the fresh plant into 100ml of cold water; bring to the boil and allow to simmer for 15-30 minutes. Soak a cloth and apply once or twice a day to the painful areas.

IF SYMPTOMS PERSIST, CONSULT A DOCTOR

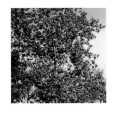

Pygeum

Pygeum africanum Rosaceae

Found across the entire continent of Africa, pygeum is a tall evergreen that thrives at altitudes of 1000m or more. The trunk can grow as wide as 1m in diameter and the leaves are thick and leathery.

Parts used

Bark

- Pygeum bark yields an extract that can be turned into tablets.
- It is also used to make infusions.

Constituents

The active constituents of pygeum bark include phytosterols such as betasitosterol that have an anti-inflammatory effect on the prostate. The pentacyclic triterpenes have decongesting properties, and substances called linear alcohols that reduce prolactin levels and block the accumulation of certain steroids in the prostate.

Medicinal uses

In the 18th century, African tribes-people showed European explorers how to treat 'old man's disease' with a tea made from powdered pygeum bark. Since then, numerous experiments have been conducted using pygeum bark extract, all of which confirm it as an effective remedy for prostate problems.

Today, pygeum is the most widely used medicine in France for treating benign prostatic enlargement – a condition that affects up to half of all men between 40 and 60, and whose symptoms can include difficulty urinating.

Recent pharmacological studies have shown that pygeum can be used to treat water retention and inflammatory swellings, increase the elasticity of the bladder, stimulate secretions from the prostate gland and modify its cells.

Studies performed in 1985 showed that pygeum's phytosterols exerted anti-inflammatory effects and reduced swelling: in particular, the constituents betasitosterol and pentacyclic triterpenoid acids are thought to be the active agents.

In 1998 clinical trials conducted at three Central European laboratories demonstrated that the plant helps in cases of excessive urination at night and reduces other symptoms resulting from an enlarged prostate.

The advantage of pygeum over other treatments for prostate problems is that it does not stimulate production of the female hormone oestrogen – which interferes with male sexual function. Taken as a preventive measure, pygeum inhibits the formation of cysts and protects the testicles and seminal sacs.

Cultivation

More suited to equatorial climates, pygeum is not a tree that could be easily cultivated in Britain.

CAUTIONS

- Do not give to children.
- Do not take if pregnant.
- Do not take if suffering from high blood pressure.
- Some individuals have reported nausea, constipation and diarrhoea.
- Do not self-prescribe for prostate problems – seek professional advice.

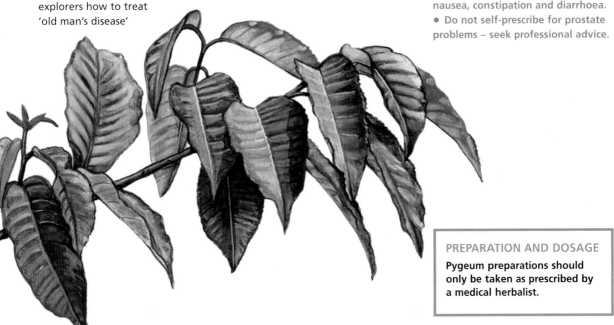

PREPARATION AND DOSAGE

Pygeum preparations should only be taken as prescribed by a medical herbalist.

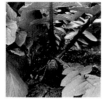

Radish, black

Raphanus sativus niger Cruciferae

This garden vegetable is a biennial that can grow to a height of 1m. The black species has a swollen taproot that is black on the outside while the inner flesh is white. Its leaves are rough to the touch, deeply lobed and serrated. The pale lilac flowers grow in clusters and are followed by short, swollen seedpods. Radish was grown by the ancient Egyptians and the Romans. The name radish derives from the Latin word 'radix', meaning root.

Parts used

Root

- The plant is pulled up in autumn when its roots contain the maximum amount of active substances.
- The roots are then used to make liquid or dry extracts.

Constituents

Radish contains an essential oil rich in sweet-smelling sulphur compounds called glucosinolates. Raphanin is also present and possesses antiseptic properties. The plant contains vitamin C, group B vitamins, minerals (calcium and arsenic) and sugars.

Medicinal uses

Radish has been used to treat disorders of the gastrointestinal tract. It promotes the secretion of bile and so can alleviate indigestion. It further stimulates intestinal contractions and can be taken to remedy constipation.

Radish may relieve abdominal distension. In 2002 Hungarian scientists fed radish to mice that had been given a high fat diet. They found that mice given radish had fewer symptoms such as bloating.

Due to the raphanin in the essential oil, radish is capable of killing bacteria and studies have also indicated antiviral activity.

PREPARATION AND DOSAGE

For internal use

TO TREAT bile flow problems, constipation

JUICE OF THE FRESH ROOTS

Drink 1 tablespoon of juice diluted in a glass of water three times a day.

CAPSULES (100mg dry extract)

Take 2 capsules in the morning before eating.

IF SYMPTOMS PERSIST, CONSULT A DOCTOR

CAUTIONS

- Do not use radish if you have gastritis, stomach ulcers, gallstones or an obstruction of the bile tract as there could be unpleasant side effects, such as irritation of the lining of the stomach, heartburn and diarrhoea.
- The sulphur compounds in radish may cause inflammation of the thyroid gland.
- Radish is not recommended for people with thyroid problems.
- Do not use radish continuously for more than a month at a time.

Radish has also been used to treat minor skin burns and irritation, such as nappy rash.

Radish is high in glucosinolates and according to a 2002 American review, the consumption of vegetables containing glucosinolates may be related to a lower incidence of cancers.

Cultivation

Grow in moist, well-drained soil in a sunny spot. Sow the seeds in spring.

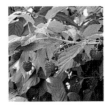

Raspberry

Rubus idaeus Rosaceae **Also called** Garden raspberry, European red raspberry

Native to both Europe and Asia, raspberry has long been grown for its sweet red berries. This deciduous biennial shrub with pale green leaves can reach a height of 2m. Clusters of white flowers appear in the second year of growth.

Parts used

Leaves and fruit
- The leaves are used in infusions, liquid extracts and tablets.
- The berries, used in decoctions, are ready from summer to early autumn.

Constituents

The leaves contain polypeptides, flavonoids and tannins including anthocyanins, while the fruit contains pectin, fruit sugars and acids, and vitamins A, B₁ and C.

Medicinal uses

A tea made from the leaves can be taken to treat diarrhoea, urinary problems, kidney stones, gallstones, and fluid retention. Traditionally the leaves have been used just before and during labour to stimulate the uterus and bring on childbirth.

External applications of the leaves are used to treat eye inflammation, skin irritations and wounds, and excessive vaginal discharge. The berries also have an astringent action which helps to heal wounds. This may be due to the anthocyanins, which American scientists showed in 2001 could inhibit enzymes involved in the body's inflammatory response.

Cultivation

Plant young plants in moist, well-drained soil, in sun or partial shade.

CAUTIONS

- Not recommended in pregnancy, except at the onset of labour.
- If using during childbirth, medical supervision is strongly recommended.
- Do not combine with drugs that lower blood sugar levels or the drug Antabuse.

PREPARATION AND DOSAGE

For internal use
TO TREAT diarrhoea, urinary infections
INFUSION Steep 1 teaspoon of dried leaves in a cup of boiling water for 10 minutes, strain and drink three times a day.
LIQUID EXTRACT Take 4-8ml in water three times a day.
TINCTURE (1:4 in 25% alcohol) Take 20 drops in water three times a day after meals.
TABLETS (raspberry leaf 900mg): Take 1 tablet twice a day with water.

For external use
TO TREAT skin ailments
COMPRESS Soak a cloth in the infusion or diluted tincture and apply to affected area.

IF SYMPTOMS PERSIST, CONSULT A DOCTOR

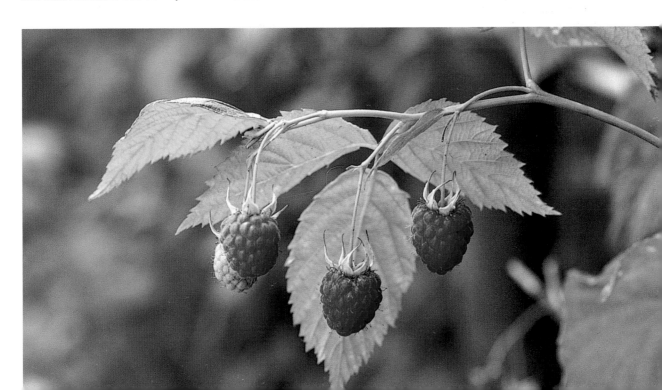

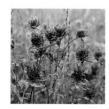

Red clover

Trifolium pratense Leguminosae/Papilionaceae **Also called** Purple clover, Wild clover, Trefoil

A short-lived perennial that grows to a height of 40cm, red clover is common throughout Europe, particularly in sandy meadowland. It has long-stalked leaves along its hairy stems, usually made up of three, pointed, oval leaflets marked with a white crescent. Its fragrant, globular, pink-purple flowers appear in late spring and summer.

Parts used
Flowerheads
- The flowerheads are picked as soon as they open, in late spring and early summer.
- The flowerheads are dried and used to prepare infusions, liquid extracts, tinctures and ointments.

Constituents
Red clover contains isoflavones that mimic the action of oestrogen. Anti-inflammatory salicylates and phenolic glycosides and saponins are also present. Another constituent is sitosterol, which research indicates may help to treat certain cancers.

Medicinal uses
Red clover is used both internally and externally for treating skin ailments, such as the inflammatory conditions eczema and psoriasis.

CAUTIONS
- Red clover should be avoided by women trying to conceive, as research on livestock has shown that it can act as a contraceptive.
- Red clover is not recommended for people with a history of tumours that are stimulated by the presence of the hormone oestrogen.
- The plant should not be taken at the same time as drugs that thin or inhibit the clotting of the blood.
- Avoid fermented clover, which can sometimes cause internal bleeding.

The plant is also known to be helpful in relieving sore throats and mouth ulcers. Recent studies have shown that this anti-inflammatory action is partly due to the isoflavones, some of which are also reputed to help ease menopausal symptoms, because of their oestrogenic effect.

The plant's anti-inflammatory action, combined with its ability to act as a diuretic and so help the body to eliminate toxins, make it useful for treating gout. In addition, the saponins act as an expectorant and the plant is prescribed for soothing spasmodic coughs.

The plant is also thought to stimulate the liver and gall bladder, helping to keep the digestive system in a healthy state.

Cultivation
Red clover can be grown from seeds, sown in spring. Plant in moist well-drained soil in a sunny spot.

PREPARATION AND DOSAGE
For internal use
TO TREAT skin ailments, gout, coughs, sluggish digestion
INFUSION Infuse 2 teaspoons of flowerheads in 1 cup of boiling water for 10 minutes. Strain. Drink 3 cups a day.
LIQUID EXTRACT (1:1 in 25% alcohol) Take 1.5-3ml a day.
TINCTURE (1:10 in 45% alcohol) Take ½-1 teaspoon a day.

For external use
TO TREAT Skin ailments, gout
COMPRESS Soak a clean cloth in the infusion (see above) and apply to affected areas.
TO TREAT Sore throats, mouth ulcers
MOUTHWASH, GARGLE Use the infusion (see above).

IF SYMPTOMS PERSIST, CONSULT A DOCTOR

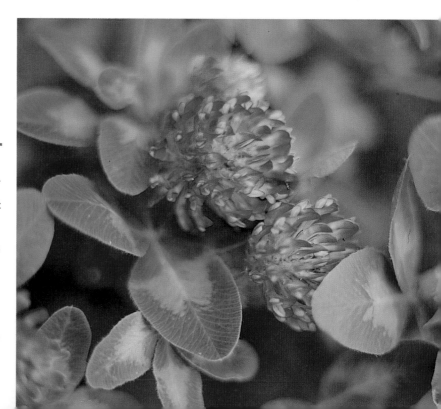

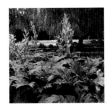

Rhubarb

Rheum palmatum Polygonaceae **Also called** Chinese rhubarb

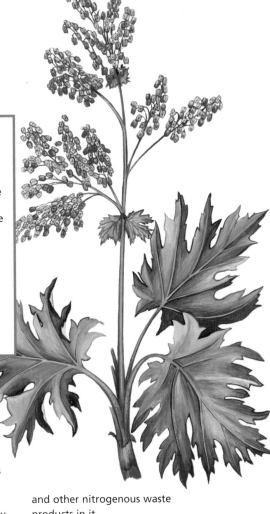

Native to north-east Asia, this species of rhubarb — unlike the more familiar garden variety — is used as a herbal remedy. A tall herbaceous plant, it has very thick, fleshy leafstalks and wide, jagged, palm-shaped leaves. Loose clusters of tiny, star-shaped, white, greenish or reddish flowers appear in July and August, followed by dry, winged fruits. Only the bulky rhizome is of medicinal value.

Parts used

Rhizome
- Although grown in Europe, the rhizome used in herbal medicine usually comes from China and Korea.
- Rhizomes of plants between six to ten years old are dug up in autumn.
- Dried rhizome is used to prepare infusions, decoctions, tinctures and powders, or is sold in fragments.

Constituents

The components in Chinese rhubarb that are responsible for its laxative action are anthracene derivatives,

mainly consisting in the dried rhizome of anthraquinone glycosides. Flavonoids and tannins are also present. The latter are thought to be responsible for the constipation sometimes induced by low doses of rhubarb.

Medicinal uses

Rhubarb is an extremely effective laxative, although very low doses have sometimes been known to cause constipation. Numerous studies have revealed how the plant stimulates the intestinal muscles and increases the absorption of water and electrolytes. However, rhubarb preparations should not be used for longer than ten consecutive days, because of the danger of developing laxative-induced illnesses, such as colitis, diarrhoea, electrolyte imbalances and hypokalemia (a reduction of potassium in the blood).

Recent studies in China have shown that rhubarb preparations can actually help to cleanse the blood by reducing excessive amounts of urea

and other nitrogenous waste products in it.

It is thought that this is due to direct action by the plant on the kidneys, which further research has revealed may also help to limit inflammation in cases of chronic renal failure.

Chinese scientists have also shown that the plant can inhibit the chain of reactions in the body that leads to the constriction of blood vessels.

Rhubarb is also used to stimulate the appetite and improve digestion, as well as to treat liver and gall-bladder problems and to soothe inflammation and oral infections.

Cultivation

Chinese rhubarb can be grown from seeds, sown in late winter, or from root cuttings planted in late autumn. It prefers moist, well-drained soil, rich in humus, and exposure to plenty of sunshine.

CAUTIONS

- Chinese rhubarb should not be taken at the same time as other laxatives, and it is advisable to combine the treatment with exercise and changes in diet.
- People suffering from an intestinal obstruction, arthritis, kidney disease or urinary problems should not use Chinese rhubarb preparations.
- The plant is not recommended as a laxative for children aged between ten and fifteen, and should never be given to children under ten.
- It is not advisable to take rhubarb when pregnant or breastfeeding.
- People with known allergies should be cautious when using Chinese rhubarb preparations in case they are sensitive to the plant.

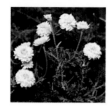

Roman chamomile

Chamaemelum nobile Asteraceae/Compositae

A small perennial, common in the dry areas of western and southern Europe, Roman chamomile has widely spreading stems that are covered in tiny jagged leaves. In summer, a single, daisy-like flower, its yellow centre surrounded by a ring of white petals, opens at the tip of each stem. The whole plant gives off a powerful, pleasant scent.

Parts used

Flowerheads

• The flowers are collected in spring, just as the buds begin to open. The harvesting is now largely mechanised but the flowers should be carefully examined to remove any insects.

• The flowers can be used fresh, but their constituents will remain active for up to a year if they are properly dried in a dark, dry place.

• Roman chamomile is mainly used for infusions and extracts and is a constituent of eye lotions, throat sprays, mouthwashes and pastilles.

Constituents

The plant contains coumarins and flavonoids, which have a digestive, antispasmodic and anti-inflammatory action, and sesquiterpene lactones, which give it its bitter taste. There is also some essential oil.

Medicinal uses

Roman chamomile has long been used to treat digestive problems, such as sluggish digestion, bloating, belching and flatulence. The bitter sesquiterpene lactones stimulate the digestive juices, and the flavonoids and coumarins have antispasmodic and anti-inflammatory powers.

Recent studies have also shown that the essential oil has the ability to ease inflammation, too, as well as having an antidiuretic and sedative effect. Because of this soothing action, it is often included in

preparations that are applied externally to treat skin ailments such as eczema, which can cause severe itching. It is also found in medicines used for treating eye irritations, sore throats, rhinitis and sinusitis, and in mouthwashes.

Some herbalists also recommend the use of the plant's soothing action for insomnia, haemorrhoids and even menstruation problems.

Cultivation

Roman chamomile can be grown from seed, rootstock or young bought plants. Plant in spring in well-drained, light soil, preferably in a warm, sunny position.

PREPARATION AND DOSAGE

For internal use

TO TREAT digestive problems
INFUSION Add 1 dessertspoon of flowerheads to a cup of boiling water, and leave to infuse for 10 minutes, then strain. Drink 3-4 cups a day.

For external use

TO TREAT eye irritations
EYE LOTION Use only commercially available sterile eye lotions. Follow directions given.

TO TREAT sore throat
THROAT SPRAY Prepare an infusion (see above). Cool. Spray the back of the throat, two or three times a day.

TO TREAT rhinitis, sinusitis
INHALATIONS Prepare an infusion (see above) two or three times a day. While it is still hot, inhale the steam rising from it.

IF SYMPTOMS PERSIST, CONSULT A DOCTOR

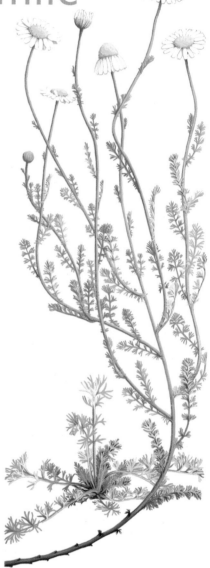

CAUTIONS

• Roman chamomile should not be taken when pregnant.

• It is not advisable to use Roman chamomile when breastfeeding.

• Do not use this plant if you are taking anticoagulants.

• Asthma sufferers and individuals with a history of allergies to related plants, such as marigold and arnica, may also have an adverse reaction to Roman chamomile preparations, so should avoid them.

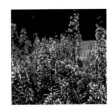

Rose bay willow-herb

Epilobium parviflorum, E.angustifolium Onagraceae

Among the ten or so varieties of rose bay willow-herb that grow in Europe, only two are used for their medicinal properties. One of these is Epilobium parviflorum, *a small plant with tiny, pale pink flowers and hairy, spear-shaped leaves.* E. angustifolium, *the other variety, is a tall, handsome plant, with stems that are covered in long, smooth, narrow leaves and crowned by a spike of striking, pink-purple flowers in summer. Both varieties can be found in woodland or hilly areas, and on wasteground.*

Parts used
Flowers and leaves
• The leaves and flowers are picked in September, at the end of the flowering season.
• They are dried, and then used in infusions, powders and tinctures.

Constituents
The beneficial effects of rose bay willow-herb stem largely from the flavonoids and tannins. The major flavonoid in *E. parviflorum* is myricitroside; the main one in *E. angustifolium* is quercetol-gluceronide. Both plants also contain betasitosterol and gallic acid. The tannins – oenotheines A and B – are present in both their flowers.

Medicinal uses
Rose bay willow-herb is noted for its ability to reduce inflammation – largely as a result of its flavonoids and tannins. It is often prescribed to relieve the symptoms of benign prostate enlargement, although it is essential to have a thorough medical examination before using the plant for this purpose, to ensure that the swelling really is benign. There is also some debate over choosing which variety of the plant is best to prescribe for this condition. While *E. angustifolium* is known to contain highly active inflammation-reducing tannins, those in *E. parviflorum* appear to be especially successful in treating an enlarged prostate gland.

The plant's soothing powers have also been employed to treat irritable bowel syndrome, diarrhoea, sore throats, mouth ulcers and skin irritations such as eczema. The leaves are known to improve urinary flow and are beneficial in the treatment of cystitis and an irritable bladder.

Cultivation
Rose bay willow-herb is a common weed, and is therefore not usually cultivated, but simply gathered from the wild. Occasionally, gardeners plant *E. angustifolium* for its decorative value.

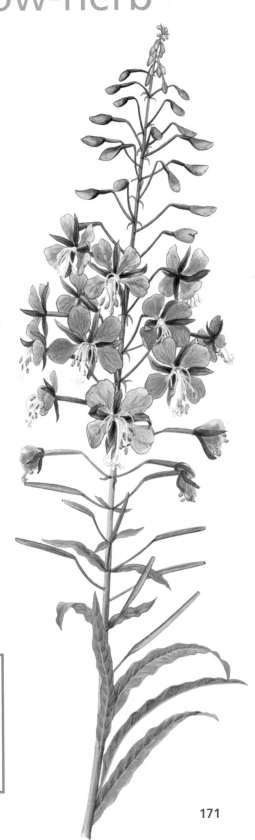

CAUTION
• Although no adverse side effects have been noted when using rose bay willow-herb preparations, the plant should only be used under close medical supervision.

> ### PREPARATION AND DOSAGE
> **It is not advisable to use any preparation made with rose bay willow-herb, from simple infusions to more complex commercial products, unless they have been prescribed by a a doctor or medical herbalist.**

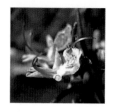

Rosemary

Rosmarinus officinalis Lamiaceae

From medieval times rosemary – a symbol of love and fidelity – was often worn in bridal wreaths and given to wedding guests. Rosemary is a bushy, aromatic evergreen shrub found all over the Mediterranean. Spikes of pale blue or lilac flowers bloom in May and June. They yield an essential oil that is one of the ingredients of eau de cologne.

Parts used

Flowers and leaves

- The flowers are gathered in full bloom and then dried.
- The evergreen leaves can be collected at any time of year.
- The leaves are scalded and dried.
- Rosemary is used in infusions, tinctures and as an essential oil.

Constituents

Rosemary contains many active constituents. Its flavonoids are stimulant and antioxidant; its phenols – in particular rosmarinic acid – are antiseptic and reduce inflammation; its astringent tannins fight infection; and rosmaricine has been shown to have stimulant and analgesic properties. The volatile oil has a sharp, stimulating fragrance and several active compounds including cineole and camphor.

Medicinal uses

The flavonoids in rosemary stimulate the circulation by strengthening the capillaries and improving venous blood flow – benefits that justify rosemary's traditional medicinal

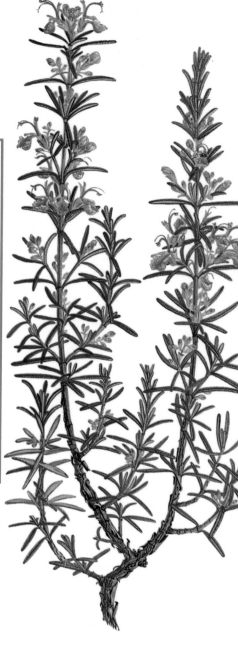

application for improving memory and concentration, easing headaches and stimulating hair growth.

The herb also calms the digestion, and is prescribed for gut problems such as dyspepsia, stomach cramps, bloating and constipation.

Animal studies conducted in 1987 found that an extract of rosemary increased the flow of bile, important in the digestion of fats. And research published in 1995 found the plant to be diuretic and to have a detoxifying effect on the liver.

Rosemary is an effective anti-inflammatory. It has expectorant and antibacterial properties and can be used to treat bronchial, ear, nose and throat infections. It is also a good tonic for people suffering from general fatigue.

Externally, rosemary oil is diluted in a neutral oil, such as sunflower oil, and used as a rub to ease muscular pain, sciatica and rheumatic pain and inflammation. An infusion added to bath water is said to help to ease rheumatism. Rosemary extract also stimulates hair follicles and scalp circulation, and is applied to the head as a preventive against premature baldness. Its antiseptic and astringent actions make it useful for treating dandruff.

Cultivation

Rosemary is easily grown from cuttings. Once rooted, plant in a warm sheltered spot, ideally in well-drained sandy soil.

> ## PREPARATION AND DOSAGE
>
> ### For internal use
>
> **TO TREAT dyspepsia, stomach cramps, bloating, constipation, and bronchial and ear, nose and throat infections**
> INFUSION Put 2-4g of dried plant into 1 cup of boiling water, cover and leave to infuse for 10 minutes. Drink 3 cups a day after meals.
>
> ### For external use
>
> **TO TREAT rheumatism**
> INFUSION Put 50g of herb into a litre of boiling water. Cover and leave to infuse for 30 minutes and add to the bath water.
> ESSENTIAL OIL Dilute, allowing 3 drops to 10ml of carrier oil. Rub on painful joints.
>
> IF SYMPTOMS PERSIST, CONSULT A DOCTOR

CAUTIONS

- Do not take the essential oil by mouth.
- Do not give to children.
- If pregnant or breastfeeding, do not consume more than would be found in the diet.

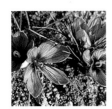

Saffron

Crocus sativus Iridaceae **Also called** Autumn crocus, Saffron crocus

A native of India and the eastern Mediterranean, saffron was brought to England in the Middle Ages and was cultivated around Saffron Walden near Cambridge, hence the town's name. Today, most saffron is imported. It takes around 75,000 flowers, harvested by hand, to obtain 500g of saffron. This makes saffron very expensive. Its name comes from zafaran, the Arabic word for yellow.

Parts used
Stigmas
- Stigmas are gathered in autumn when the flowers are in full bloom.
- They are grasped between thumb and index finger and detached – a delicate and time-consuming job.
- After drying, they are used whole as flavouring, or powdered.
- Extracts are made into tinctures, syrups and gels for medicinal use.
- Saffron should be used within a year of picking.

Constituents
Saffron contains a bitter substance called picrocrocin, which stimulates the appetite and aids digestion. The plant's essential oil is rich in safranal, a compound that gives saffron its characteristic aroma, and which could be responsible for the plant's sedative effect. The stigmas contain yellow and red carotenoid pigments – crocin and gentiobiose – that have antioxidant properties.

Medicinal uses
Saffron has been used as a kitchen herb for centuries, both for its bright orange-yellow colour and for its strong, intense flavour and aroma. The ancient Greeks, Egyptians and Romans valued saffron for its aphrodisiac properties. However, the high cost of this spice means that it is rarely used as a natural medicine.

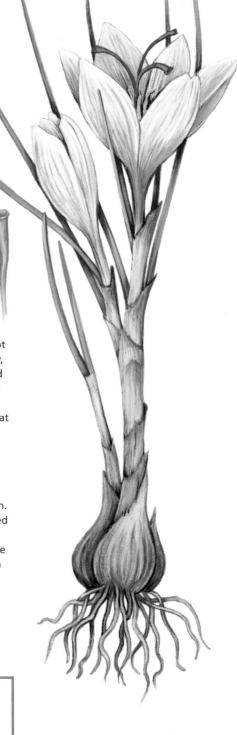

Saffron was traditionally used to treat teething pain in infants. It is thought to regulate menstruation, and aid conception; it is also reputed to remedy colic and lower blood pressure. Saffron is prescribed for nervousness as it is believed to be a sedative. This attribute has not yet been confirmed experimentally, but research in Iran, in 2002, found extracts of saffron to be both anti-inflammatory and analgesic.

Researchers have been looking at the cancer-fighting antioxidant action of saffron. In 1996 Spanish scientists found that saffron inhibited the growth of human tumour cells, a property that they attributed to the carotenoid, crocin. And in 1999, further studies showed that crocin suppressed the development of colon cancer. These findings could open up a new area of medicinal use for the plant.

Cultivation
Plant the corms in summer in a well-drained soil. Saffron likes full sun and a warm environment.

PREPARATION AND DOSAGE
For internal use
TO TREAT menstrual disorders
TINCTURE (1:5 in 60% alcohol) Take 5-15 drops in water three times a day.

IF SYMPTOMS PERSIST, CONSULT A DOCTOR

CAUTIONS
- Large doses of saffron are poisonous and can damage the kidneys and central nervous system.
- Do not use when pregnant or breastfeeding.

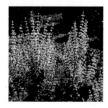

Sage and clary sage

Salvia officinalis and *S. sclarea* Lamiaceae

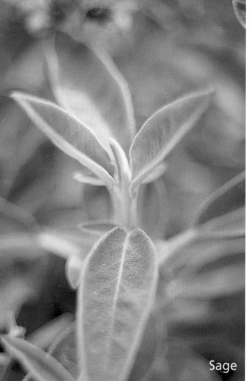

Sage

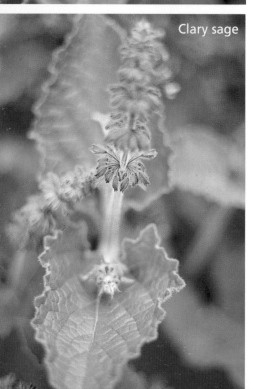

Clary sage

Native to the Mediterranean, common sage is a woody aromatic shrub. Its small grey-green leaves are thick and downy. Clary sage looks different, having much larger leaves, but has similar medicinal properties. German wine merchants used to add extracts of clary sage to Rhine wines to improve their aroma, and its essential oil is used in perfume manufacture.

Parts used

Leaves

- The leaves are collected in summer before flowers appear, or in autumn.
- They are dried under cover and away from daylight.
- Both forms of sage yield an aromatic essential oil.
- Sage is used for infusions, decoctions, liquid extracts and tinctures. Powdered sage is available in capsule form.

Constituents

Common sage leaves contain flavonoids – antioxidants that improve the circulation, phenols such as caffeic and rosmarinic acid, and tannins which have antimicrobial and anti-inflammatory properties.

The main constituents of common sage essential oil are substances called thujones, along with terpenes, cineole and camphor. Clary sage oil has a scent similar to ambergris and contains linalyl acetate and linalool.

CAUTIONS

- Sage leaves should not be used over a long period of time.
- Do not take sage essential oil internally.
- Do not give to children.
- Avoid sage if pregnant or breastfeeding.
- Sage may interfere with hypogly-caemic and anticonvulsant therapy.

Medicinal uses

Sage suppresses sweat secretion and is especially useful for reducing night sweats, hot flushes and other symptoms of menopause. Common sage and clary sage are prescribed for digestive ailments such as indigestion and bloating. Sage is also a tonic, helping to combat fatigue, especially after illness.

In vivo tests published in *Planta Medica* in 1988 found sage oil to be antispasmodic. It may, therefore, prove to be beneficial for period pains and stomach cramps. And researchers at Middlesex University and at King's College, London are studying the possible benefits of sage for treating Alzheimer's disease.

Used externally, a strong infusion of the fresh herb makes a soothing antiseptic mouthwash and gargle.

Cultivation

Sage is easily grown from cuttings. Plant in full sun in a well-drained, neutral to alkaline soil.

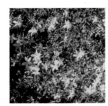

St John's wort

Hypericum perforatum Hypericaceae/Guttiferae

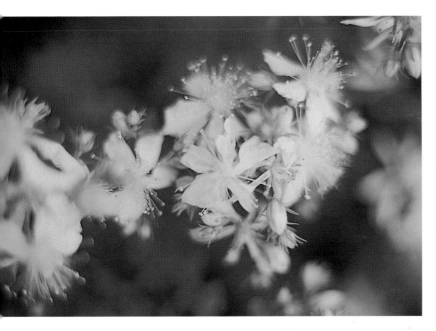

The scent of St John's wort was thought by the ancient Greeks to ward off evil spirits. The plant grows wild throughout Europe, thriving in woods, hedgerows, roadsides and meadows. Its bright yellow flowers bloom from June to September. St John's wort has been used as a remedy for nervous disorders for more than 2000 years.

Parts used

Flowering tops
● Flowers are gathered in summer and dried in bunches.
● There are many similar-looking plants; St John's wort is distinguished by black spots on its flower petals and translucent spots on its leaves.
● St John's wort is used in infusions, tinctures and as a liquid extract.

Constituents

The yellow flowers of St John's wort yield a deep red oil – the colour comes from hypericin, a red pigment believed to be one of the substances responsible for the plant's medicinal effects in addition to hyperforin. The plant also contains flavonoids and tannins.

Medicinal uses

Because of its wound-healing properties, St John's wort has traditionally been used to treat burns and skin irritations. However, it has also been shown to have a positive effect on less serious cases of depression and today is now widely prescribed in Europe as a mild antidepressant.

Recently, the plant's mood-lifting properties have attracted great attention, and extensive clinical trials have been carried out to enable this use to be officially recognised. The mechanism by which the plant exerts its antidepressant action, however, remains unclear.

In vitro studies in 1984 suggested that hypericin acted in a similar way to monoamine oxidase inhibitor antidepressants (commonly known as MOAIs). And German research published in 1998 documents the antidepressant activity of hyperforin in the plant, which appears to have a beneficial effect on serotonin activity in the brain.

St John's wort is also prescribed for depressive symptoms including nervous fatigue, negativity and sleeping difficulties.

Externally, St John's wort is recommended for minor burns and scalds and to ease neuralgia, sciatica and other painful inflammations.

Cultivation

St John's wort is a perennial weed. Once established, it is hard to get rid of. Plant seeds in a well-drained soil. in a sunny or lightly shaded location.

CAUTIONS

● Avoid sunbathing as external use may cause photosensitivity.
● Taken internally, the plant may react with certain drugs including: oral contraceptives, theophylline, digoxin, antidepressants, and protease inhibitors used in HIV therapy. Check with your doctor if you are taking any medicines.
● Do not take if pregnant or breastfeeding.

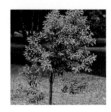

Sandalwood

Santalum album Santalaceae

A small tree grown mainly in India, sandalwood is the source of a valuable oil used in perfumes, soaps and incenses. Sandalwood oil has long been used to scent and purify the air in the home and in places of worship: when burned as joss sticks or in an oil burner it releases a sweet, soothing aroma. The wood itself is prized for woodcarving.

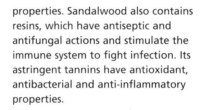

Parts used

Heart of the trunk
• The heartwood is yellowish and has a subtle scent.
• It can be gathered at any time of year but is at its best in summer.
• Powdered sandalwood is used in the perfume industry and to make capsules, infusions, decoctions and extracts for use in aromatherapy.
• Its essential oil is an ingredient in many creams and balms.

Constituents

Sandalwood contains a pigment called santalene, which is the source of its red colour. Its essential oil is rich in terpenes – specifically santalol – which give it its pleasing aroma and are thought to have sedative properties. Sandalwood also contains resins, which have antiseptic and antifungal actions and stimulate the immune system to fight infection. Its astringent tannins have antioxidant, antibacterial and anti-inflammatory properties.

Medicinal uses

Sandalwood's essential oil was used for a long time as a cure for gonorrhoea, cystitis and other urinary infections. It was also prescribed for skin diseases and acne. Traditional Chinese practitioners use sandalwood oil as a sedative.

Today, antibiotics are used to treat most genitourinary infections. However, modern herbalists still prescribe sandalwood as a diuretic, to combat water retention and oedema (swelling) in the lower legs.

And Chinese practitioners use it as a painkiller for gum pain, toothache, gastric problems and migraines.

Japanese studies published in 2000 found that the terpene, santalol, had analgesic effects on rats. It is believed to relieve abdominal pain and chest pain.

The scent of sandalwood is reputed to calm the mind, and it is often used in Buddhist monasteries as an aid to meditation; it is used for the same purpose in some British monastic communities.

Sandalwood may have cancer-fighting properties: American research carried out in 1997 suggested that the oil slows down the development of skin tumours. It also inhibits the proliferation of viruses: an *in vitro* study conducted in Argentina in 1999 showed that sandalwood oil acted against the herpes viruses responsible for genital herpes and coldsores.

Cultivation

Sandalwood, rarely cultivated outside the tropics, is parasitic and needs a host tree nearby for its roots to suck on. It likes light shade and moist, well-drained, fertile soil.

PREPARATION AND DOSAGE

For external use

TO TREAT abdominal and chest pains
ESSENTIAL OIL Dilute, allowing 3 drops to 10ml of carrier oil. Massage into affected areas.

TO TREAT skin infections
ESSENTIAL OIL Dilute a few drops in 180ml of water and apply to the affected area three times a day.

IF SYMPTOMS PERSIST, CONSULT A DOCTOR

CAUTIONS
• Do not take sandalwood essential oil internally unless advised to do so by a medical herbalist or doctor, and then for no longer than six weeks.
• Internal use is not recommended for people with kidney disorders, for for children, or for pregnant or breastfeeding women.

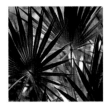

Saw palmetto

Serenoa repens Palmae **Also called** Shrub palmetto

A small, palm-like plant, saw palmetto is native to North America. Native American Indians and early American settlers used the berries to treat genitourinary problems. Its therapeutic effect on the neck of the bladder and the prostate in men was so effective that it became known as the 'plant catheter'. Its fruit is an oval, fleshy purplish black berry.

Parts used
Berries
● Berries are gathered in autumn when they ripen.
● They are used in tinctures and various pharmaceutical products.

Constituents
The active constituents of saw palmetto are a volatile oil, steroidal saponins, tannins, flavonoids, fatty acids and polysaccharides. The plant is a tonic, and is one of the few herbal remedies considered to be anabolic – which means that it strengthens and builds body tissues.

Medicinal uses
Saw palmetto extract is prescribed for benign enlargement of the prostate gland in men, as long as the growth is not large enough to need surgery. In 1996 French scientists demonstrated saw palmetto's effectiveness in reducing benign prostate enlargement. It works by preventing testosterone from being converted into dihydrotestosterone, the hormone thought to cause prostate cells to multiply, leading to an enlarged prostate gland.

In clinical trials conducted over the past 20 years, men taking saw palmetto felt less urgency and got up less often at night to urinate, or had greater urine flow. Research suggests that, while the conventional prescription drug finasteride is better at increasing the rate of urine flow and shrinking the prostate, saw palmetto causes fewer problems with sex drive and performance.

The herb stimulates the appetite and improves digestion, making it a useful supplement for convalescents. Saw palmetto has hormonal effects, and women have used it to stimulate breast enlargement and lactation. It has also been prescribed for reduced sex drive and impotence.

Cultivation
Saw palmetto does not tolerate temperatures below 10°C. Grow in a heated greenhouse or indoors.

PREPARATION AND DOSAGE
For internal use
TO TREAT benign enlargement of the prostate
TINCTURE (1:5 in 75% alcohol)
Take 10-20 drops in water two or three times a day.

IF SYMPTOMS PERSIST, CONSULT A DOCTOR

CAUTIONS
● No adverse side effects have been recorded to date.
● Saw palmetto has hormonal effects and may interfere with oral contraceptives and hormone replacement therapy.
● Do not take if pregnant or breastfeeding.
● Do not use if you are taking prescribed prostate drugs or any anticoagulants.

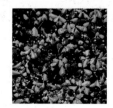

Schisandra

Schisandra chinensis Schisandraceae **Also called** Chinese magnolia vine

Native to north-east China, schisandra is a woody climbing plant. Fragrant pink flowers are followed by small red berries, known in Chinese herbal medicine as 'fruit with five flavours'. These flavours correspond to major human organs: sour to liver, bitter to heart, sweet to spleen, pungent to lungs and salty to the kidneys.

Parts used
Berries
- Berries are gathered when they ripen in autumn.
- They are dried and used to make powders, dry extracts and tinctures.

Constituents
Schisandra contains essential oils, phenols and lignans. The active components are all lignan derivatives. Lignans are thought to help to protect against prostate, colon and breast cancers.

Medicinal uses
Schisandra was traditionally valued by Chinese women as a youth tonic. Recent research suggests that the berries may have important protective effects against certain forms of cancer, and have a healing and cleansing action on the liver.

Scientists are focusing on the actions of lignans. Lignans are often thought of simply as a type of fibre, but they are also phytoestrogens – plant compounds with oestrogen-like activity and cancer-fighting properties. In 1992 Japanese scientists showed that a lignan isolated from schisandra protected against inflammation and chemically induced tumour development.

Schisandra has been shown to promote liver regeneration and detoxification. And in 2002 Chinese scientists found that schisandra protects against the oxidation of lipids in the liver. The Chinese researchers also observed that the extract enhanced concentration and may be helpful in improving memory. In addition, it strengthens and quickens reflexes and increases efficiency in stress-related tests.

It has an overall protective effect on the body's cells and muscles and can help to lower blood cholesterol.

Cultivation
If you want berries, you will need male and female plants. Schisandra does best in rich, well-drained, moist soil, ideally with its roots in the shade and its top in the sun.

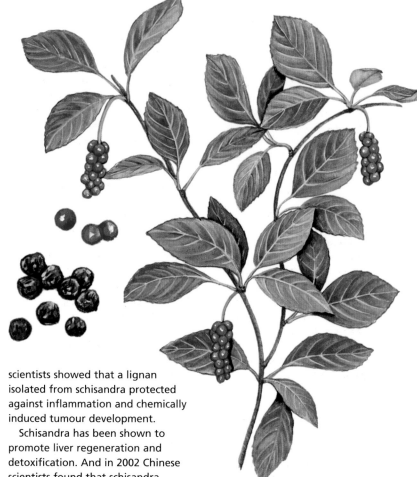

CAUTIONS
- No adverse side effects or toxicity have been recorded to date.
- However, as the plant treats serious illnesses, it is advisable to consult a doctor or medical herbalist.
- Do not use during pregnancy.

PREPARATION AND DOSAGE
For internal use
TO TREAT high blood cholesterol levels
TO PROTECT cells and muscles
POWDER Take 3-9g a day, divided into three smaller doses.
DRY EXTRACT Take 1-3g a day, divided into three or six smaller doses.
TINCTURE Put 20-40 drops into a glass of water. Take this dose three times a day.

IF SYMPTOMS PERSIST, CONSULT A DOCTOR

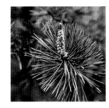

Scots pine

Pinus sylvestris Pinaceae

Native to the mountainous regions of Europe and north and west Asia, Scots pine can reach a height of 30m or more. In the Highlands, the trees were once used as dramatic markers for the burial places of warriors, heroes and chieftains. Druids used to light large bonfires of Scots pine at the winter solstice to celebrate the passing of the seasons and to draw back the sun.

Parts used

Cones, resin and needles

- Cone buds are picked in spring.
- The essential oil is extracted or the buds are dried.
- The needles are the source of essential oils used in disinfectants.
- The resin, collected from cuts in the trunk, is distilled and provides turpentine oil for ointments and liniments.
- Scots pine extracts are used in many pharmaceutical products.

Constituents

Scots pine buds contain an essential oil rich in pinene, limonene and resin. Pine needle oil is distilled from the fresh needles and branch tips. The needles also contain flavonoids and a small amount of vitamin C. Scots pine resin is rich in terpenes, which give it its aroma.

Medicinal uses

Pine has long been recognised as a powerful bronchial disinfectant. According to Egyptian papyruses, physicians treating the pharaohs used to prescribe pine resin for pneumonia and lung problems. It has a soothing effect on mucous membranes making it a good inhalant for respiratory problems.

Scots pine has antiseptic, diuretic and antirheumatic properties. It exerts a decongestant effect on the upper respiratory tract and is prescribed for chronic (long-term) bronchitis, coughs and laryngitis.

Its powerful antiseptic action helps to eliminate respiratory and urinary tract infections. Finnish studies performed in 2000 found Scots pine to be effective against several species of bacteria as well as *Candida albicans*, the fungus responsible for causing thrush.

Externally, turpentine oil rubbed into the skin stimulates circulation in the peripheral blood vessels, which helps to remove toxins and supply vital nutrients to the cells.

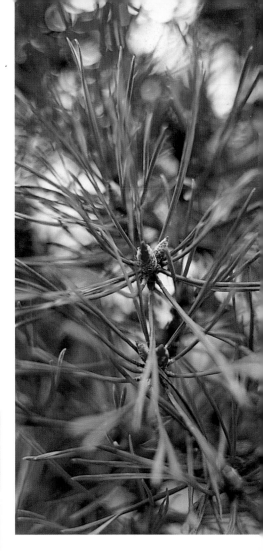

PREPARATION AND DOSAGE

For internal use

TO TREAT bronchitis, coughs
INFUSION Put 20g of buds into 1 litre of boiling water. Infuse for 10 minutes and strain. Drink 4-5 cups a day.

For external use

TO TREAT laryngitis
INFUSION (see above) Use as a gargle four or five times a day.

TO TREAT colds, chills
INFUSION (see above) Inhale the steam from an infusion three or four times a day.
BATH Put 250g of dried pine needles into a fabric bag into a warm bath. Or put about 250g of pine needles into 2 litres of boiling water and let them infuse for 20 minutes. Strain and add to a warm bath.

TO TREAT rheumatic pains
OINTMENTS, LINIMENTS Apply several times a day as directed.
ESSENTIAL OIL Dilute, allowing 3 drops of essential oil to 10ml of carrier oil, and massage into affected areas.

IF SYMPTOMS PERSIST, CONSULT A DOCTOR

Pine needle oil is used in vapour rubs that are recommended as a supplementary treatment for colds and chills. Drops of the essential oil added to boiling water make a refreshing decongesting steam vapour for blocked nose or sinuses.

Cultivation

The Scots pine grows very tall and can quickly dominate a small garden. It likes any well-drained soil and prefers a sunny location.

CAUTIONS

- No adverse side effects from the use of Scots pine buds have been recorded to date.
- Do not use essential oils internally without professional advice.
- Do not use external applications if you are prone to skin allergies.

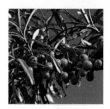

Sea buckthorn

Hippophae rhamnoides Elaeagnaceae

A deciduous, thorny shrub that can reach a height of 5m, sea buckthorn grows on dry, sunny slopes all over Europe, but mainly beside fast-flowing streams in the Alps, along the Rhine and on Scandinavian coasts. It is sometimes planted to bind soils together and to help to prevent soil erosion, especially in coastal areas. It has long been important in Tibetan medicine and is used traditionally in China, Mongolia and Russia. Sea buckthorn has long, narrow silvery leaves that are similar to those of the willow. Small, yellow-green flowers appear before the leaves in spring and are followed by orange berries on the female plants.

Parts used

Berries

● The berries are rich in vitamin C and have a very high oil content.
● When pressed, the berries produce a juice that can be drunk just as it is or made into a syrup.
● The oil is used in cosmetics.

Constituents

The amount of vitamin C contained in the pulp is high: 200-600mg per 100g (ten times the amount present in lemons). The pulp is also a source of flavonoids, betacarotene, vitamin E and a small quantity of oily substances, mainly saturated fatty acids including palmitic acid (known for its benefits to the skin), and also monounsaturates.

The seeds possess oil rich in polyunsaturated fatty acids (mainly linoleic and alpha-linoleic acids).

CAUTION
● Avoid if taking anticoagulants.
● Avoid taking sea buckthorn juice or syrup at the end of the day as it can have a stimulating effect.

Medicinal uses

Sea buckthorn juice is a natural source of vitamins, particularly vitamin C; three dessertspoons of the juice provide an adult's daily needs. Vitamin C promotes resistance to infection, and is especially recommended for exhaustion and during convalescence. Pregnant women, sportsmen and smokers are also advised to take it. Vitamin C also facilitates the synthesis of collagen (necessary for healthy skin) and helps the body to absorb iron.

Vitamin C is an antioxidant and together with other antioxidants found in sea buckthorn berries (vitamin E, carotene and flavonoids) it helps to defend the body from free radicals. Indian research published in the *Journal of Ethnopharmacology* in 2002 verified this activity, showing that leaf and fruit extracts of sea buckthorn inhibited the generation of free radicals *in vitro*.

Finally, the oil is valuable for treating dry skin and it also helps to heal cuts and wounds. It calms skin irritations and cures infections. In 2002 Chinese researchers found that sea buckthorn's seed and pulp oil demonstrated both preventative and curative effects against gastric ulcers induced experimentally in rats.

Cultivation

Sea buckthorn can be grown from young plants or seeds sown in autumn. It thrives in well-drained, sandy soil with plenty of sunshine.

PREPARATION AND DOSAGE

For internal use
TO TREAT exhaustion, lack of vitality
PURE JUICE OR SYRUP Drink 1-3 dessertspoons a day in a glass of water.

For external use
TO TREAT dry skin, cuts and wounds
SEED OR PULP OIL Apply the oil, or a preparation with a base of the oil to the affected area once or twice a day.

IF SYMPTOMS PERSIST, CONSULT A DOCTOR

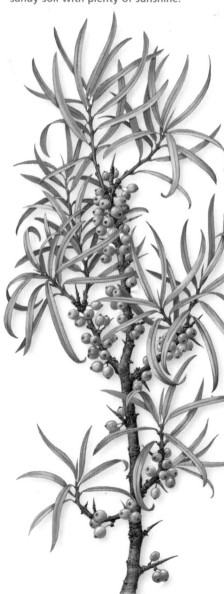

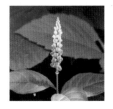

Senega snakeroot

Polygala senega Polygalaceae **Also called** Rattlesnake root

The herb is made up of several 20-30cm high stems, rising from a root that widens into a knotty crown. Senega snakeroot owes its name to a tribe of Native American Indians, the Senecas, who used it to treat snakebites and other poisons. The erect stems bear lance-shaped leaves and spikes of white flowers. The fruit is a papery capsule.

Parts used
Root
• In autumn the plant is pulled out of the ground.
• The root is separated from the plant, then dried before being used for decoctions, infusions, tinctures, liquid extracts and powders. It is also an ingredient in syrups.

Constituents
The plant has an abundance of triterpenoid saponins, which are derivatives of presenegin. These are thought to be helpful in expelling phlegm. It also contains methyl salicylate, phenolic acids and lipids.

Medicinal uses
Because of the properties of its saponins, senega snakeroot is well known as an expectorant. It is prescribed for coughs and bronchitis and is given as a syrup to children with wet, phlegmy coughs.

Senega snakeroot is also used to treat mild constipation, and has a diuretic action. It also encourages perspiration. In 1996, Japanese scientists demonstrated that the roots lower blood sugar levels without altering insulin levels. In the same year another Japanese research group found that senega snakeroot lowered the levels of both cholesterol and triglycerides in the blood of normal, cholesterol-fed and hyperlipidemic mice.

This plant is also indicated in the treatment of ailments with an inflammatory component such as eczema, psoriasis, snakebites and sore throats.

Cultivation
Senega snakeroot can be grown from seeds. They should be planted in autumn, in moist, well-drained soil, in either a sunny or lightly shaded location.

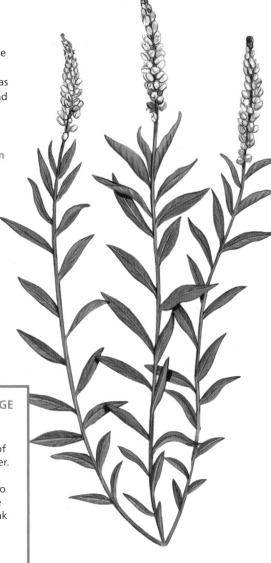

PREPARATION AND DOSAGE
For internal use
TO TREAT coughs, bronchitis
DECOCTION Put 1 teaspoon of dried root into 750ml of water. Drink 2-3 cups a day.
INFUSION Put 10g of root into 1 litre of boiling water. Leave to infuse for 10 minutes. Drink 3-4 cups a day.
CAPSULES (40mg) Take 3-6 capsules a day.
TINCTURE Put 30-40 drops into a glass of water. Take three to six times a day.
LIQUID EXTRACT Take 20 drops two to four times a day.

TO TREAT mild constipation, wet, phlegmy coughs in children
SYRUP Administer 3-4 teaspoons a day.

IF SYMPTOMS PERSIST, CONSULT A DOCTOR

CAUTIONS
• Do not use during pregnancy.
• Very occasionally, and only as a result of excessive or prolonged use, senega snakeroot may cause nausea.
• Excessive use of the plant can also result in diarrhoea.
• Senega snakeroot should not be taken by people with gastritis or a gastric ulcer.
• The root can be used fresh, but it may irritate the mouth.

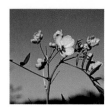

Senna

Cassia angustifolia (*Senna alexandrina*) Caesalpiniaceae

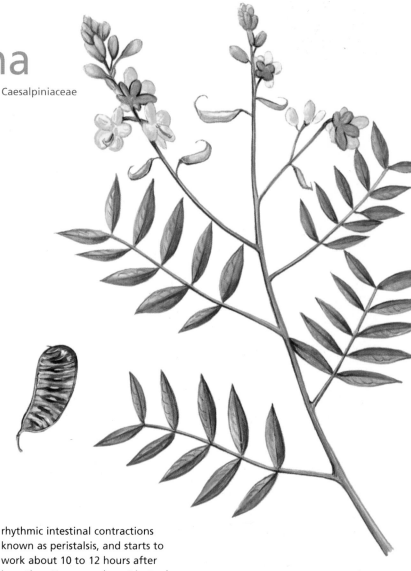

The laxative effects of senna were first discovered by Arab physicians in the 10th century. The shrub, which grows to about 1m in height, is native to hot, barren regions and is cultivated in India and Pakistan. Its yellow flowers are followed by flat papery pods containing six to eight seeds.

Parts used

Leaves and pods
- The leaves are picked before the plant flowers.
- The pods are harvested in autumn.
- Leaves and pods are sun-dried.
- They are used in decoctions, laxative medicines and tablets.

Constituents

Senna's main laxative components are anthraquinones known as sennosides. The plant also contains flavonoids and mucilage.

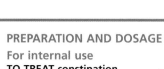

Medicinal uses

Senna is a powerful laxative and the main active ingredient in many proprietary brands of constipation remedy. It works by stimulating rhythmic intestinal contractions known as peristalsis, and starts to work about 10 to 12 hours after ingestion. However, do not just rely on laxatives, deal with the cause of the constipation. This usually involves eating high-fibre foods such as fruit, vegetables and wholegrains (for example, wholemeal bread or brown rice), drinking plenty of fluids and taking exercise.

A clinical study conducted in the UK in 1993 found senna to be more effective than the commonly prescribed laxative, lactulose, in treating chronic constipation in elderly individuals.

Cultivation

Senna can be grown from seeds, planted in well-drained soil. It will not tolerate frost, needing a warm location with plenty of sunshine.

CAUTIONS

- Do not take senna for more than eight to ten days at a time. Excessive or prolonged use can cause severe digestive problems.
- Repeated use of strong laxatives may aggravate constipation.
- Do not give senna to children under 12 years of age.
- Do not take at the same time as drugs that contain anthraquinones.
- Do not take when pregnant or breastfeeding.
- Consult a doctor before use if taking the heart drug digitalis.
- Do not take if you have any intestinal blockage or inflammation, or suffer from haemorrhoids.

PREPARATION AND DOSAGE

For internal use
TO TREAT constipation
DECOCTION Steep 3-6 pods in 150ml of water for 6-12 hours. Drink one dose a day.
LIQUID EXTRACT (1:1 in 25% alcohol) Take 0.5-1ml a day.
TABLETS (7.5mg sennosides) Take 1-2 tablets at bedtime. Do not take more than 2 tablets in a 24-hour period.

IF SYMPTOMS PERSIST, CONSULT A DOCTOR

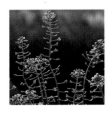

Shepherd's purse

Capsella bursa-pastoris Brassicaceae

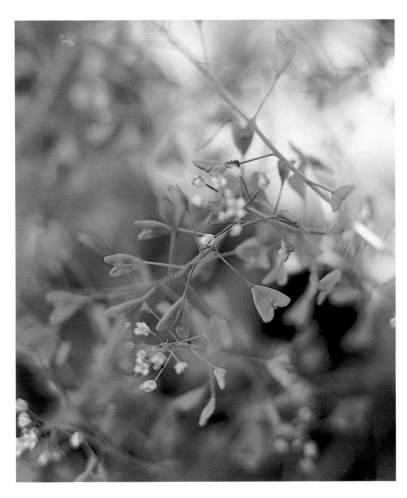

The plant has antiseptic, diuretic and urinary properties. which make it a useful remedy for cystitis, and is also astringent and anti-inflammatory.

Shepherd's purse can also cause the uterus to contract. This effect was demonstrated in 1969 in a study that observed the stimulating effect of the plant's alkaloids on the uterus.

Cultivation
Shepherd's purse will flourish in even the poorest soils. Plant in a sunny or lightly shaded spot.

CAUTIONS
• No toxicity or undesirable side effects have been recorded to date, but shepherd's purse may have a sedative effect.
• Do not used the herb at the same time as anticoagulants.
• Consult a doctor before use if you are taking drugs for blood pressure, heart problems or thyroid disorders.
• Shepherd's purse should not be used when pregnant.

Common throughout Europe, shepherd's purse is a weed that thrives on waste ground. Fragile, upright stems bear clusters of little white flowers followed by seedpods shaped like small pouch purses – from which the plant gets its name.

Parts used
Aerial parts
• The plant may be harvested from March to November.
• Its active components lose some of their potency when stored.
• It is used for infusions, tinctures and in pharmaceutical products.

Constituents
The plant contains a powerfully active essential oil, choline, acetylcholine, tyramine and flavonoids.

Medicinal uses
Traditionally shepherd's purse was used to treat haemorrhaging after childbirth and for all forms of internal bleeding. In the First World War, it was employed to staunch bleeding when supplies of other styptic medicines, such as ergot, ran low. Today, it is prescribed as a gentle remedy for heavy periods, and can be used to stop nosebleeds.

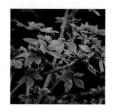

Siberian ginseng

Eleutherococcus senticosus Araliaceae

As its name suggests, this thorny shrub comes from Siberia. It forms a bush, 2-3m in height, its grey stems and branches bearing palmate leaves. The small, globular flowers are held singly or in groups of two or three on smooth leaf stalks. The female flowers are yellow, while the males are purple.

Parts used

Roots

- The roots are collected when they are rich in active constituents either in autumn just before the leaves fall or in spring as new growth begins.
- Certain Russian researchers advocate the use of the leaves as well but this is currently under debate.
- The root is used as a dry extract, a powder or a tincture. It can also be prescribed as an infusion.

Constituents

The constituents in the root of Siberian ginseng include poly-saccharides and eleutherosides A to G and I to M, which are thought to stimulate the immune system.

CAUTIONS

- Before using the plant, it is best (though not essential) to consult a doctor or medical herbalist.
- It should not be given to children before they reach puberty, or to pregnant and breastfeeding women, or those taking oral contraceptives.
- It is not suitable for people who are suffering from insomnia, high blood pressure, nervous tension, obesity, heart palpitations and benign breast disease.
- Hyperactive, schizophrenic or manic individuals should avoid it.
- Stimulants, alcohol and spicy foods should be avoided while using ginseng.

Medicinal uses

Siberian ginseng is described as being an adaptogen because it helps the body to adapt to physical and psychological stress. Russian doctors, who were the first to draw attention to its therapeutic value, have used it to ameliorate the effects of stress.

The herb has been similarly prescribed in Western Europe and also as a treatment for fatigue and high blood pressure. An American paper published in the *Journal of Ethnopharmacology* in 2000 reviews the research on the adaptogenic nature of Siberian ginseng, including its cancer-fighting properties and the plant's ability to stimulate the immune system.

Its positive effect on the immune system means that the plant can help to protect against viral infections. Its potential as an immune stimulant was supported by a study performed in Germany in 1987 which showed that Siberian ginseng increased the total number of lymphocytes.

It is described as being beneficial for maintaining good health rather than treating illnesses per se, and is reputed to be a tonic for all organs of the body. The root has been shown to stimulate the central nervous system and the adrenal gland, as well as being beneficial in the treatment of impotence.

It is also reputed to lower blood sugar levels and treat inflammation.

Cultivation

Plant in well-drained, rich soil in a sunny or slightly shady location.

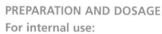

PREPARATION AND DOSAGE

For internal use:

TO TREAT stress, fatigue, viral infections

CAPSULES (150mg powder)
Take 1 capsule, three times a day with a large glass of water.

CAPSULES (50mg dry extract)
Take 4-6 capsules a day with a large glass of water.

TINCTURE (1:3 in 25% alcohol)
Take 10-20 drops with water after meals three times a day.

Do not use Siberian ginseng for more than a month, followed by a break of at least two months before restarting.

IF SYMPTOMS PERSIST, CONSULT A DOCTOR

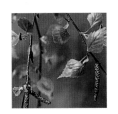

Silver birch

Betula pendula Betulaceae **Also called** European white birch

This elegant deciduous tree is distinguished by its smooth, papery, silver bark and long, drooping catkins in spring. In folklore the silver birch is held to have sacred powers against evil spirits and witchcraft. The tree can reach a height of 25-30m. Its leaves are triangular with serrated edges and its fruits are winged seedpods.

Parts used

Young leaves and bark

• Newly formed leaves are collected in spring.

• After drying, the leaves are used for infusions, powders, capsules or tinctures.

• The bark, collected from felled timber, is mainly used for decoctions.

PREPARATION AND DOSAGE

For internal use

TO TREAT minor inflammation of the urinary tract, urinary or kidney stones, oedema
INFUSION Put 2-3g of dried leaves cut up into small pieces in a cup of boiling water. Leave to infuse for 10-15 minutes. When the temperature lowers to 40°C, add sodium bicarbonate (1g a litre). Take 3 cups a day, 30 minutes before meals.
CAPSULES (50mg dry extract) Take 1 or 2 capsules, one to three times a day.
TINCTURE (1:4 in 25% alcohol) Put 15 drops into a glass of water. Take three times a day after meals.

For external use

TO TREAT skin inflammations
INFUSION Use 50g of dried leaves to 1 litre of water. Bathe skin with the infusion two or three times a day.

IF SYMPTOMS PERSIST, CONSULT A DOCTOR

Constituents

As much as 3 per cent of the silver birch leaf is made up of flavonoids (hyperoside and rutoside mostly), which have anti-inflammatory and diuretic effects. The leaf and bark contain phenolic acids, tannins, plus vitamin C and methyl salicylate.

Medicinal uses

Because of the large amount of flavonoids present in the plant, the silver birch leaf is an effective diuretic and anti-inflammatory agent, besides being a urinary and renal antiseptic. Such properties make it useful for treating minor infections of the urinary tract such as urethritis and cystitis. It is also used to treat urinary or kidney stones as well as oedema.

A further use for the anti-inflammatory action of silver birch is in the treatment of rheumatic pains, where it is often combined with spiny restharrow, nettle or meadowsweet. Externally, an ointment containing silver birch can ease eczema and psoriasis.

The silver birch is reputed to be able to cure warts. A small, moistened piece of fresh bark, which is changed every day, is placed on the skin over the wart. Alternatively, a decoction made of ground-up bark can be used. The effect is thought to be due to the tree's antiviral compounds (betulinic acid) and its salicylates. Extensive research of a betulinic acid derivative, reviewed in 2002, highlights its effective antiviral activity against HIV.

Cultivation

Suited to well-drained acidic soil. Position in the sun or shade. Birch is grown from cuttings, grafting and by seed. A young specimen can also be planted.

CAUTIONS

• To date, silver birch has revealed no toxic effects when taken in therapeutic doses. However, it could cause certain allergies, especially in people who are sensitive to celery and mugwort pollen.

• Caution should be taken by hayfever sufferers.

• Silver birch is not recommended for individuals with kidney or heart disorders.

• Because of its methyl salicylate content, children should not take it.

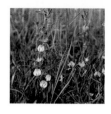

Spiny restharrow

Ononis spinosa Leguminosae

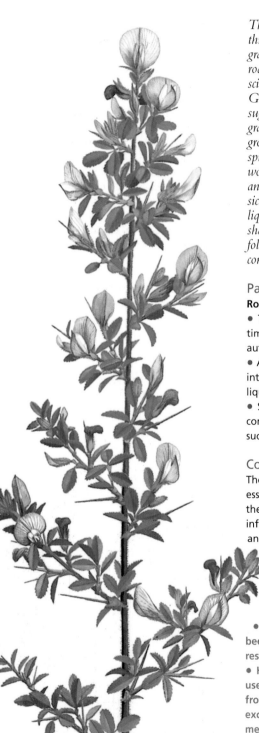

This herbaceous perennial grows throughout Europe in dry grassland, hedgerows and by roadsides. Spiny restharrow's scientific name comes from the Greek word onos (donkey), suggesting that donkeys and other grazing animals like to eat it. It grows to a height of 30-60cm, its spiny branches held erect from a woody base. The woody roots emit an unpleasant aroma and have a sickly sweet taste similar to liquorice. Pinkish white butterfly-shaped flowers emerge in summer, followed by hairy, oval-shaped pods, containing up to three round seeds.

Parts used
Roots
• The roots can be collected at any time of year, although spring and autumn are best.
• After drying, the roots are crushed into fragments for use in infusions, liquid extracts or tinctures.
• Spiny restharrow is often combined with other diuretic plants, such as juniper and parsley.

Constituents
The root contains a small amount of essential oil. Other constituents of the root are phenols, which reduce inflammation, lectins, medicarpin and triterpenoids such as onocerin.

CAUTIONS
• No adverse side effects have been reported when taking spiny restharrow in therapeutic doses.
• However, the plant must not be used to treat fluid retention arising from cardiac and kidney disorders, except under the supervision of a medical herbalist as complementary to any prescribed medical treatment.

PREPARATION AND DOSAGE
For internal use
TO TREAT urine retention, gout, nephritis, cystitis, rheumatism
INFUSION Add 1 heaped teaspoon of the root to 1 cup of boiling water. Infuse for 15 minutes, then strain. Drink 1 cup three times a day.
TINCTURE Put 40 drops into a glass of water and take three times a day between meals.

For external use
TO TREAT eczema and other skin complaints
DECOCTION Simmer 20g of dried root with 750ml of water until it has reduced by roughly a third. Allow to cool. Apply topically two to three times a day.

IF SYMPTOMS PERSIST, CONSULT A DOCTOR

Medicinal uses
Spiny restharrow has a diuretic effect, which is thought to be due to the essential oil, flavonoid derivatives including a-onocerin. Taken orally, the spiny restharrow root is used to treat fluid retention, nephritis (kidney inflammation) and cystitis, as well as to prevent bladder and kidney stones.

The plant also has an anti-inflammatory action and is used for treating rheumatism and gout.

Decoctions of the root can be applied to the skin to treat eczema and other skin disorders.

Cultivation
Spiny restharrow can be grown from seed. It prefers a well-drained soil in full sun.

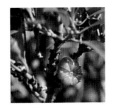

Star anise

Illicium verum Illiciaceae **Also called** Chinese anise

Native to southern China and northern Vietnam, this evergreen can grow to a height of 18m. Star anise has white, aromatic bark and its leaves taper to a point. The single flowers are greenish or whitish yellow and followed by star-shaped fruit, hence its common name. The fruit has a strong aroma and a sweet, sugary flavour. A single fruit is made up of 8 to 12 seedpods, each containing a brown, shiny seed.

Parts used
Fruits
● The tree can live for 80 years but the fruit is not harvested during the first ten years. The fruits are picked when still green and not fully ripe.
● After being dried in the sun the fruits turn a reddish brown colour.

Constituents
The fruit contains a large quantity of essential oil (5-10 per cent), which is rich in anethole. This is mainly in the form of E-anethole.

Medicinal uses
Anethole is thought to be the source of many of the therapeutic properties associated with star anise. Traditionally, the plant is used to relieve digestive and intestinal problems and is particularly useful for treating colic.

CAUTIONS
● Care must be taken not to confuse the fruit of star anise with the poisonous fruit of Japanese anise. Although the fruits are quite similar in appearance, the fruit of Japanese anise is smaller and more irregular than that of star anise. The fruit also has a sharp, bitter odour, whereas star anise smells and tastes like aniseed.

PREPARATION AND DOSAGE
For internal use
TO TREAT digestive problems
INFUSION Put 1 teaspoon of dried fruit into a cup of boiling water and leave to infuse for 10 minutes, then strain. Drink 2 cups a day before meals.

IF SYMPTOMS PERSIST, CONSULT A DOCTOR

The effects of the fruits vary according to the amount of anethole present. In small doses it stimulates the appetite, promotes digestion, helps to expel wind and calms intestinal spasms. In large doses it can **stimulate** the central nervous system to such a degree that it causes trembling and convulsions.

Like anise, star anise possesses oestrogenic effects: it promotes menstruation, eases childbirth and stimulates milk secretion. A study published in the *Journal of Ethnopharmacology* in 1980 suggests that the active ingredients are based on anethole polymeric units. Star anise is also believed to increase libido in both men and women.

The plant is reputed to possess stimulant and diuretic properties and can be beneficial in conditions such as lumbago. Like anise, it is often present in cough remedies. Japanese and Indian researchers have found that star anise is effective against various strains of bacteria, yeast and fungi and could therefore be useful in fighting off infections.

Cultivation
Plant in moist, well-drained, neutral to acid soil in a slightly shaded position.

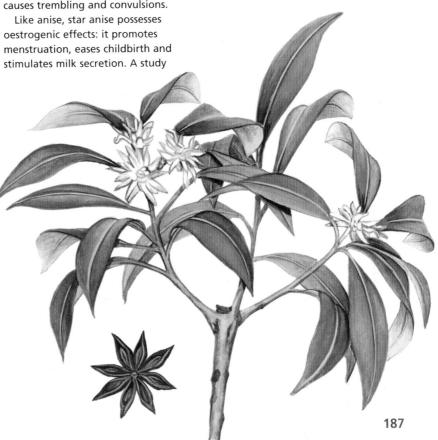

187

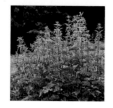

Stinging nettle

Urtica dioica Urticaceae

Until the 17th century, nettle stalks were widely used for their fibres which make a hardwearing linen-like fabric. And the Germans used nettle fabric to make army uniforms in the First World War when cotton ran short. The word 'nettle' comes from an old Scandinavian word, noedl, meaning needle, from the plant's needle-sharp stinging hairs. Stinging nettles colonise ditches, clearings and waste ground.

PREPARATION AND DOSAGE

For internal use

TO TREAT rheumatic pain, fatigue, poor appetite
INFUSION Put 2-4g of dried herb into 1 cup of boiling water. Drink 3 cups a day.
FRESH JUICE Drink 10-15ml three times a day.
CAPSULES (500mg) Take 3-6 capsules a day.
DRY EXTRACT Take 250mg two or three times a day.
TINCTURE (1:4 in 25% alcohol) Take 20 drops in water three times a day after meals.

TO TREAT urination difficulties linked to prostate problems
INFUSION Put 2-4g of dried herb into 1 cup of boiling water. Drink 3 cups a day.
CAPSULES (300mg) Take 3-6 capsules a day.
LIQUID EXTRACT Put 30-60 drops into a glass of water. Take three to six times a day.

For external use

TO TREAT skin and scalp conditions
STEWED LEAVES OR ROOTS Apply as a poultice twice a day.

IF SYMPTOMS PERSIST, CONSULT A DOCTOR

Parts used

Leaves and roots
- The plant is harvested in May and June before flowering when the stinging hairs are rich in histamine and serotonin.
- The leaves are used fresh or dried to make infusions.
- The roots may be dried and powdered for capsules or used fresh.
- Both leaves and roots are crushed to yield juices.

Constituents

The leaves contain both iron and vitamin C – which aids iron absorption. They also contain other minerals, especially calcium, potassium and silicic acid, as well as phenols and flavonoids.

The roots are rich in poly-saccharides, lecithin, several phenolic compounds and sterols.

Medicinal uses

'Urtication', or flogging the affected parts with nettles, was an old remedy for painful rheumatic joints. Today, treatment is less brutal. Nettle is prescribed internally as a diuretic as it can increase elimination of sodium and urea, thus helping to ease rheumatic and arthritic conditions. And the leaves are also strongly anti-inflammatory, as shown by German *in vitro* studies in 1999.

CAUTIONS

- If taken over a long period, nettle leaves can cause skin rashes.
- May cause gastric inflammation.
- Do not self-prescribe for prostate problems – seek medical advice.
- Do not use if taking medication to treat diabetes, high or low blood pressure, or to depress the central nervous system.
- Do not take if pregnant or breastfeeding.

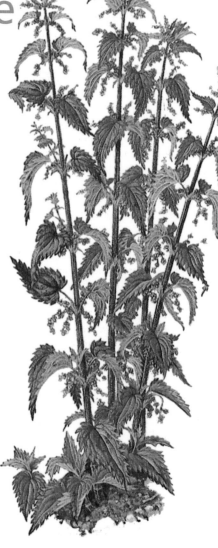

A nettle infusion is a good tonic: it stimulates the appetite, provides iron and fights fatigue.

The fresh root may help prostate and urination problems: German research in *Planta Medica* in 2000 observed that the root inhibited the growth of prostate tissue. Italian research in 2002 suggests that root extracts may be useful in reducing blood pressure.

Externally, nettle is used for acne, eczema, greasy skin and dandruff.

Cultivation

Nettles can be cultivated from seed planted in spring in a moist, loamy soil and in sun or light shade.

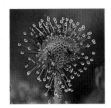

Sundew

Drosera rotundifolia Droseraceae

A small aquatic plant, sundew is now rare in the UK. It can be seen in damp peaty areas, especially in Wales, in summer. The plant eats insects. The leaves, which lie flat on the ground, are covered in fine, red, insect-trapping sticky hairs. Each hair is tipped with a small fluid-filled gland that looks like a dewdrop, hence the plant's name.

Parts used

Whole plant

● Sundew is collected from June to September when in flower.

● It can be used fresh.

● It can also be dried and powdered for use in infusions and tinctures.

● Sundew is often combined with other plants that relieve coughs.

Constituents

Sundew contains naphthaquinones, including an antibacterial and antispasmodic called plumbagin. It also contains flavonoids that improve the circulation by strengthening blood vessels, astringent tannins, which have antioxidant, antibacterial and anti-inflammatory properties, and mucilage – which soothes inflamed mucous membranes.

Medicinal uses

Sundew tea has long been used in European traditional medicine to treat lung ailments and dry coughs.

CAUTIONS

● Sundew can irritate the skin and mucous membranes.

● It may cause nausea and blood-specked diarrhoea.

● Do not take on an empty stomach.

● Sundew is least likely to cause adverse effects when combined with other ingredients.

● Do not use when pregnant or breastfeeding.

PREPARATION AND DOSAGE

For internal use

TO TREAT bronchitis, dry, tickly or nervous coughs, whooping cough

INFUSION Add 1-2g of dried plant to 1 cup of boiling water. Infuse for 10 minutes and strain. Drink 3 cups a day.

For external use

TO TREAT warts

FRESH SAP Apply directly to warts once or twice a day.

IF SYMPTOMS PERSIST, CONSULT A DOCTOR

The main active constituent in sundew is a compound called plumbagin, which has an antispasmodic effect, particularly in the respiratory and intestinal tracts. This effect was demonstrated by Swiss research conducted in 1993.

The herb also exerts soothing and expectorant actions, and sundew is prescribed to treat respiratory tract illnesses such as bronchitis and pertussis (whooping cough), dry, tickly or nervous coughs and other respiratory conditions that cause the production of sticky mucus. It is often combined in syrups with other cough remedies such as thyme.

The usefulness of sundew in treating chest infections is reinforced by the fact that plumbagin inhibits the proliferation of germs such as streptococcus, staphylococcus and pneumococcus, as well as certain disease-causing fungi.

Externally, the juice of the raw, untreated plant has been used as an effective treatment for warts.

Cultivation

Sundew can be cultivated from seed but needs to be planted in wet peat in a spot that receives full sunshine.

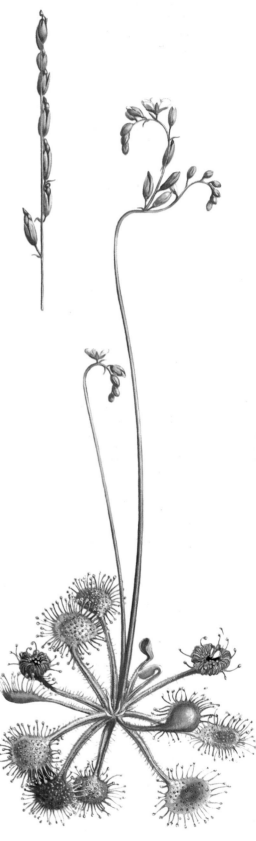

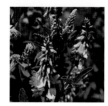

Sweet clover

Melilotus officinalis Fabaceae **Also called** Melilot

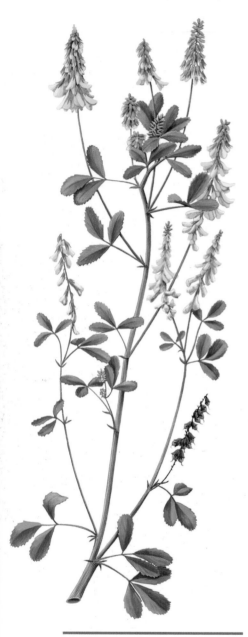

Found throughout Europe and northern Asia, sweet clover thrives in dry, chalky areas in fields, on wasteland, and along embankments. An annual, or sometimes biennial, it is about 30-90cm tall. Its fluted, erect stems bear leaves made up of three oval leaflets with indented edges. In summer, small, yellow, sweetly scented flowers form in elongated clusters at the tops of the stems. These are succeeded by small, oval yellowy brown fruits.

Parts used

Stems, leaves and flowers
• The aerial parts of the plant are harvested in July and then dried.
• Dried sweet clover is used to prepare infusions, decoctions, powders, dry extracts and tinctures.
• It is often combined with plants that help to strengthen the blood vessels, such as witch hazel, horse chestnut and bilberry.

Constituents

Sweet clover contains the glucoside melilotoside. This is converted to coumarin, which gives the plant its scent. Flavonoids are also present. If contaminated by fungi sweet clover produces dicoumarol, a compound that prevents blood clotting.

Medicinal uses

Because of its melilotoside content, sweet clover can help to strengthen blood vessels, and is used for circulatory problems such as varicose veins and to relieve related conditions such as swelling due to fluid retention. A clinical trial by Italian scientists in 1999 found that sweet clover could reduce the upper-arm swelling in women who had undergone breast cancer surgery.

The plant is also known to be anti-inflammatory – an ability now substantiated by animal studies. It is used on wounds, bruises, sprains, eye irritations and for rheumatism. The flavonoids act as diuretic and help to ease digestive problems.

Furthermore, the plant may have the potential to treat thrombosis, when the anticoagulant compound dicoumarol is present. This, however, should not be used as an alternative or adjunct to properly monitored anticoagulant medication.

Cultivation

Sweet clover can be grown from seed, which is planted in autumn or spring. The plant thrives in a well-drained, neutral to alkaline soil, exposed to plenty of sunlight.

CAUTIONS

• Because dicoumarol may be present, people with blood-clotting disorders or on blood-thinning drugs should not ingest sweet clover.
• Only take the plant in small doses, as the coumarin content, in large amounts, can cause liver damage.

PREPARATION AND DOSAGE

For internal use
TO TREAT haemorrhoids, varicose veins, heavy (dead) legs, fluid retention, digestive problems
INFUSION Put 1 teaspoon of dried flowers into a cup of boiling water. Leave to infuse for 5 minutes, then strain. Drink 3-4 cups a day.
CAPSULES (50mg powder) Take 1-2 capsules, three times a day with meals.
TINCTURE Put 35 drops into a glass of water. Take three times a day with meals.

For external use
TO TREAT sprains, bruises, eyelid irritation, bleeding
COMPRESS Put 20g dried flowers into 100ml of water. Boil for 15 minutes. If using for sprains or bruises, soak a cloth in the liquid while warm, and apply to the affected area, two or three times a day. Allow liquid to cool before using for eyelid irritations or to stop bleeding.

IF SYMPTOMS PERSIST, CONSULT A DOCTOR

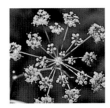

Sweet fennel

Foeniculum vulgare var. *dulce* Apiceae **Also called** Florence fennel, Finocchio

A native of southern Europe and the Mediterranean, sweet fennel can grow to a height of nearly 2m, with elegant, long, slender leaves and pretty umbrella-shaped clusters of yellow scented flowers. Some gardeners grow it purely as an ornamental plant. The tiny fruits are a yellowy green, ridged with black, and have a penetrating sugary flavour.

Parts used
Root, leaves and fruit (seeds)
● The roots are harvested in autumn and dried. Sachets of dried root, which are used for infusions, are often on sale in pharmacies.
● The leaves can be collected at any time, and are used in cookery as a flavouring and garnish.
● The fruit – usually referred to as 'seed' – is collected when ripe, then dried. Medicinally, it is used to prepare infusions, powders, capsules and liquid extracts. An essential oil is also extracted from it.

Constituents
Sweet fennel contains a large amount of essential oil, which is rich in anethole, a white crystalline substance with the odour of liquorice. About 60 per cent of this oil is found in the fruit.

CAUTIONS
● Because the anethole in sweet fennel essential oil can be toxic in high doses, the essential oil, like that of anise, should only ever be taken under prescription from a medical herbalist. Preparations should always be taken under medical herbalist supervision.
● Sweet fennel essential oil and any products containing it should never be used by pregnant women.

Medicinal uses
Essential oil of sweet fennel is traditionally used to treat digestive problems, such as sluggishness, flatulence, constipation, bloating and belching. It also has diuretic and anti-inflammatory powers and can help remedy ailments of the urinary system. It is also reputed to soothe sore throats and gums, when taken as a gargle, and can be used in an eyewash to treat conjunctivitis.

Fennel contains constituents that are thought to mimic the action of the female hormone oestrogen, which is why the plant has been used to stimulate lactation and menstruation. Research has shown that anethole polymers are responsible for this activity rather than anethole itself. It has been proved, however, that anethole can stimulate respiratory secretions and act as an expectorant.

Cultivation
Sweet fennel can be grown from seeds, which should be planted in spring. It is suited to rich, light soils and prefers a sunny position.

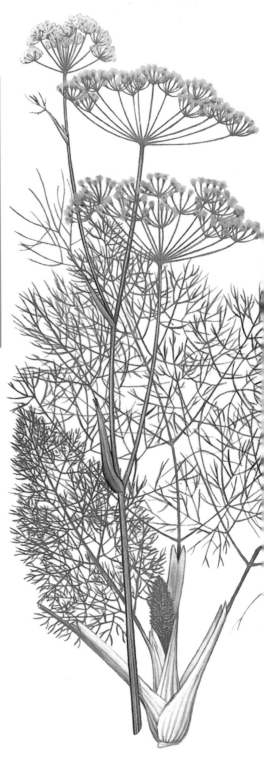

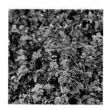

Sweet marjoram

Origanum majorana Lamiaceae

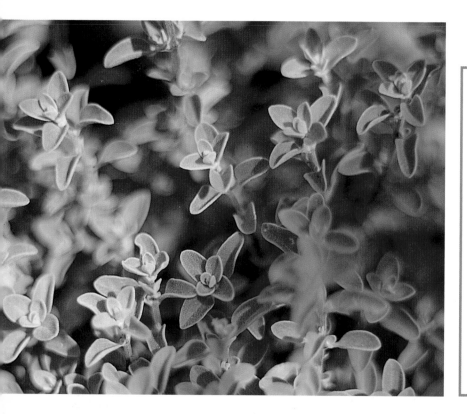

A woody perennial, sweet majoram grows to a height of about 60cm. Small velvety, oval leaves crowd its stems, with tight spikes of white or pinkish flowers opening all summer. Apart from its medicinal uses, the sweet aroma makes it a popular culinary herb. It is widely cultivated in Hungary, Spain and North Africa, as well as being picked from the wild in its native Portugal.

Parts used

Stems, leaves and flowers

• Aerial parts are collected from July to September, as the plant flowers.

• The stems and leaves are dried, then used to prepare infusions, powders and tinctures.

• A yellowy green essential oil is extracted from fresh flowers. It has a very penetrating, camphorated smell.

Constituents

Sweet majoram contains bitters, tannins, flavonoids, manganese and zinc. Its essential oil is rich in cavacrol and thymol, and sabinene, linalool and terpenes are also present.

Medicinal uses

Sweet marjoram is recognised as a useful plant for treating digestive problems, such as intestinal spasms, nausea, bloating, loss of appetite, flatulence and diarrhoea. It can also act as a sedative, so is effective in

CAUTIONS

• Always seek medical advice before using sweet marjoram essential oil.

• It is advisable to avoid all sweet marjoram essential oil preparations when pregnant or breastfeeding.

cases where indigestion is due to a nervous problem, as well as being an effective remedy for insomnia and palpitations. Researchers in Korea have recently shown that the plant's ursolic acid (a terpene) is responsible for this power to calm.

Sweet marjoram is also known to stimulate lactation and perspiration. The latter action, coupled with the plant's diuretic powers, helps to expel toxins from the body.

Applied externally, the essential oil will soothe joint and muscle ache, and can be helpful in easing the pain of toothache and mouth ulcers.

Cultivation

Sweet majoram will grow from seed. Plant in a warm, sunny position in spring. It thrives in well-drained, neutral to alkaline soil.

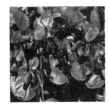

Sweet violet

Viola odorata Violaceae

A herbaceous perennial, sweet violet can be found in damp, shady places in most temperate regions of the world. About 10-15cm high, its bright green leaves form a rosette around the base of the long, erect flower stems. The young leaves are kidney-shaped, taking on their familiar heart shape and becoming slightly downy as they mature. From late February to late April single violet-blue to whitish flowers open, filling the surrounding air with their sweet fragrance.

Parts used
Whole plant
- The leaves, flowers and stems are picked in spring, and the rhizome (rootstock) in August and September.
- Sweet violet is used to prepare infusions, tinctures and syrups.

Constituents
The sweet violet plant contains phenolic glycosides, saponins, flavonoids and mucilage.

Medicinal uses
Sweet violet has long been used to treat respiratory tract illnesses and inflammation of the intestines. It has been the subject of research that has demonstrated the anti-inflammatory, analgesic and expectorant powers of its constituents in helping to dissolve mucus, loosen phlegm, reduce fever and ease pain.

These soothing powers have also been harnessed to treat mouth infections and certain skin conditions, such as cracked skin.

CAUTION
- When taken in large doses preparations containing sweet violet rhizome can cause vomiting.

Recent studies in Sweden suggest suggest its potential to treat cancer as well. Peptides from sweet violet were shown to have a cytotoxic effect, inhibiting the growth of certain types of malgnant tumours.

Cultivation
Sweet violet is grown by dividing a mature plant, or from seeds sown in spring, or from cuttings planted in autumn. It thrives in moist, well-drained, soil in a sunny location, but must have some shade in summer.

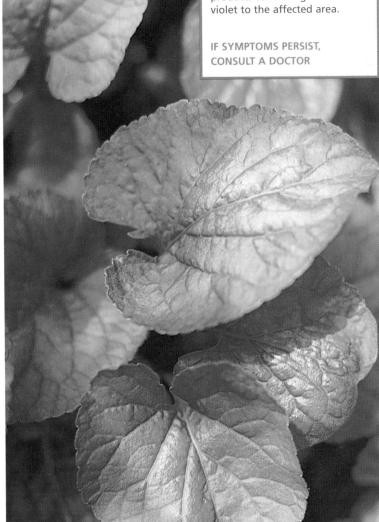

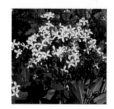

Sweet woodruff

Asperula odorata (Galium odoratum) Rubiaceae

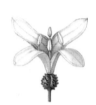

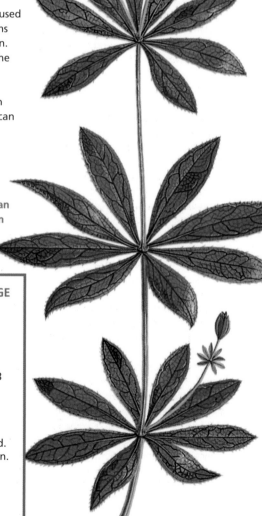

A lover of woods and shaded hedgerows, sweet woodruff is a small perennial that thrives in cool, clay soils. Star-like whorls, each made up of six to eight bright green, oval leaves, spring at intervals straight from the stem. In early summer, sprays of delicate, white flowers open on long stalks at the top of the plant. They are followed by small, round fruits, that are covered in tiny, hooked spines.

Parts used

Leaves, stems and flowers
- The aerial parts are collected when the plant flowers in May and June.
- The cut plant is tied into bunches, and left to dry. While drying, it develops a subtle aroma.
- Once dried, sweet woodruff is used to prepare infusions.

Constituents

The aerial parts of sweet woodruff contain coumarins, which have a sedative effect and are responsible for the dried plant's pleasant aroma. Asperuloside, an anti-inflammatory, is also present.

Medicinal uses

Because of the antispasmodic and sedative action of its coumarins, sweet woodruff has long been used to treat the symptoms of nervous agitation, including insomnia and irritability, as well as digestive problems that can result from anxiety, such as stomach spasms, sluggishness, bloating and belching.

The plant is also reputed to strengthen blood vessels and is used in the treatment of varicose veins and any associated inflammation. Recent animal studies confirm the beneficial effect of using sweet woodruff in such cases.

Sweet woodruff is also known to be an effective diuretic, and can help to keep the liver healthy.

Cultivation

Sweet woodruff prefers moist, neutral to alkaline soil. Mostly, it is picked from the wild, but can be grown from seeds, planted in late July or early August in a shaded area.

CAUTIONS

- Large doses of sweet woodruff can cause internal bleeding.
- Avoid sweet woodruff when using drugs to treat circulatory disorders.
- The plant is not recommended when pregnant or breastfeeding.

PREPARATION AND DOSAGE

For internal use
TO TREAT nervous agitation
INFUSION Put 10g of dried aerial parts into 1 litre of boiling water. Infuse for 10 minutes, then strain. Drink 2-3 cups a day.

TO TREAT insomnia
INFUSION (see above) Drink 1 cup, half an hour before bed. This is also suitable for children.

TO TREAT stomach spasms and digestive problems
INFUSION (see above) Drink 2-3 cups a day.

IF SYMPTOMS PERSIST, CONSULT A DOCTOR

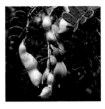

Tamarind

Tamarindus indica Caesalpiniaceae **Also called** Indian date

Native to Madagascar, the tamarind tree is cultivated in numerous other tropical regions, such as India and the Caribbean. It can reach a height of 20-25m, with branches that hang so low that they often touch the ground. The fragrant, golden-yellow flowers are streaked with red. Following them are long, dangling seedpods, that start grey-green, ripening to a rich rust. They contain a sweet, brownish yellow pulp in which sit five to ten shiny, reddish brown seeds.

Parts used

Fruit pulp
• The fruit is picked from June to October. The pulp is extracted and the seeds removed and discarded.
• The pulp can be used fresh, or to prepare a powder or dry extract.
• Sometimes the juice is used. This is obtained by soaking the pulp in hot water and then pressing it.

Constituents

Tamarind pulp is rich in pectin, simple sugars and organic acids, including tartaric and citric acid. Its slightly aromatic scent is due to terpene compounds. Contrary to a popular belief, there is no vitamin C.

Medicinal uses

Tamarind pulp is a potent laxative and is recommended as a treatment for constipation in both adults and children. It can also help to remedy other digestive ailments, such as sluggishness, flatulence, nausea and 'morning sickness' during pregnancy, while its soothing powers are known to ease sore throats, ulcers and rheumatic pain.

In India, tamarind is used to fight infections, particularly those of the intestines, as well as colds and catarrh. This use is backed up by the recent discovery in Mexico that tamarind has antibacterial powers. Also, Italian researchers have shown that tamarind gum can inhibit the spread of the rubella virus.

Tamarind has been used to treat asthma and jaundice, and is known to reduce fevers and have a general cooling effect on the body.

Cultivation

Tamarind can be grown from seeds, planted in spring, but needs a temperature of at least 18°C, so will only grow under glass in temperate regions. It will tolerate poor soil and drought, but requires plenty of light.

CAUTIONS

• Tamarind may interact adversely with aspirin and other non-steroidal anti-inflammatory drugs.
• Only take the recommended therapeutic dose of the plant, and avoid long-term use.

PREPARATION AND DOSAGE

For internal use
TO TREAT constipation
FRESH SEEDLESS PULP Eat 10-50g a day, adjusting the dose as necessary.
CAPSULES (200mg) Take 1-2 capsules with a large glass of water, after the evening meal.
POWDER Add 1-2g to a cup of boiling water, then leave for 10 minutes. Drink this after the evening meal.

IF SYMPTOMS PERSIST, CONSULT A DOCTOR

Thyme, common

Thymus vulgaris Lamiaceae

A low-lying, perennial shrub, common thyme grows wild on arid hillsides across the Mediterranean. This rugged plant was a symbol of courage to the ancient Greeks and in medieval Europe. Tiny, greyish green leaves, their edges curling inwards, coat the numerous wiry branches of the erect, woody stems. From May until August, spikes of small, white or pink flowers appear. The warm pungent taste and rich aroma of the leaves, make them a popular flavouring in a wide range of dishes and cuisines.

CAUTIONS

• To date, common thyme has shown no adverse side effects, but excessive use is not advisable.
• Do not use thyme when pregnant or breastfeeding.
• The essential oil should be used only under a doctor's supervision.

Parts used

Leaves and flower stalks
• The leaves and flowers stalks are gathered at the beginning of the flowering season and dried carefully away from sunlight.
• The dried thyme is used to prepare infusions, powders for capsules and in pharmaceutical products, such as soothing cough syrups.
• An essential oil is also extracted from the dried leaves and flower stalks. This is used in antiseptic creams and ointments. A related plant, Spanish thyme (Thymus zygis), is also used for the antiseptic power of its essential oil.

Constituents

The dried leaves and flower stalks of common thyme contain flavonoids and 0.5 to 2 per cent essential oil. The composition of the essential oil varies; thymol, methylchavicol, cineole and borneol are all present.

PREPARATION AND DOSAGE

For internal use

TO TREAT sluggish digestion, bloating, belching, flatulence, inadequate bile flow, coughs
INFUSION Put 2g of dried plant into a cup of boiling water. Cover and leave to infuse for 5 minutes. Drink 3 cups a day.
CAPSULES (325mg) Take 3 a day, with a large glass of water.

For external use

TO TREAT wounds, aching muscles
INFUSION (see above) Use to wash affected areas, several times a day.
OINTMENT Apply to affected areas, several times a day.

IF SYMPTOMS PERSIST, CONSULT A DOCTOR

Medicinal uses

Research has shown that the flavonoids in thyme – methylchavicol and thymol – have a muscle relaxing effect. As a result the plant is widely used as an antispasmodic to treat digestive problems, such as bloating, belching, flatulence, sluggish digestion and poor bile flow.

Thyme is also effective for soothing coughs and can help to relieve nasal congestion due to colds, hayfever and asthma.

Studies have demonstrated that thyme's essential oil is antiseptic, and it is often recommended for minor cuts and wounds, as well as for insect bites and stings. The plant is also sometimes prescribed to treat gum disease and tonsillitis.

Cultivation

Grow from seed, sown in early April, or summer cuttings. A warm, sunny plot with rich, dry, light soil is ideal.

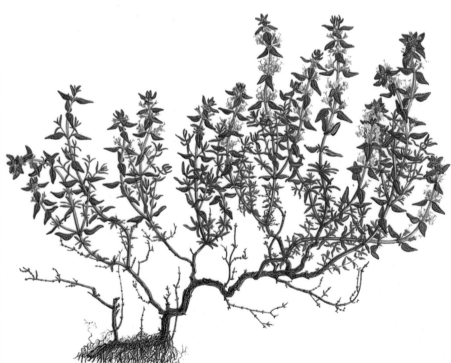

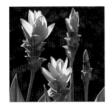

Turmeric

Curcuma longa Zingiberaceae

Cultivated in Asia, Africa and the West Indies, turmeric is a tropical perennial. Its pointed, lance-shaped leaves can be up to 70cm long. Low clusters of flowers spring up from the middle of the plant in summer. The rhizome is cylindrical, often with finger-like protuberances, and is a rich yellowy orange on the inside. It has a warm, slightly acrid taste. When powdered, it is widely used to colour and flavour food.

Parts used

Rhizome

● The rhizome is dug up in winter, when it is dormant. It is cut into pieces, boiled and then dried.

● In herbal medicine, turmeric rhizome is mainly used to prepare powders and tinctures, and occasionally for making infusions.

Constituents

Turmeric rhizome contains a number of curcuminoids, which are mainly responsible for its colour and are known to be anti-inflammatory. It is also rich in essential oil.

Medicinal uses

Turmeric rhizome is prescribed as a treatment for lack of appetite, indigestion and stomach acidity, as well as liver and gall-bladder problems. It has been found to have a protective effect on the liver,

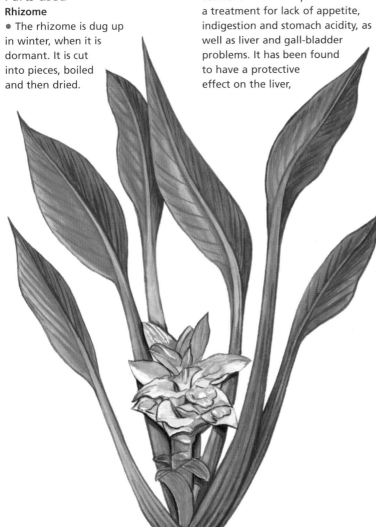

and the essential oil is known to stimulate the secretion of bile. Scientists have also demonstrated that the curcuminoids can have a powerful anti-inflammatory effect, which underlies the traditional use of turmeric in treating rheumatism, arthritis, eczema, asthma, psoriasis, and other inflammatory conditions.

Turmeric has also displayed antioxidant and antibacterial properties, and is believed to help to lower blood cholesterol and inhibit blood clotting. This suggests that it could be beneficial in preventing hardening of the arteries and heart attacks. There is also evidence that it may be useful in the treatment of circulatory and menstrual disorders.

Cultivation

Turmeric can be grown from seeds, planted in autumn, or rhizome cuttings, planted in early summer. It thrives in moist, well-drained soil. Because it needs plenty of sunshine, temperatures in excess of 15°C and high humidity, it is best cultivated in a greenhouse in temperate regions.

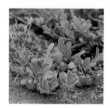

Uva-ursi

Arctostaphylos uva-ursi Ericaceae **Also called** Bearberry

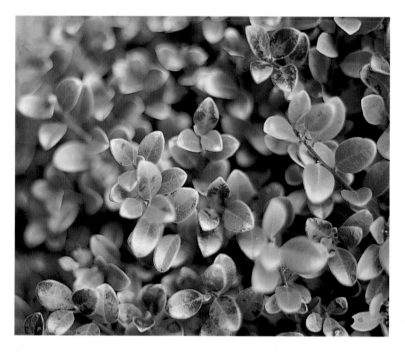

Found in the mountainous parts of Europe, Asia and America, uva-ursi is a small, low-growing shrub, with woody branching stems that trail along the ground. Its leathery, evergreen leaves are spatula-shaped, and are joined in early summer by clusters of pretty, waxy-looking flowers – white lightly marked with red. Glossy bright red berries follow them in autumn.

Parts used
Leaves
• As they are evergreen, the leaves can be picked at any time, though only the youngest are chosen.
• Once dried in the open air, the leaves are used to make infusions or dry extracts for use in various powders, tinctures and capsules.

Constituents
Uva-ursi contains phenolic glycosides, mainly arbutin, which the body are converts into antibacterial hydroquinones. Healing tannins and allantoin, and diuretic flavonoids are also present.

Medicinal uses
A number of recent research projects have clearly demonstrated that when the phenolic glycosides in uva-ursi, especially arbutin, are converted to hydroquinone inside the body, they act as a powerful antibiotic. Uva-ursi has been shown to be effective for treating urinary tract infections, such as cystitis and urethritis, boils and abscesses infected with the *Staphylococcus aureus* bacterium, and also food poisoning and diarrhoea.

Uva-ursi is thought to be more effective in fighting the bacteria that cause urinary infections when the patient's urine is more alkaline than acidic. Therefore, during treatment with the plant, it is advisable to follow a strict diet, containing plenty of fresh fruit and vegetables and only a small quantity of meat and dairy products. An alternative would be to take a regular dose of bicarbonate of soda.

Animal research into uva-ursi has also demonstrated it ability to reduce inflammation.

Cultivation
Uva-ursi can be grown from seeds planted in autumn, or cuttings planted in summer. Use moist, peaty to sandy soil. The plant will thrive in a sunny or lightly shaded plot.

CAUTIONS
• Because uva-ursi is rich in tannins, which, in high doses, can cause liver damage, any course of treatment using the plant should not last longer than a week. Also, no more than five such courses should be taken in a single year.
• The plant is not recommended as a treatment for people suffering from kidney disease.
• The high tannin content of the plant can also cause nausea.
• Avoid uva-ursi when pregnant or breastfeeding.
• Children under 12 years old should not be treated with uva-ursi.

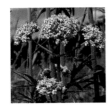

Valerian

Valeriana officinalis Valerianaceae

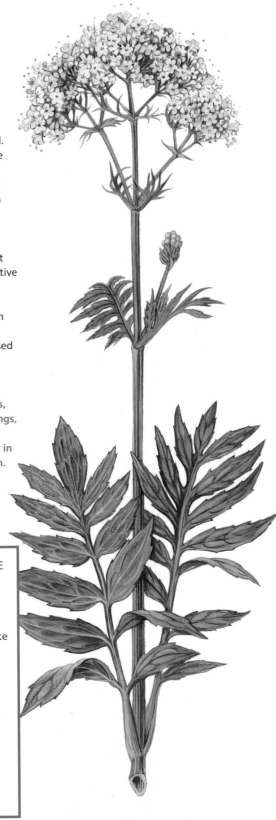

Found throughout Europe and northern Asia, valerian is a herbaceous perennial. It prefers damp places, but can survive in dry ground. The erect, fluted stems can grow as tall as 2m, with indented leaves forming a rosette around the base of the plant. Throughout the summer, umbrella-shaped clusters of white, pink or red flowers open at the very top of the main stems.

Parts used
Rhizome
• The rhizomes of plants over two years old are dug up in autumn.
• They are washed, then left to dry at a low temperature to preserve their active constituents.
• The dried rhizome is used to make powders, dry extracts, aqueous or alcohol extracts, suspensions and drinkable solutions.

Constituents
The main compounds in valerian are valepotriates, valerenic acid, and valeranone, which have a sedative effect and can calm muscle spasms. Gamma-aminobutyric acid (GABA), which can block the tranmission of signals in the brain, is also present.

Medicinal uses
Valerian is one of the best known herbal tranquillisers, and is frequently prescribed to both adults and children as a remedy for minor nervous disorders and sleeping difficulties. Because of this, it has been the subject of a number of studies in many parts of the world. These have confirmed the sedative and antispasmodic powers of the valepotriates and valerenic acid in the plant. Its antispasmodic action may be the basis of its purported ability to lower blood pressure.

Recent clinical trials conducted in Brazil demonstrated clearly that valerian was not only highly effective in remedying insomnia, but could also improve the quality of sleep enjoyed. In addition, extracts from the plant showed great potential in the treatment of disorders caused by extreme anxiety.

Cultivation
Valerian can be grown from seeds, planted in April, or rhizome cuttings, planted in late summer. It grows best in moist, rich soil, preferably in a sunny or lightly shaded location.

CAUTIONS
• It is not advisable to take valerian when pregnant or breastfeeding.
• Valerian should never be used at the same time as other drugs that have a sedative effect.
• Do not drive, or engage in any activity where lack of concentration could be dangerous, for up to 2 hours after ingesting valerian.

PREPARATION AND DOSAGE

For internal use
TO TREAT minor nervous disorders and sleeping difficulties
CAPSULES (240mg powder) Take 1-2 capsules a day. If treating sleeping disorders, take 1-2 hours before retiring.
CAPSULES (50-100mg dry extract) Take 2 capsules, three times a day.
LIQUID EXTRACT (1:1 in 60% alcohol) Take 0.3-1ml of liquid extract three times a day.

IF SYMPTOMS PERSIST, CONSULT A DOCTOR

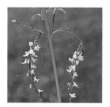

Vervain

Verbena officinalis Verbenaceae **Also called** Verbena, Simpler's joy, Turkey grass

A herbaceous perennial, found by roadsides and in sunny pastures in Europe and parts of Asia, vervain grows to a height of 30-70cm. Magical powers were attributed to it by the ancient Germans and Celts, and it was used in Druid ceremonies. Pairs of lobed, oval leaves grow opposite each other along the erect, branched stems. Long, slender spikes of pale lilac flowers hang from the top of the plant in July and early August. Sometimes known as verbena, the plant should not be confused with lemon verbena (Aloysia triphilla).

Parts used

Leaves, stems, flowers
• The aerial parts are picked in July, when the flowers are in bloom.
• Vervain must be dried promptly to preserve the power of its active compounds. It is used mostly to prepare infusions and tinctures.

Constituents

Vervain flowers and stems contain iridoid glycosides, including verbenalin and aucubin, which are known to be both anti-inflammatory and antispasmodic.

Medicinal uses

Vervain has been used for centuries for a variety of infections, but the ability of its extracts to soothe, heal and relax has only recently been demonstrated by researchers in India. The plant will treat conditions such as sunburn, nappy rash and cracked or chapped skin, and, taken internally, is known to relieve muscle cramps and the symptoms of colds and influenza. It is especially noted for its calming effect on the uterus, providing relief from menstrual cramps. It has also proved effective in combating nervous tension and fatigue and digestive problems, as well as acting as a diuretic.

New studies indicate that vervain helps boost immunity and certain hormonal secretions, including those involved in breast-milk production.

Cultivation

Vervain can be grown from seed. Plant in any moist well-drained soil in spring or autumn, in a sunny spot.

CAUTIONS

• Vervain preparations should not be taken during pregnancy.
• It is not advisable to use vervain when taking any drugs to raise or lower blood pressure.

PREPARATION AND DOSAGE

For internal use
TO TREAT nervous tension, cramps, fatigue, influenza
INFUSION Put 2g of dried plant into a cup of boiling water and infuse for 10 minutes. Strain. Drink 1 cup three times a day.
TINCTURE (1:1 in 40% alcohol) Take 30-50 drops in a glass of water, three times a day.

For external use
TO TREAT rashes, sunburn, cracked and chapped skin
COMPRESS Add a handful of dried plant to 150ml of boiling water. Infuse for 10 minutes. Apply on a soaked cloth, two or three times a day.

IF SYMPTOMS PERSIST, CONSULT A DOCTOR

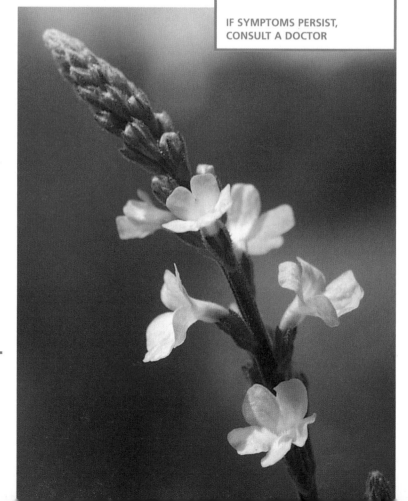

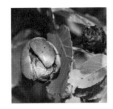

Walnut

Juglans regia Juglandaceae

Native to Anatolia, walnut trees are now found across Europe, the Middle East and in parts of India. They grow to 25m in height, with a massive trunk and widely speading boughs. In early spring, long catkins, or male flowers, hang from the previous year's branches, while the new branches sport small spikes of female flowers. The leaves, each made up of five to nine leaflets are first red, then gradually turn green. The fruit, a woody nut, has a smooth coating that changes from green to brown as it ripens.

Parts used

Leaves

● The leaves are picked in June and July, and dried rapidly at a temperature of 40°C.
● Dried leaves are used for infusions, tinctures and liquid extracts. Each must contain at least 2 per cent of the flavonoid, hyperoside.

Constituents

Walnut leaves are rich in healing tannins. Napthaquinone, juglone, and the flavonoids, hyperoside and quercetin are also present, together with ascorbic acid and essential oil.

Medicinal uses

Because the plant's nut is similar in shape and appearance to a human brain, it was traditionally believed that eating it would help to improve concentration and memory.

However, the real medicinal value of walnut stems mainly from its leaves, with their astringent, healing tannins and antibacterial juglone. Leaf preparations are used to treat diarrhoea and intestinal infections, and are reputed to boost immunity and improve the circulation.

Walnut leaf can also strengthen the protein, keratin, found in the surface of the skin. It is therefore an effective treatment for problems, such as acne, eczema and ulcers.

Cultivation

Buy a ready-grown small tree or plant seeds under cover in rich, well-drained acidic soil. The trees thrive in full sunlight.

CAUTION

● Although walnut has no known toxic side effects, it is not advisable to exceed the recommended dosage.

PREPARATION AND DOSAGE

For internal use

TO TREAT diarrhoea, disorders involving the bacteria of the intestinal tract

INFUSION Put 10g of dried leaves into 1 litre of boiling water. Infuse for 15 minutes, then strain. Drink 3-5 cups a day.

For external use

TO TREAT acne, eczema, skin infections and ulcers

CREAMS, GELS, SOAPS (containing 1-3% tincture or liquid extract) Use one of these preparations regularly on affected areas.

IF SYMPTOMS PERSIST, CONSULT A DOCTOR

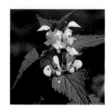

White deadnettle

Lamium album Lamiaceae **Also called** Archangel

A common weed of wasteground, roadsides and hedgerows, white deadnettle is seen throughout Europe, except in the hotter climes of the Mediterranean region. Its hollow, square stems grow to 60cm tall, bearing serrated, heart-shaped leaves. All parts of the plant are finely hairy, but unlike the common nettle they do not sting. In spring, white, two-lipped flowers cluster in whorls around the points where the leaves join the stem.

Parts used
Flowers
- The flowering tops are gathered in April and May.
- The flowers are dried quickly to preserve their colour.
- White deadnettle is used in infusions, tinctures and powders.

Constituents
The plant contains phenylpropanoid esters, iridoids (lamalbide), tannins, mucilages, saponins, organic acids and triterpenoids.

Medicinal uses
White deadnettle has traditionally been used to treat excessively heavy menstruation, bleeding after childbirth and vaginal discharge. Its decongestant properties can also be used to treat blocked sinuses. It is also prescribed to treat high blood pressure, haemorrhoids and varicose veins and as a remedy for digestive disorders such as diarrhoea, flatulence, gastritis and bloating.

Used externally, white deadnettle is beneficial in the treatment of itchy, flaky scalps and other irritations of the skin and mucous membranes. The anti-inflammatory activity of white deadnettle was confirmed experimentally in 1983, when researchers discovered that the effect was due to the plant's triterpenoid constituents.

White deadnettle is also taken to remedy insomnia.

Cultivation
White deadnettle can be grown from seed in a wild area of the garden in moist but well-drained soil in sun or light shade.

PREPARATION AND DOSAGE
For internal use
TO TREAT gynaecological disorders, diarrhoea, insomnia
INFUSION Put 2 teaspoons of dried flowers into a cup of boiling water. Infuse for 5 minutes, then strain. Sweeten with honey. Drink 3 cups a day.
TINCTURE (1:4 in 25% alcohol) Take 20 drops in a little water three times a day.
POWDER Take ¼-½ teaspoon three times a day with food or water.

For external use
TO TREAT inflammation of the skin or mucous membranes
COMPRESS Put 2 teaspoons of dried flowers into 100ml of boiling water. Infuse for 10 minutes. Soak a cloth with this infusion and apply to affected area two or three times a day.

TO TREAT vaginal discharge
DOUCHE Use an infusion (above) once or twice a day.
SITZ BATH Put 3 tablespoons of dried flowers into 500ml of boiling water. Infuse for 10 minutes. Strain and add to bath.

IF SYMPTOMS PERSIST, CONSULT A DOCTOR

CAUTION
- Do not use if suffering from intestinal obstruction.

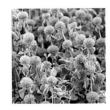

White horehound

Marrubium vulgare Lamiaceae **Also called** Common horehound

A native of the Mediterranean, white horehound is seen throughout Europe, preferring warm, sunny locations, often by roadsides. Its erect, hairy stems reach 30-60cm in height and bear wrinkly leaves with scallop-shaped indentations. In summer, small white flowers appear where the leaves join the stem. The plant has an apple-like smell.

Parts used

Flowering tops
- Harvesting begins in May and June, when the plant is in bloom.
- After drying and fragmentation, the plant is used in infusions, decoctions, tinctures and extracts.

Constituents

The flowers contain bitter diterpenes, including marrubiin, premarrubiin and marrubic acid. Other constituents include flavonoids, alkaloids and a small amount of essential oil.

Medicinal uses

The plant is traditionally used to treat coughs and it is one of the most effective herbal expectorants known. It works by breaking up and releasing phlegm, exerting an anti-spasmodic action and relieving inflammation in the respiratory tract. The expectorant activity of white horehound has been verified by experiments performed in 1976.

Due to its bitter constituents (in particular marrubiin), white horehound stimulates the appetite and aids digestion.

When used externally, white horehound is a treatment for ulcers and wounds that exude pus or that are slow to heal.

An animal study in 2001 highlighted the potential of white horehound for treating high blood pressure.

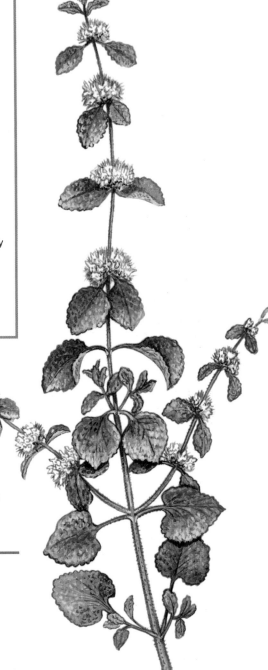

PREPARATION AND DOSAGE

For internal use

TO TREAT minor digestive problems, stubborn coughs
TINCTURE (1:4 in 25% alcohol)
Put 10-20 drops into a glass of water. Take two or three times a day before meals.

TO TREAT poor appetite
INFUSION Put 1-2g of dried plant into a cup of boiling water. Infuse for 10 minutes. Drink 3 cups a day.

For external use

TO TREAT ulcers, wounds discharging pus
COMPRESS Put 30-60g of dried plant into 1 litre of boiling water. Boil for 3 minutes and infuse for 10 minutes. Soak a cloth in this decoction and apply to the affected area once or twice a day.

IF SYMPTOMS PERSIST, CONSULT A DOCTOR

Cultivation

Plant in well-drained, neutral to alkaline soil in a sunny location. Choose a wild part of the garden as the plant can be invasive.

CAUTIONS

- High doses of marrubiin can adversely affect the heart.
- Pregnant women should avoid this herb, while those who are breastfeeding should limit consumption to small amounts.

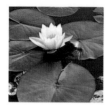

White & yellow water lily

Nymphaea alba, Nuphar luteum Nymphaeaceae

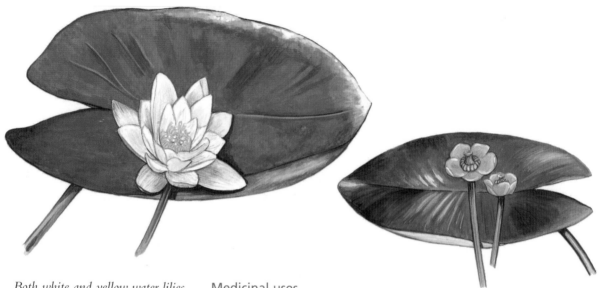

Both white and yellow water lilies are aquatic with floating leaves, submerged stems and rhizomes that anchor them to the pond floor. They have sweet-smelling flowers and large, long-stalked leaves. The white water-lily flower grows to a diameter of 12cm, while the yellow water-lily flower is 4-5cm across.

Parts used

Rhizome (both); **flowers** (white water lily)

• The flowers and rhizomes (lifted when dormant) are dried and used for infusions and decoctions.

Constituents

The rhizomes contain sesquiter-penoid alkaloids (nupharine, nymphaeine, nuphacristine, thiobinupharidine), astringent tannins, flavonoids and vitamin C.

CAUTION

• White water lily is best taken as directed by a medical herbalist as excessively high doses over a long period of time could cause an irreversible loss of libido.

Medicinal uses

The white water lily has sedative properties and relieves diarrhoea and intestinal inflammation. It is also able to reduce blood pressure.

The yellow water lily, traditionally known as the 'destroyer of pleasure and poison of love', has long been used in potions and cordials intended to reduce sexual desire and send the imbiber to sleep. In fact both white and yellow water lily share this ability to calm the libido.

The plants are used to treat inflammation of the skin, mouth and throat, and to treat catarrh. Yellow water lily is also prescribed to treat vaginal discharge and fungal infections. Studies published in *The Journal of Pharmaceutical Sciences* in 1973 verified the antifungal activity of the plants, attributing it to a sesquiterpenoid alkaloid found in the rhizomes.

Cultivation

Submerge in water up to 45cm deep and plant in moist, nutrient-rich soil.

PREPARATION AND DOSAGE

For internal use

White water lily

TO TREAT excessive sexual arousal or libido, diarrhoea
INFUSION Put 5g of dried flowers into 250ml of boiling water. Leave to infuse for 20 minutes. Strain. Drink 2-3 cups a day.
DECOCTION Put 5g of dried rhizome into 200ml of boiling water. Boil for 15 minutes. Drink 2-3 cups a day.

Yellow water lily

Use only as prescribed by a medical herbalist

For external use

White and yellow water lily

TO TREAT cracked, chapped skin, burns, sunburn, nappy rash
COMPRESS Soak a cloth with the decoction (above). Apply to affected area three to six times a day.

IF SYMPTOMS PERSIST, CONSULT A DOCTOR

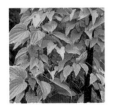

Wild yam

Dioscorea villosa Dioscoreaceae **Also called** China root, Colic root, Rheumatism root

A relative of the edible yam, wild yam is native to Mexico and the southern USA. It is a large climbing plant with dense tuberous roots and twining stems that can reach a height of 6m. Its heart-shaped leaves are held on long stalks and its yellowy green flowers form small clusters.

Parts used

Rhizome

• The plant's rhizome measures 5-10cm in diameter. Once cleaned, it is dried, crushed or ground to a powder.

• Wild yam is most frequently used in decoctions.

Constituents

Wild yam's rhizome contains steroidal saponins (dioscin, gracillin), tannins, phytosterols and starch. Wild yam is also the source of diosgenin.

Medicinal uses

Wild yam has been used to treat rheumatism and arthritis. This anti-inflammatory action is thought to be imparted by dioscin. Wild yam is also antispasmodic and is used as a treatment for colic, irritable bowel syndrome and other types of painful muscular spasms. This has led to its use in relieving menstrual cramps and labour pains. There is much folklore connected with wild yam's use in treating women's hormonal problems, but no scientific evidence to prove this. In an Australian clinical trial performed in 2001, patients were given a wild yam-based cream to rub into their bodies, while other patients received a placebo. The researchers did not observe any relief of menopausal symptoms with either the placebo or the wild yam.

PREPARATION AND DOSAGE

For internal use

TO TREAT digestive problems
DECOCTION Put 1-2g of rhizome into a cup of water. Boil for 15-20 minutes and strain. Drink 1-2 cups a day.

TO TREAT rheumatic pain
CAPSULES (powdered root, 500mg) Take 1-2 capsules up to three times a day.

IF SYMPTOMS PERSIST, CONSULT A DOCTOR

CAUTION

• Women who are pregnant or breastfeeding should avoid using wild yam.

Cultivation

Plant in well-drained, nutrient-rich soil in sun or light shade.

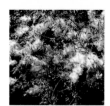

Willow

Salix alba Salicaceae **Also called** White willow

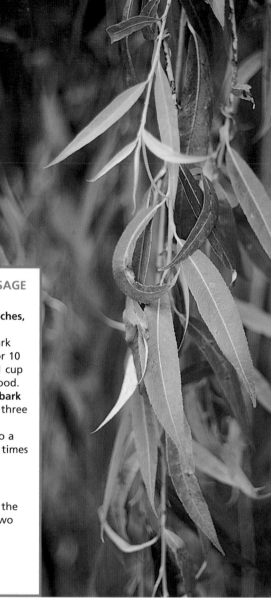

This deciduous tree is characterised by its graceful branches bearing silky, lance-shaped leaves. It grows to a height of 10-15m and is found throughout Europe in damp places, especially on riverbanks. Its flowers are catkins that appear in spring. The supple young twigs are traditionally used as a material for fences and basketwork.

Parts used
Bark
- The bark is taken from young branches collected in March from trees that are 2-5 years old.
- The bark is cut into small pieces or crushed for use in decoctions.
- It is also used in powder capsules, tinctures and liquid extracts, often in combination with other anti-inflammatory plants such as devil's claw and blackcurrant.

Constituents
Willow bark contains salicin, which the body converts into salicyl alcohol and subsequently to the known anti-inflammatory agent salicylic acid (a natural form of aspirin). It also contains flavonoids and proantho-cyanidins (condensed tannins) that are well known for their astringent and wound-healing properties.

Medicinal uses
Willow bark combats inflammation, rheumatism, pain, headaches and fever. Japanese scientists carried out experiments in 2002 which demonstrated that salicylic acid (produced from the conversion of salicin in the intestines), reduced fever without damaging the stomach.

Willow bark is also known to have an antiseptic effect and is used externally to treat wounds and ulcers. It has been used in the treatment of diarrhoea and for intestinal infections. For its ability to reduce fever, it is also indicated in the treatment of influenza.

A trial carried out in Germany in 2001 found that willow exerted a moderate analgesic effect on people who were suffering from osteoarthritis.

Cultivation
Suited to moist or wet soil and a sunny location. Willow will take up a lot of space in a smaller garden.

PREPARATION AND DOSAGE
For internal use
TO TREAT fever, flu, headaches, pains, rheumatism
DECOCTION Put 1-3g of bark into a cup of water. Boil for 10 minutes and strain. Drink 1 cup three times a day before food.
CAPSULES (200mg willow bark powder) Take 2-4 capsules three times a day with water.
TINCTURE Put 40 drops into a glass of water. Drink three times a day.

For external use
TO TREAT ulcers, wounds
COMPRESS Soak a cloth in the decoction (above). Apply two or three times a day.

IF SYMPTOMS PERSIST, CONSULT A DOCTOR

CAUTIONS
- When taken in large doses, willow can cause nausea, gastrointestinal discomfort, dizziness and a rash.
- Willow bark is not recommended for pregnant or breastfeeding women, children or people with asthma, stomach ulcers, diabetes, or kidney or liver disorders.
- Individuals who are allergic to salicylates must not take willow.
- It should not be taken in combination with diuretics, drugs that lower blood pressure or thin the blood, or non-steroidal anti-inflammatory drugs.
- Excessive use of a decoction of the plant can cause mouth sores.

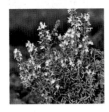

Winter savory

Satureja montana Lamiaceae

This small, woody perennial grows wild as a small bush in well-drained, chalky areas of southern Europe and bears tough, shiny, lance-shaped leaves. Winter savory has been grown as a culinary herb in Britain since the Middle Ages. Its flowers are pure white or speckled with pink.

Parts used

Non-woody flowering tops
● The herb is harvested just after the flowers come into bloom in summer.
● The crop may be dried for use as a seasoning or as an infusion or it may be processed for its essential oil.

Constituents

The essential oil is rich in carvacrol and thymol but also contains other monoterpenes. The exact mix of compounds varies according to the time of year and the weather.

Medicinal uses

Winter savory owes its therapeutic properties mainly to its essential oil. The plant is traditionally used for its tonic and digestive qualities. Today it is used in pharmaceutical products that relieve intestinal spasms as well as fungal and bacterial infections.

Externally, the herb's antiseptic properties mean it is useful for treating minor wounds, fungal skin infections, mouth ulcers, thrush and sore throats.

In 1998 in vitro studies performed by Japanese scientists found that winter savory demonstrated potent activity against HIV type 1.

Cultivation

Plant seeds in spring in a sunny spot. Use well-drained, preferably alkaline soil.

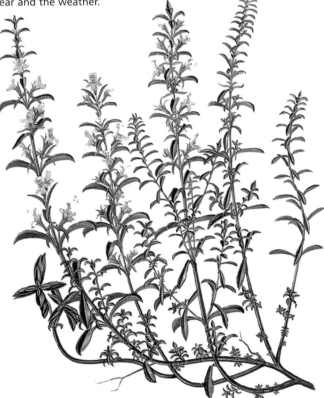

PREPARATION AND DOSAGE

For internal use

TO TREAT belching, flatulence, diarrhoea
INFUSION Put 20g of dried flowering tops into 1 litre of boiling water. Infuse for 10 minutes and strain. Drink 2-3 cups a day.

TO TREAT bronchitis, cystitis
ESSENTIAL OIL Requires the supervision of a trained herbalist or doctor.

For external use

TO TREAT minor wounds
INFUSION Put 30g of dried flowering tops into 1 litre of boiling water. Infuse for 10 minutes, then strain. Apply directly onto the wound to clean it.

TO TREAT fungal skin infections
COMPRESS Soak a cloth in the infusion (above) and apply to the affected areas two times a day.

TO TREAT mouth ulcers, thrush, sore throats
GARGLE Use the infusion (above) three or four times a day.

IF SYMPTOMS PERSIST, CONSULT A DOCTOR

CAUTIONS

● Only take the essential oil internally under the supervision of a medical herbalist or doctor.
● When the essential oil is used externally, there is a risk that it will irritate the skin.
● Winter savory is not recommended in any form for pregnant women.

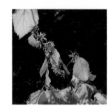

Witch hazel

Hamamelis virginiana Hamamelidaceae

A North American tree, witch hazel is widely grown for the ornamental appeal of its spidery flowers and large oval leaves. Its yellowish flowers grow in clusters at the junction of branches and leafstalks in winter. It bears brown fruit consisting of small capsules, which split to release the seeds.

Parts used

Leaves and bark

- The leaves are gathered during summer before they turn brown.
- The bark is harvested in autumn or spring.
- Once dried, witch hazel leaves and bark are used for infusions, powders, dry and liquid extracts, and tinctures.
- Witch hazel is an ingredient in mouthwashes, gels and ointments.

Constituents

Tannins constitute more than 10 per cent of the dried leaf. They impart vasoconstrictive and anti-inflammatory effects. Witch hazel also contains flavonoids – which are anti-inflammatory and strengthen the blood vessels – and a small proportion of essential oil.

Medicinal uses

Experiments have demonstrated that the extract made from witch hazel leaves strengthens veins, reduces the permeability of capillaries and has anti-inflammatory properties. It has also been shown to constrict blood vessels. In 2002 German trials showed that witch hazel can reduce erythema, which is the reddening of the skin due to dilated blood vessels. The plant's anti-inflammatory activity supports its use in treating eczema.

Witch hazel can be taken orally or applied as an ointment to treat circulatory problems such as heavy, aching legs, varicose veins and haemorrhoids.

Further German research in 2002 has demonstrated the plant's anti-microbial activity. A formulation containing witch hazel was found to be effective against the bacterium *Staphylococcus aureus* and the yeast *Candida albicans*.

The plant's antibacterial and soothing qualities account for its use in mouthwashes and eye drops.

Cultivation

Plant young specimens in moist, rich neutral to acid soil.

CAUTION

- Witch hazel appears to have no toxic effects but it might cause contact allergies.
- Pregnant or breastfeeding women should avoid taking witch hazel internally.

PREPARATION AND DOSAGE

For internal use

TO TREAT circulatory problems, haemorrhoids
INFUSION Put 10g into 1 litre of water. Leave to infuse for 5-10 minutes. Drink 1-2 cups a day.
CAPSULES (dried leaf) Take 2g three times a day.
LIQUID EXTRACT (1:1 in 45% alcohol) Take up to 2ml three times a day.

TO TREAT poor oral hygiene
INFUSION Put 2g of dried leaf into 1 cup of boiling water. Allow to infuse for 10 minutes, then strain. Rinse the mouth, then swallow, or use as a gargle. Repeat once or twice a day.

For external use

TO TREAT circulatory problems, haemorrhoids, inflammation
GELS, OINTMENTS Massage into affected area once a day.
WITCH HAZEL WATER Apply once or twice a day.
TINCTURE Add 200g of broken up dried bark to l litre of 40% alcohol and store in sterilised dark-coloured bottle. Mix 20ml tincture with 100ml water and apply to varicose veins.

IF SYMPTOMS PERSIST, CONSULT A DOCTOR

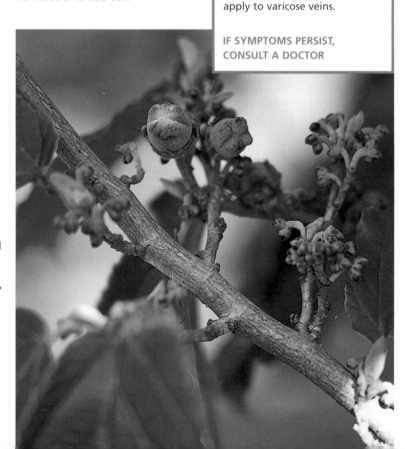

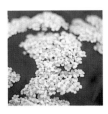

Yarrow, common

Achillea millefolium Compositae/Asteraceae **Also called** Milfoil

This European herb grows on rough ground in meadows and on roadsides. Its thin dark green leaves are divided into many segments, reflected in its Latin name of 'millefolium', which means 'a thousand leaves'. Flat heads of numerous tiny white, or sometimes pink, flowers appear in summer.

Parts used

Flowerheads, non-woody parts of the plant and seeds
- The plant is harvested just after flowering from June to October.
- Yarrow is usually dried for use as an infusion but it can also be used fresh. It is also available as a liquid extract, a tincture or as a powder.

Constituents

The flowers contain 0.2-0.5 per cent essential oil, whereas the leaves contain 0.02-0.07 per cent. The oil contains sesquiterpenes, namely azulene and lactone achilleine, which have an anti-inflammatory action. Anti-inflammatory flavonoids are also present as well as tannins, alkaloids and bitter compounds.

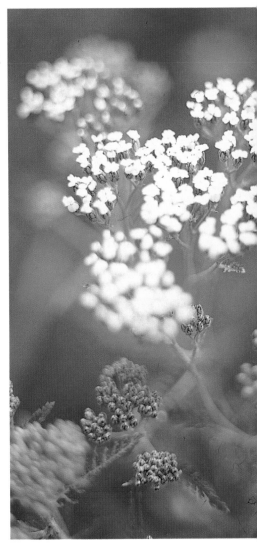

Medicinal uses

As a result of its numerous active components, yarrow has many medicinal uses. Its antispasmodic, carminative (ability to relieve the build-up of trapped wind), its anti-inflammatory and anthelminthic (capacity to destroy intestinal worms) actions are mostly due to its essential oil. Animal studies published in 1982 in *Economic Botany* established the anti-inflammatory action of the constituent azulene. Azulene also possesses antibacterial qualities, as reported in the *Journal of Ethnopharmacology* in 1986.

The plant is commonly used for the relief of digestive disorders including stomach ailments, inflammation of the intestinal walls, constipation and flatulence.

Used externally, yarrow's anti-inflammatory action relieves rheumatic pains and haemorrhoids. It is also used to treat mouth infections, conjunctivitis, eczema and other conditions including fevers.

Yarrow is diuretic, it lowers blood pressure and is also indicated for treating thrombotic diseases, and hypertension. In addition, it can be used to combat urinary tract infections.

The plant has traditionally been used to soothe uterine cramps during menstruation and childbirth. Taken regularly in small doses it can also help to regulate the menstrual cycle, particularly when menstruation is scant or infrequent.

It is used to reduce phlegm and treat conditions of the respiratory tract. Common yarrow can also cleanse greasy skin and is often found in cosmetic products.

PREPARATION AND DOSAGE

For internal use
TO TREAT digestive disorders
LIQUID EXTRACT Take up to 2ml three times a day.
INFUSION Put 1 teaspoon of the dried plant into 250ml of boiling water. Leave to infuse for 5 minutes, then strain. Drink 3-4 cups a day.

For external use
TO TREAT uterine pains
SITZ BATH Put 100g of the dried plant into 20 litres of hot water.

IF SYMPTOMS PERSIST, CONSULT A DOCTOR

Cultivation

Plant in well-drained soil and position in a sunny location.

CAUTIONS

- Common yarrow may cause contact allergies.
- It is not advisable to use it when pregnant or breastfeeding.
- Exposure to sunlight is not recommended. Yarrow may act as a photosensitiser.
- Large doses may produce vertigo and headaches.

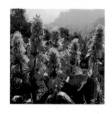

Yellow gentian

Gentiana lutea Gentianaceae **Also called** Great yellow gentian, Bitterwort

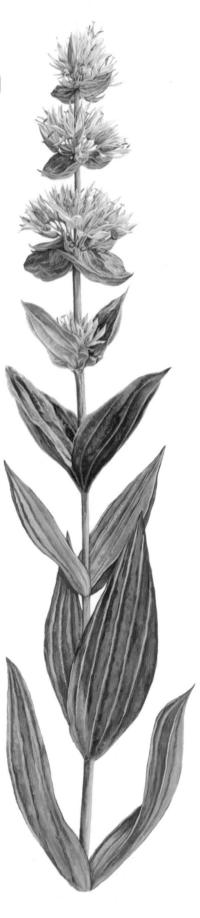

This large, upright perennial is commonly found in the Alps and other mountainous areas south of Europe. Yellow gentian's large leaves have five to seven prominent veins on the underside. The plant's showy flowers are a golden yellow and grow at the points where the leaves meet the stem. The thick, wrinkly roots have a bitter taste.

Parts used

Roots

• At the end of summer the roots are collected from wild plants that are preferably 7-10 years old.

• The roots are washed, cut up and dried in the open air.

• They are used to make powders, tinctures or extracts that are included in numerous pharma-ceutical products such as drinkable solutions, medicinal wines, tablets, capsules and syrups.

Constituents

The bitter taste of the yellow gentian root is due to secoiridoids, principally amarogentin and also gentiopicroside (from the Greek pikros, meaning bitter). When they are taken internally these substances provoke a reflex action that stimulates salivary and gastric secretions.

Medicinal uses

The substances in yellow gentian stimulate the flow of saliva and gastric juices even in very small amounts. A simple experiment proves it: merely grinding the root will cause one to salivate.

The root is traditionally used to remedy a lack of appetite and has long been an ingredient in aperitif drinks. It acts as a tonic on the whole digestive system, relieving gastric pains and improving sluggish digestion. A clinical study published in 1967 verified yellow gentian's digestive qualities, observing that the herb promoted the secretion of gastric juices.

Yellow gentian is also reputed to lower fevers and treat inflammation.

Cultivation

Plant in well-drained, humus-rich soil in a sunny or lightly shaded location.

PREPARATION AND DOSAGE

For internal use

TO TREAT gastric pains, sluggish digestion, loss of appetite
INFUSION Add 0.6-2g of dried root to 1 cup of boiling water. Infuse for 10 minutes, then strain. Drink 3 cups a day.
DRINKABLE SOLUTIONS, MEDICINAL WINES, SYRUPS Take 1-4 tablespoons before main meals.
TINCTURE Take 2-5 drops with water before eating.

IF SYMPTOMS PERSIST, CONSULT A DOCTOR

CAUTIONS

• Yellow gentian could cause some side effects, such as headaches, if used in excess of prescribed doses.

• Pregnant or breastfeeding women should not use yellow gentian.

• Individuals with gastroduodenal ulcers or high blood pressure should also avoid yellow gentian.

• The plant should only be harvested by specialists because there is a danger of confusing it with white veratrum, and also because unsustainable harvesting has made it scarce in some areas.

Yohimbe

Pausinystalia yohimbe Rubiaceae

A native of the forests of tropical Africa, yohimbe is a tall tree that can grow as high as 30m. Its reddish bark is crisscrossed with furrows and cracks, while the silky inner surface is fawn coloured and grooved lengthways. Yohimbe has large, oval, pointed leaves that are 30-40cm long. Its green, yellow or pinkish buds develop into sweet-smelling white flowers that turn yellow and then red. The tree's fruit is a flat, shuttle-shaped capsule, with two valves that open to release numerous little winged seeds.

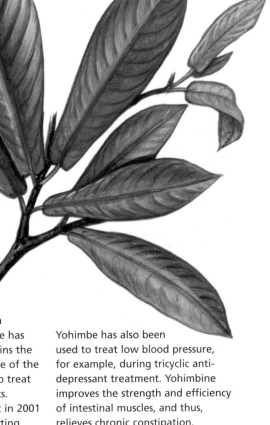

Parts used

Bark

• Bark from the trunk is picked off in the dry season, cut into pieces and then dried in the sunshine. The bark from the branches is not collected, because it contains fewer active constituents.

• The bark is odourless but has a bitter, astringent taste. It is used in pharmaceutical products.

Constituents

The plant's principal constituents are indole alkaloids, for example, yohimbine. The bark also contains another active constituent, ajmalicine.

CAUTIONS

• In no circumstances whatever should yohimbe bark be used except under medical supervision.

• The dosage has to be precisely correct, otherwise the effects can be the opposite of those intended and cause an increase in blood pressure, digestive and nervous problems.

• People with high blood pressure, kidney or liver disorders should not take yohimbe.

• Do not use yohimbe if pregnant or breastfeeding.

Medicinal uses

Yohimbe's traditional use as a treatment for male impotence has long been debated and remains the subject of active research. One of the plant's most popular uses is to treat impotence in diabetic patients.

Studies performed in Egypt in 2001 go some way towards supporting this use. Researchers found that yohimbine prevented an increase in blood sugar in both diabetic and non-diabetic rats through inhibition of alpha-2 adrenreceptors. These nerve receptors are also responsible for constricting blood vessels, and so their inhibition results in a widening of the vessels – a key to its potential for treating impotence. If further studies can verify this effect in humans, it is possible that yohimbe may one day be considered as a natural alternative to Viagra.

Yohimbe has also been used to treat low blood pressure, for example, during tricyclic anti-depressant treatment. Yohimbine improves the strength and efficiency of intestinal muscles, and thus, relieves chronic constipation.

Cultivation

Plant in moist soil. Yohimbe does not tolerate temperatures below 15°C, so must be grown in a greenhouse in the UK.

PREPARATION AND DOSAGE

Preparations that contain yohimbe should only ever be taken in consultation with a qualified medical herbalist.

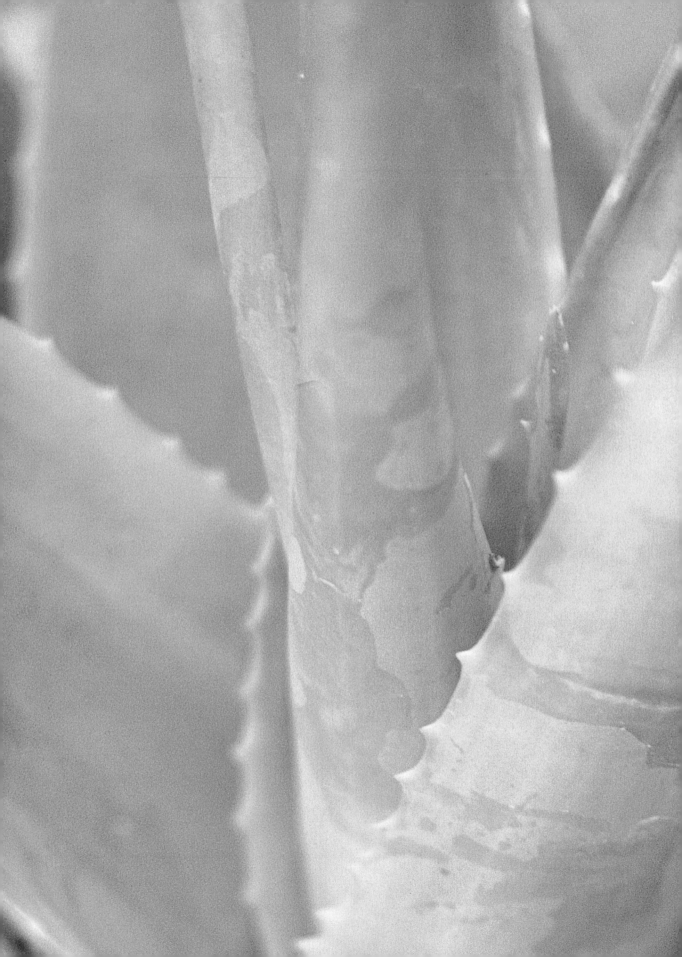

A to Z of Ailments

Addiction
Alcoholism

Characterised by the frequent and excessive consumption of alcoholic drinks, alcoholism is a state of both physical and psychological dependence. The quantity of alcohol consumed is not necessarily a determining factor, as tolerance varies according to the individual.

The British Medical Association recommends a limit of 3-4 units a day for men and 2-3 units a day for women who are not pregnant. A unit is: 25ml spirits (40% alc.vol.); 50ml sherry or port (20% alc.vol);125ml wine (8% alc.vol); or 1 small can (275ml) beer, lager or cider (3.5% alc.vol.).

The threshold of alcoholism has been defined as a daily intake in excess of 1ml pure alcohol per kilo of body weight, or 750ml (one bottle) of wine with an alcohol content of 10% for a person weighing 75kg (165lb).

Symptoms
- Trembling – sometimes known as DTs (*delirium tremens*) – until an alcoholic drink is consumed
- Redness and enlarged capillaries in the face
- Weight loss
- Blackouts
- Aggressive behaviour
- Emotional behaviour: excessive laughing or crying
- Memory problems
- Pain (polyneuritis) in the legs
- Sexual impotence

Consult your doctor or medical herbalist
- Withdrawal from excessive alcohol consumption should be carried out under medical supervision and may even require hospitalisation.

Causes
Alcoholism is often caused by depression or other psychological problems. Belonging to certain professions or social groups who drink habitually can encourage a lifestyle that leads to alcoholism. Though once an adult problem, alcoholism is beginning to affect more and more younger people.

WHICH PLANTS?
WARNING Use only one of the following at any given time

Internal usage
For anxiety and depression
Lemon balm (capsules, 200mg powder) Take 1 capsule before meals three times a day.

As a sedative
Valerian (capsules, 240mg) Take 1-2 capsules at bedtime.

Other measures
- Begin individual or group psychotherapy.
- Join a society such as Alcoholics Anonymous.
- Take vitamins B_1, B_2, B_6, nicotinamide, C, D, and E to correct the deficiencies linked to alcoholism.
- Avoid plant extracts or cosmetic products containing alcohol (such as aftershave).

See *also* Hepatitis, Cirrhosis

DID YOU KNOW?
Alcoholism

Japanese arrowroot can aid withdrawal from alcohol.

A number of studies have shown that saponins in the plant protect the liver and also combat alcohol cravings.

Japanese arrowroot is also believed to help treat symptoms of drug withdrawal.

Drug withdrawal problems

Using certain drugs that act on the brain, such as sleeping tablets or antidepressants, can create a dependency. When the course of treatment ends, it may prompt problems known collectively as 'withdrawal syndrome'.

Withdrawal from particular sedatives, such as benzodiazepines is especially difficult. If they are withdrawn too quickly, anxiety may recur, either because the condition is still present and the drugs have been withdrawn too soon, or because withdrawal itself provokes an acute reaction.

Sleeping tablets, particularly diazepam-based preparations, can also create withdrawal problems.

Symptoms
- Rapid aggravation of the condition being treated (anxiety, depression, insomnia)
- Aches and pains with no apparent cause
- Insomnia or an overwhelming desire to sleep
- Shaking, sweating and inability to concentrate
- Fatigue, irritability, depression, greatly increased or decreased sexual urges
- Convulsions (if a long-term sedative treatment is suddenly discontinued)

Consult your doctor or medical herbalist
- Some treatments must be followed for a specified period of time in order to be effective.
- Patients should never discontinue a course of treatment on their own initiative, though they may feel normal for 24 hours before experiencing symptoms of withdrawal syndrome.
- Only the prescribing doctor can help a patient through a successful withdrawal.

WHICH PLANTS?
WARNING Use only one of the following at any given time

A qualified medical herbalist can advise on the time-scale for the withdrawal and usually prescribe specific doses of plant-based treatments to ease the process.

Internal usage
Withdrawal from tranquillisers
Use plants with sedative proper-ties, such as Passionflower (tincture,1:8 in 25% alcohol). Take 25-75 drops in water at bedtime.

Withdrawal from opiates
Use plants with sedative proper-ties, such as Lavender. Infuse 2-3g of flowers in 1 cup of boiling water for 5-10 minutes, drink 3-4 cups a day between meals.

Withdrawal from anti-depressants
St John's wort (fluid extract), whose effects should take over from the antidepressant after about a week. Take 2-4ml three times a day (1:1 in 25% alcohol). The withdrawal symptoms are likely to be less pronounced and the St John's wort should help to combat any residual depression.

Other measures
- Acupuncture and yoga can help people to get through this difficult period.
- Remember that a healthy lifestyle and regular exercise can help to prevent stress.

Nicotine addiction

Nicotine addiction is a form of drug addiction resulting from the habitual use of tobacco. Its dangers are linked to both the components of the tobacco and their chemical effects on the body.

It is now known that heavy smoking can cause premature skin ageing, cancers of the mouth, lung and bladder, cardiovascular diseases (atherosclerosis, deteriora-tion of the cardiac muscle, cerebral haemorrhage), respiratory diseases (chronic bronchitis, emphysema) and impotence. It can also cause pre and postnatal prob-lems, such as miscarriage, compli-cations in pregnancy, foetal growth defects, sudden infant death syndrome and increased susceptibility to infection.

Symptoms
- An urge to smoke, especially after a meal or when taking another stimulant (eg coffee)
- When unable to smoke: diffi-culty in concentrating, irritability, a sense of deprivation, increased appetite, sleep disorders, etc.

Consult your doctor
- Sometimes nicotine addiction can require medical treatment, especially if there is any kind of associated problem.
- The practice nurse at your local surgery should be able to help with advice and even free supplies of nicotine replacement devices – these are also available from your local chemist.

Causes
The nicotine contained in tobacco is the main cause of the addiction. It modifies the chemistry of the brain and has both a stimulatory and a relaxing effect. But smoking is also a habit that often has pleasurable associations with, for example, the first cup of tea or coffee of the day, or a sociable evening or meal with friends.

WHICH PLANTS?
WARNING Use only one of the following at any given time

A programme for giving up smoking, which above all requires strong motivation, must be adapted to each individual case by the herbalist and take account of the individual's personality and lifestyle.

Internal usage
To alleviate withdrawal symptoms
Red clover (1:10 in 45% alcohol) Take 20-30 drops in a glass of water, three times a day.

To treat nervous anxiety and sleep disorders
Valerian (capsules, 500mg dried extract) Take 1-2 capsules at bedtime.

To reduce short-term stress
Siberian ginseng (capsules, 150mg) Take 1-3 capsules with water daily.

External application
To prevent voice loss, hoarseness and sore throat associated with giving up smoking
Tamarind Gargle with a decoction of the fruit pulp prepared by boiling 40g fresh pulp with 750ml of water and reducing to 500ml.
Myrrh (1:5 in 90% alcohol) Add 1 teaspoon of tincture to water and gargle. Repeat three times a day.

Ageing

Ageing is a natural process, which begins to take effect as soon as we reach adulthood and stop growing. It is caused largely by the progressive degeneration of the non-renewable tissues throughout the body and usually becomes more noticeable after the age of 60.

Symptoms

- Ageing skin
- Insomnia
- Blood, heart and circulatory problems
- Deterioration associated with the brain and nervous system and memory loss, mental fatigue and slowing down of psychomotor skills
- Breathing difficulties, chronic coughs, frequent mouth infections
- Deterioration of kidney function
- Various eye ailments
- Reduction of muscular mass and osteoporosis
- Reduced resistance to cold
- Fear of confronting new situations, irritability

Consult your doctor or medical herbalist

- Ageing is inevitable but it is important to see your doctor about troubling symptoms in case they are signs of a more serious disorder.
- GPs are advised to offer annual health checks to all patients over the age of 75, which should uncover most of these symptoms and conditions.
- A medical herbalist can suggest which herbs may prevent over-rapid ageing and limit its more harmful effects.

Causes

Disorders associated with ageing are a result of general wear and tear on the body, the ageing of tissues as cellular proteins break down, and a gradual decrease in general metabolic rate.

WHICH PLANTS?

WARNING Use only one of the following at any given time

Internal usage

To improve energy levels

Sea buckthorn Take 1-3 dessert-spoons a day of juice or syrup.
Dog rose Infuse 2-2.5g fragmented dried rosehips in a cup of boiling water for 10 minutes. Strain. Drink 3-4 cups a day.
Fenugreek (tincture, 1:3 in 25% alcohol) Take 20 drops in water three times a day.
American ginseng (capsules, 380mg) Take 2 capsules a day.

To prevent cardiovascular disorders

Garlic (capsules, 300mg) Take 1-3 capsules a day.
Ginkgo (tincture, 1:4 in 25% alcohol) Take 15 drops in water three times a day.

To alleviate anxiety

Lime tree Infuse 5g of dried flowers in 1 litre of boiling water for 5 minutes, then strain. Drink 1 cup in the evening.
Valerian (capsules, 240mg) Take 1-2 capsules a day.

To prevent digestive disorders

German chamomile Infuse 1 sachet of German chamomile flowers in a cup of boiling water for 5-10 minutes. Drink 3 cups a day before meals.
Anise Heat 1 dessertspoon of seeds in 250ml of milk, for 10 minutes. Strain. Drink after meals.

To relieve chronic coughs

Eucalyptus (tincture) Take 50 drops in a glass of water, four to six times a day.
Hyssop Infuse 1-2 teaspoons of dried flowers in a cup of boiling water for 5-10 minutes. Drink 3 cups a day.
Elecampane Boil 10-15g of dried root in 1 litre of water for 10 minutes, then strain. Take 1 dessertspoon every 2 hours.

External application

For mouth infections

Roman chamomile Infuse 1 teaspoon of dried flowers in a cup of boiling water, allow to cool. Strain and use as a mouthwash.
Myrtle Infuse 10g of dried leaves in 1 litre of boiling water for 10 minutes and strain. Cool and use as a mouthwash.
Cloves Chew a clove three or four times a day.

Other measures

- Eat small, regular meals that are nutritionally balanced and not too spicy or rich.
- Eat plenty of red fruit (bilberries, redcurrants, blackberries, raspberries) and fruit containing vitamin C (oranges, clementines, lemons, mangoes, kiwi fruit). Kiwi fruit is rich in antioxidants (thought to slow the destructive action of free radicals), vitamins, calcium and iron.
- Take as much exercise as possible as it promotes good circulation. Regular massages will also help circulation.
- Keep your mind and memory active: read, take up a hobby, join in with social activities.
- Try to reduce your stress levels through relaxation and other techniques. Stress can have an adverse effect on the liver and the digestive system.

Ageing skin

As a person ages all the elements of the skin begin to change, the surface dries and there is less tone and elasticity. This transformation is unavoidable but the speed at which it takes place varies from person to person depending on genetic make-up and lifestyle factors such as smoking and over-exposure to the sun.

Symptoms

- Wrinkles and acne rosacea to a greater or lesser degree
- Age spots on the face and hands
- Finer, more transparent skin, which turns a yellowish grey colour
- Dehydrated, flaky skin
- Dry skin due to a lack of sebum
- Flabby, itchy skin

Causes

Skin ageing is a normal part of the general ageing process. It can be accelerated by dehydration caused by exposure to the sun or wind, by a lack of the vitamins A and D, and by excessive alcohol consumption and smoking.

WHICH PLANTS?

WARNING Use only one of the following at any given time

Internal usage

To improve skin condition
Evening primrose (soft capsules, 500mg) Take 1-2 capsules a day with a glass of water at mealtimes.

External application

To treat dry, rough skin
Evening primrose Mix 3 drops of essential oil to every 10ml of carrier oil. Apply once or twice a day.
Marigold Apply a marigold-based cream as directed on the label.

Other measures

- Reduce your use of alcohol and stop smoking.

- Prevent dehydration by drinking 1.5-2 litres of water every day and, if possible, do not use diuretics such as dandelion.
- Take cod-liver oil capsules (1 capsule a day) and brewer's yeast (2g a day).
- Avoid overexposure to sun and sunbeds and protect your skin against ultraviolet radiation with products suited to your skin type.

Memory loss

Memory is the product of a network of millions of neurons communicating with each other and transmitting information received through the five senses. There are two kinds of memory. Short-term memory retains practical information that is useful more or less immediately (the time of an appointment, for example). Long-term memory stores recollections of past events.

The problems of each type of memory-loss, therefore, have different consequences. Memory loss can affect anyone over 60, and in some cases younger people too.

Symptoms

- Short-term memory loss: inability to recall recent events; poor attention span; appearing withdrawn; disturbed sleep
- Long-term memory problems: no sense of time or place; difficulty in recognising others, or of remembering past events; depression

Consult your doctor or medical herbalist

- Consult your doctor if the symptoms occur persistently. Medical advice is essential as it can indicate the development of Alzheimer's disease and other causes of dementia.

Causes

Ageing is one of many factors that can cause memory problems. Other causes include: stress, physical exertion, certain medications (such as antidepressants), arterial hypertension, hypothyroidism, syphilis, alcoholism, lack of sleep, lack of vitamins B_1, B_{12}, epilepsy, concussion, stroke or cranial trauma.

WHICH PLANTS?

WARNING Use only one of the following at any given time

Internal usage

To improve the blood supply to the brain
Ginkgo (capsules, 50-100mg) Take 1 capsule three times a day before meals.
See also Cerebral circulation

External use

Sage and lemon balm (essential oils) have both been shown to inhibit an enzyme that causes the breakdown of acetylcholine (a key chemical involved in memory storage). Recent UK research has shown that sage and lemon balm have great potential for reducing memory loss, and it is possible that both essential oils from the plant could be used to beneficial effect in an aromatherapy massage.

Other measures

- Keep up intellectual and social activities.
- Take regular physical exercise which will help you to relax, improve your sleep and develop your concentration.
- Take care to eat a healthy, well-balanced diet.

Ageing

Wrinkles, bags under the eyes

The first visible signs of ageing usually appear on the face as wrinkles and shadows under the eyes. There may also be swelling and reddening of the upper eyelids.

Symptoms
- Wrinkles: creases of varying depths in the skin
- Bags under the eyes: puffy, darkened skin below the eyes

Causes
Wrinkles are due to the loss of elasticity in the skin that occurs with age. Premature wrinkling can be caused by overexposure to the ultraviolet rays in sunlight.

The first lines to appear are usually 'crows'-feet', more generously termed 'laughter lines', which occur at the corners of the eyes as a result of repeatedly contracting the facial muscles. Frown lines may occur between the eyebrows and furrows may crease the forehead.

Bags under the eyes are due to a congestion of the area beneath the lower eyelid, when there are localised problems with the circulation of lymph. They often appear in cases of acute or long-term insomnia. Stress, headaches and fatigue can accentuate the problem.

WHICH PLANTS?
WARNING Use only one of the following at any given time

Internal usage
To combat wrinkles
Evening primrose (soft capsules, 500mg) Take 1-2 capsules a day during meals with a glass of water.

External application
To combat wrinkles
Marigold Apply marigold-based cream daily as directed on the label.

To treat bags under the eyes
Green/black tea Infuse two sachets of dried leaves in boiling water for 5 minutes, allow to cool and then place one over each eye for 5-10 minutes.
Roman/German chamomile Follow directions for green/black tea (see above).

Other measures
- Don't smoke; moderate your alcohol intake.
- Avoid stress and learn to relax.
- Eat a healthy diet.
- Drink 2 litres of water a day.

Allergies

Allergies result from an abnormal reaction of the body's immune system when it comes into contact with a particular substance. The substance (known as an allergen) does not provoke the same reaction among non-allergic people. Allergic reactions may occur rapidly after contact with the allergen or can be delayed by several hours.

Symptoms
- Difficulty breathing, wheezing (asthma), coughing
- Rash, itching, urticaria
- Runny nose, blocked nose, sneezing
- Conjunctivitis: sore, red eyes that are watery or itchy
- Diarrhoea (in the case of food allergies)
- In rare cases, a person may develop such an extreme sensitivity to a substance that they suffer anaphylactic shock when they come into contact with it. This life-threatening condition is characterised by swelling of the lips, tongue and throat. The airway may become blocked and there may be a loss of consciousness. The most common triggers are insect stings, shellfish and nuts

Consult your doctor
- Medical advice is needed to determine the cause of an allergy and to evaluate its degree of severity. A doctor may suggest skin or blood testing to try to identify the allergen.
- Seek immediate emergency medical attention for cases of swelling of the lips, throat and upper body, or if there is any difficulty in breathing.
- Some susceptible people are advised to carry adrenaline injections or antihistamine tablets for protection against future attacks.

Causes

Contact hypersensitivity may be due to plants, metal, fabric, etc. Respiratory allergies are triggered by pollen (see hay fever), animal hair, mould, house dust. Food allergies are caused by numerous types of food and by certain food colorants. They can affect specific parts of the body. For example, people who are allergic to lactose may have an allergic reaction of the digestive tract.

Susceptibility to allergies often runs in families. Stress and alcohol intake may aggravate the symptoms of an allergy.

WHICH PLANTS?

WARNING Use only one of the following at any given time

Internal usage

To ease digestive allergic reactions

Globe artichoke Infuse 30-40g of dried leaves in 1 litre of boiling water for 10 minutes, then strain. Drink 3 cups a day 15-20 minutes before meals.
Peppermint Infuse 1 dessertspoon of dried leaves in 150ml of boiling water for 10-15 minutes. Strain. Drink 1 cup after every meal.

To combat eye symptoms

Greater plantain Put 1-2 drops of sterile eye lotion in each eye two or three times a day.

To combat nasal symptoms

Common elder (tincture, 1:5 in 25% alcohol) Take 20 drops in water three times a day after meals.

Other measures

- Avoid all contact with known allergens as far as possible.
- Pay attention to your diet: milk, tomatoes, chocolate and eggs are the foods most frequently implicated in chronic food allergies; shellfish and nuts are commonly associated with violent and sudden allergic reactions. You can try to find the culprits by following an elimination diet: cut out one, and only one, suspect food from your diet completely for two weeks, observe any changes in your symptoms, then start eating the food again and observe what happens. Then try another suspect.
- Take supplements that can ease the symptoms of allergic reactions: vitamin C, flavonoids, vitamin E, group B vitamins (particularly pantothenic acid B_5); but also calcium, magnesium and especially manganese which are often deficient in people who have allergies. Essential fatty acids omega-3 and omega-6 are important, as are vitamin A and zinc.

See also Eczema

Hay fever

One of the most common allergies is triggered by pollen. Hay fever is suffered by nearly 10 per cent of the UK population, who are affected in the respiratory tract and eyes. The allergy tends to start during adolescence or early adulthood and is associated with a family history of allergies (including eczema and asthma).

Symptoms

- Blocked nose
- Frequent sneezing
- Nasal discharge, initially runny and clear and then thick and greenish yellow
- Itching in the nasal area, eyes, and throat
- Sometimes wheezing in the chest, or worsening of an already existing asthma

Consult your doctor

- If breathing becomes difficult, asthma symptoms worsen, or there is swelling of the lips, mouth or throat, seek immediate medical attention.

Causes

There is a hypersensitive reaction to grass and tree pollens, or sometimes the spores of certain fungi. The histamine released from the lining of nasal, eye, or lungs leads to inflammation and swelling, with excessive production of mucus.

WHICH PLANTS?

WARNING Use only one of the following at any given time.

Internal usage

German chamomile Add 1 teabag to 1 cup of boiling water. Infuse for 10 minutes. Drink 3 cups a day before meals.
Ginger (tincture, 1:5 in 60% alcohol) Take 30 drops of tincture a day in a glass of water.

Other measures

- Increase your fluid intake to maintain the water content of the mucous membranes.
- Testing can be arranged through your GP to try to isolate the exact allergen that is causing the hay fever – desensitising injections are sometimes recommended but these occasionally produce dramatic reactions, and are not always effective.
- Try to avoid areas where there is a lot of your particular allergen in flower, especially when the pollen counts are high (as announced by the Met Office)

See also Common cold and allergic rhinitis, Asthma, Eye disorders

Insect stings and bites

When insects sting or bite, the wound can vary from a small skin lesion to a large angry swelling – as the body reacts against the irritant or toxin.

Symptoms
- Redness
- Bruising (haematoma)
- Swelling
- Appearance of blisters
- Itching

Consult your doctor or medical herbalist
- Insect bites are usually innocuous but some people are more sensitive than others and can have a serious allergic reaction. If this happens seek immediate emergency medical attention.

Causes
The bite or a sting causes a localised reaction. The insect may also inject poison through its sting, further irritating the skin.

WHICH PLANTS?
WARNING Use only one of the following at any given time

External application
Lavender Soak 100g of lavender flowers in 0.5 litres of alcohol that is 30% proof. Apply two or three times a day.
Common thyme Dilute the essential oil, allowing 5 drops to 10ml carrier oil. Apply to the affected area two to three times a day.
Marigold Infuse 5g of dried flowerheads in 1 litre of boiling water for 5 minutes. Soak a cloth in this infusion and apply three or four times a day.
Greater plantain Rub fresh leaves directly onto the affected area or apply a cream containing 4% of the extract.

Other measures
- Wear clothes that cover most of your body when you are in a badly infested area.
- Use an insect repellent. This can include using citronella, lavender, common thyme and peppermint essential oil in a vapouriser or oil burner. Or add drops of the oils to strips of material and hang by open windows and doors.
- Lemon juice and vinegar can help to reduce the irritation of wasp stings; alkalis (bicarbonate of soda, diluted ammonia) are better for bee stings.

Urticaria

Urticaria (hives) is an allergic skin reaction which looks very similar to nettle rash. It is characterised by raised white or yellow areas surrounded by red inflammation. The weals are extremely itchy and vary in size. Normally urticaria lasts a few hours, but it can be persistent. If it lasts longer than six weeks, it is termed chronic.

Symptoms
- A rash that forms rapidly and can cover the entire body
- Inflamed, sensitive skin with raised itchy white or yellow lumps
- General malaise

Consult your doctor
- Urticaria is never benign. It can spread rapidly in a very short time and always requires medical attention.

Causes
Urticaria can be caused by an allergy to food (such as lemons, nuts and tomatoes), medication or an insect bite or sting. It can arise after contact with a wide variety of plants, including primulas and, of course, stinging nettles.

Urticaria can also be caused by certain viral and parasitic infections or it can occur as part of an autoimmune disorder. In some cases it may be a reaction to cold, water or sunlight.

WHICH PLANTS?
WARNING Use only one of the following at any given time

Internal usage
To reduce inflammation
German/Roman chamomile Infuse 1 teaspoon of dried flowerheads in a cup of boiling water for 10 minutes, then strain. Drink 3 cups a day.

To soothe the liver
Milk thistle (tablets, 200mg) Take 1-2 tablets a day with meals.
Globe artichoke (capsules, 50-100mg) Take 1-2 capsules two or three times a day.

External application
To soothe the rash
German/Roman chamomile Soak a flannel in a bowl of tepid water to which has been added 2 drops of essential oil. Apply to the affected area.
Lavender Prepare a compress as for German chamomile (see above).
Thyme Prepare a compress as for German chamomile (see above).

As directed by a medical herbalist
- Liquorice, Fumitory, Greater plantain

Other measures
- Try to identify a trigger for the urticaria and avoid contact with it.
- Consult an acupuncturist. Chronic urticaria may respond to this therapy.

Blood, heart & circulatory problems

Anaemia

When the level of oxygen-carrying haemoglobin in the blood is below normal a person is said to be anaemic. Anaemia is often due to a deficiency of iron (the mineral needed to make haemoglobin), but there are numerous other causes. Anaemia is often a symptom of other underlying disorders or ailments.

Symptoms

- Fatigue, exhaustion
- Pale or grey tinged skin
- Dizziness when moving from a seated to a standing position
- Rapid heart rate and breathlessness at the slightest exertion
- Headaches

Consult your doctor

- Anaemia should not be taken lightly: it may not be serious, but equally it can signify the onset of a serious illness. A medical consultation is required for a proper diagnosis and to determine the origin of the anaemia.

Causes

Menstruation (in particular abnormally heavy periods) is the main cause of iron deficiency in women, together with pregnancy which drains the body's reserves. Disorders of the intestine, where there is loss of blood or malabsorption of iron and vitamins, may lead to anaemia. It can also result from long-term, usually inflammatory diseases such as rheumatoid arthritis, in which case the anaemia cannot be treated by diet or vitamin supplements alone.

WHICH PLANTS?

WARNING Use only one of the following at any given time

Internal usage

Stinging nettle Infuse 2-4g of dried leaves in a cup of boiling water. Strain. Drink 3 cups a day.
Stinging nettle Drink 10-15ml of fresh juice three times a day.
Stinging nettle (capsules, 500mg) Take 3-6 capsules a day.
Stinging nettle (tincture, 1:4 in 25% alcohol) Take 20 drops in water three times a day after meals.
Fenugreek Take 2g of seeds that have been crushed to a powder with a small amount of water each day. Flavour with a twist of lemon or dried mint leaves.

Other measures

- As a preventative measure, adopt a diet that is rich in iron and vitamins.
- Reduce your consumption of all foods likely to impair the absorption of iron, such as bran, foods rich in phosphorus (such as fizzy drinks), or stimulants (tea and coffee).

Angina

A strangling or constrictive pain in the chest is a classic symptom of angina. It is caused by a lack of oxygen in the heart muscle, usually due to an insufficient blood supply. The pain usually coincides with periods when the heart is working hard, such as during exercise, and diminishes with rest.

However, attacks may also occur when the person is inactive or even during sleep. Angina is sometimes the precursor of a heart attack (myocardial infarction) which accompanies death of part of the heart muscle.

Symptoms

- Intense and varying pain in the chest around the sternum (breastbone), radiating up to the neck and face, shoulders and arms (commonly the left arm)
- Dizziness and a tendency to faint
- Palpitations
- Breathlessness during exertion
- Nausea sometimes accompanied by vomiting
- Anxiety caused by the symptoms experienced

Consult your doctor

- If you regularly experience any of the above symptoms, especially if there is a history of cardiovascular disease in your family, consult a doctor.
- Herbal remedies should be used to complement conventional treatments and cannot replace regular medical supervision.

Causes

The most frequent causes are stress, tobacco, alcohol and excess blood cholesterol. Angina pectoris can also be caused by poor blood supply due to a lesion on a coronary artery (arteritis), or may occur following the constriction of an artery as a result of stress.

WHICH PLANTS?

WARNING Use only one of the following at any given time

The following may be recommended as a complementary treatment to conventional medicine:

As directed by a medical herbalist

- Hawthorn, Valerian, Garlic, Ginkgo, Ginger

Other measures

- Introduce foods containing antioxidants into your diet (including most fruit and fresh vegetables).
- Stop smoking (see Nicotine addiction).
- Adopt a low-cholesterol diet.
- Avoid stressful situations.
- If you have a sedentary lifestyle, take up physical activity gradually after an attack of angina.
- In place of sporting activity, go for a brisk daily walk of around 45-90 minutes duration.

Arrhythmia

Abnormalities in the rhythm or rate at which the heart beats are collectively termed arrhythmia. The rhythm of the heart is created by the contractions of the cardiac muscle which has a normal frequency of about 70-75 contractions a minute. When the heart beat is faster than normal, the arrhythmia is termed tachycardia, and when slower than normal it is termed bradycardia.

Symptoms

- Difficulty in breathing, breathlessness
- Blue lips and extremities (cyanosis)
- A trembling feeling beneath the sternum, or a feeling that the heart is pounding or beating too fast in the chest
- Tiring easily
- Oedema (water retention)
- Sometimes a cough

Consult your doctor

- An abnormal heartbeat rhythm can constitute a medical emergency. Contact your doctor as there are several types of arrhythmia, of varying degrees of severity, and only a GP or a specialist can determine the correct form of treatment.

Causes

Abnormal heartbeat rhythms are caused by a disruption of the electrical impulses within the heart muscle. Abnormal heartbeat rhythms are often the result of a heart condition such as coronary artery disease or myocardial infarction, may be due to a disorder concerning the valves of the heart, or to hormonal disorders (such as hyperthyroidism).

WHICH PLANTS?

WARNING Use only one of the following at any given time

The following plants may be recommended as a supplement to conventional medicine:

As directed by a medical herbalist

- Hawthorn, St John's wort, Lemon balm, Black horehound, Passionflower, Valerian

Other measures

- Learn to control anxiety, which increases heartbeat rhythms.
- Avoid all unnecessary fatigue and take time out to rest.
- Take trace elements, especially selenium, daily as directed by your doctor or medical herbalist.
- Reduce stimulants such as tea, coffee, chocolate.

Atherosclerosis, arteritis

Affecting the large and medium arteries, atherosclerosis is characterised by the build-up of fatty deposits, complex starches, blood platelets, fibrous and calcium-containing tissue on the artery wall. The arteries gradually harden and are eventually obstructed by the accumulation of the deposits.

Arteritis is the term given to inflammation of the arterial walls causing a narrowing or complete obstruction. Although the symptoms of arteritis are similar to atherosclerosis, treatment differs and usually involves strong anti-inflammatory medication or steroids. Complementary herbal medicine for the condition is best taken as advised by a competent medical herbalist.

Symptoms

These only appear when the condition is serious enough to affect blood flow. Symptoms vary according to the area of the body affected and can include:

- Circulatory problems of the brain, angina or heart attack and renal failure
- Pins and needles in the legs
- Intermittent pain in the calf occurring, for example, after walking a limited distance on level ground or climbing a short flight of stairs
- Cold feet
- Reduced hair growth on the legs
- Dead tissue, poorly healing wounds or even leg ulcers, and risk of gangrene

Consult your doctor

- It is best to consult a doctor about treatment although herbal medicines can play a useful complementary role.
- Atherosclerosis is a natural part of ageing, but it can be delayed and the severity of accompanying symptoms can be reduced by following a special diet and with the aid of medical herbalism.
- A competent medical herbalist should be able to suggest which plants to take for your particular condition and symptoms.

Causes

Atherosclerosis is partly due to the natural ageing of the arteries, but is also associated with obesity, diabetes, high blood pressure and

---

DID YOU KNOW?

Atherosclerosis

Garlic acts on arterial blood by reducing the level of lipids it contains. It also acts on the arterial walls causing the smooth arterial muscles to relax so that the blood vessels dilate. In this way garlic helps to combat hypertension and atherosclerosis.

high cholesterol. Those who have poor eating habits, smoke or drink alcohol to excess are most at risk.

WHICH PLANTS

WARNING Use only one of the following at any given time

The aim of the treatment is to rejuvenate the arteries and tackle problems due to high blood cholesterol, high blood pressure or diabetes.

Internal usage

As a preventative measure
Garlic (capsules, 300mg) Take 1-3 capsules a day or 900mg fresh garlic.
Ginger (tincture, 1:5 in 60% alcohol) Take 60-100 drops a day with water.
Ginkgo (tincture, 1:4 in 25% alcohol) Take 15 drops with water three times a day before meals.
Bilberry (tablets, 60mg) Take 1-3 tablets a day with water.
Sweet clover (tincture) Take 35 drops in a glass of water three times a day with meals.
Globe artichoke (capsules, 50-100mg) Take 1-2 capsules, two or three times a day.

Other measures

- Make sure your diet contains sufficient polyunsaturated fats (use vegetable and olive oils in cooking) and antioxidants such as vitamin C.
- Avoid a sedentary lifestyle, be physically active: a daily brisk walk of at least half an hour is recommended.
- Limit your intake of processed sugary foods.
- Eat fresh fruit.
- Limit your consumption of alcohol.
- Take a course of selenium.

See also Diabetes, Hypertension, Angina, Lipid disorders, Obesity

Chilblains

The excessive constriction of blood vessels just beneath the skin during cold weather can lead to the itchy, purple-red swellings known as chilblains. The condition generally affects the extremities (nose, hands, feet and ears).

Symptoms

- Initially, the skin becomes white and stiff and loses feeling
- Next, the skin turns intensely red or purple and is very painful
- Blisters and cracks appear

Consult your doctor

- In extreme cases, if sores and ulcers develop, it is best to consult your GP
- For minor cases, a medical herbalist, pharmacist or chiropodist will be able to advise which lotions or creams will help circulation problems, prevent itching and promote healing.

Causes

Exposure to natural or artificial cold or contact with a very cold surface such as ice or snow may inhibit the circulation of the blood. If this continues, it can lead to the death of the affected skin and to deep sores. Those most at risk include elderly people with circulation problems and people suffering from anaemia.

WHICH PLANTS?

WARNING Use only one of the following at any given time

Internal usage

Blackcurrant Infuse 5g of dried leaves in 1 litre of boiling water for 5 minutes, then strain. Drink 2-3 cups a day.
Blackcurrant (capsules, 340mg) Take 2 capsules three times a day.
Ginger (tincture, 1:5 in 60% alcohol) Take 60-100 drops a day in a glass of water.

Ginkgo (tincture) Take 15 drops in water three times a day before meals.

External application

Black mustard Mix 50g of fresh black mustard powder with 200g of flax powder. Add enough luke-warm water to make a thick paste and then wrap it in a thick cloth. Place the poultice wherever the pain occurs for about 10 minutes. When treating a child, do not apply the poultice for more than 3-5 minutes.
Capsicum Apply capsicum-based ointment to the affected area three to four times a day, as directed on the label.
Ginger Place fresh ginger root on unopened chilblains twice a day.
Marigold Infuse 5g of dried flowerheads in 1 litre of boiling water for 5 minutes. Soak a cloth in this infusion and apply to affected area three or four times a day.

As directed by a medical herbalist

- Lesser periwinkle

Other measures

- Protect the most exposed parts of the body from the cold.
- In cases of serious chilblains, follow a course of physiotherapy to regain mobility in the affected areas.

Haemorrhoids

The swollen veins, known as haemorrhoids or piles, occur in the lining of the anus. They may bleed or protrude outside the anus (prolapsed haemorrhoids) and cause pain on passing stools.

Symptoms

- Rectal bleeding on defecation
- Inflammation of the anus with swelling and the formation of soft, swollen veins in the lining
- Pain on defecation
- Mucous discharge and itching around anal opening (prolapsed haemorrhoids)
- Hard haemorrhoids and extreme pain, as a result of thrombosis in the veins – termed 'thrombosed external haemorrhoids'
- Occasionally, sharp pain caused by a fissure (tear) of the anus

Causes

Often hereditary, haemorrhoids are linked to chronic complaints that increase the pressure inside the abdomen (such as constipation, a chronic cough or bronchitis, pregnancy or confinement, recurrent heavy lifting and prolonged sitting). A diet lacking in fibre and digestive irritants (such as spicy food) can also be contributary.

Consult your doctor

- More serious cases, including prolapsing haemorrhoids, can require medical treatment, and sometimes surgery. A doctor can also establish that the disorder is haemorrhoids, rather than an anal fistula or a lesion that may produce similar symptoms but require different treatment.

WHICH PLANTS?

WARNING Use only one of the following at any given time

Internal usage

Grape seed (capsules, 30mg) Take 1 capsule a day.
Horse chestnut (tablets, 300mg) Take 1 tablet a day. Or use horse chestnut externally (see below).
Bilberry (tablets, 60mg) Take 1-3 tablets a day with water.
Blackcurrant Infuse 5g of dried leaves in 1 litre of boiling water for 5 minutes. Strain. Drink 2-3 cups a day.
Ginkgo (tincture) Take 15 drops of tincture in a glass of water three times a day before meals.

External application

Horse chestnut Apply horse chestnut-based ointment, cream or gel as directed.
Roman chamomile Apply chamomile flower water two or three times a day.
Lesser celandine (creams or ointments containing 3%) Apply twice a day.
Witch hazel Apply witch hazel-based ointment once a day.

Other measures

- Avoid external irritants (such as tight-fitting clothes) and internal ones (spices, alcoholic drinks).
- Observe strict hygiene.
- Avoid sitting for extended periods.
- Calm the inflammation with ice cubes wrapped in a fine cloth.
- If constipation occurs, follow an appropriate dietary regime or take gentle medication as recommended by your medical herbalist.
- Try not to carry or lift heavy weights.

See also Constipation

High blood pressure

An abnormal increase in the blood pressure of the arteries is known medically as hypertension. A permanent resting blood pressure that is greater than 140/85mm Hg is considered high. It can be symptomless or you may experience one or more of the following.

Symptoms

- Tiredness, breathlessness following effort
- Buzzing in the ears
- Occasional dizzy spells

Consult your doctor

- If you experience the above symptoms, consult your doctor to find out if you suffer from hypertension. If your blood pressure is higher than 140/85 mm Hg, it is wise to arrange to have it checked regularly.

Causes

High blood pressure can be hereditary or metabolic, or it may be associated with atherosclerosis. It is also linked to obesity and high alcohol intake.

WHICH PLANTS?

WARNING Use only one of the following at any given time

The following plants may be recommended as a complementary treatment to conventional medicine:

As directed by a medical herbalist

- **Garlic, Black cohosh, Hawthorn, Celery, Common elder, Blackcurrant, Valerian**

Other measures

- Adjust your diet if you suffer from obesity, gout, diabetes or from atherosclerosis.

- Reduce body weight to within 10 per cent of the ideal for you.
- Avoid tobacco and reduce alcohol consumption.
- Take regular physical exercise.
- Practise a relaxing hobby such as yoga, judo, meditation.
- Ensure that your diet contains as much fresh fruit and vegetables as possible.
- Reduce the amount of salt in your food. Use 'Lo-salt' as a salt substitute.

Lipid disorders

This term covers all anomalies in the balance of fatty substances (lipids) that circulate in the blood (including levels of cholesterol, phospholipids and triglycerides). An excess of these fats overloads the blood vessels and causes circulatory problems that can lead to serious illness. Blood tests are needed to identify abnormal levels of lipids in the blood. Symptoms appear as a result of circulatory problems.

Symptoms
- Dizziness, buzzing in the ears
- Pain in the chest or legs on walking (see Angina, Atherosclerosis)
- Fatty patches in the skin under the eyes or elsewhere

DID YOU KNOW?
Lipid disorders

Studies have shown that eating fewer saturated fats and replacing them with polyunsaturated vegetable oils, such as sunflower oil, will lower blood cholesterol levels more effectively than any other dietary measure.

Consult your doctor
- Monitoring and prevention are very important in this type of ailment. It is therefore essential to consult a doctor, who will make an accurate diagnosis and prescribe the appropriate tests and treatment.

Causes

In 80 per cent of cases, lipid disorders are genetic and have nothing to do with diet; in the remaining 20 per cent, a healthy diet can bring improvement. Lipid problems can be due to diabetes, obesity, age, alcohol intake, tobacco, the menopause. They can also be brought on by medication (contraceptives and some anti-HIV medicines).

WHICH PLANTS?
WARNING Use only one of the following at any given time

Internal usage
Garlic (tincture) Take 40-50 drops three times a day.
Ginger (tincture, 1:5 in 60% alcohol) Take 60-100 drops a day in a glass of water.
Globe artichoke (capsules, 50-100mg dry extract) Take 1-2 capsules, two or three times a day.

Other measures
- Stop smoking and avoid too much alcohol, although there is evidence that one glass of red wine a day is beneficial.
- Drink green tea.
- Take regular exercise.
- Adopt a diet low in saturated fats and sugar.
- Consume less meat and dairy products.

Low blood pressure

When the blood pressure is well below average the medical term is hypotension. It is most often noticed by a sufferer on moving from a seated position to standing, when there may be temporary dizziness. The normal response of the body is to raise the blood pressure a little on standing, in order to maintain a good flow of oxygen to the brain.

Symptoms
- Dizzy spells, giddiness, blurred vision, headache
- Dizziness sometimes experienced by older men when passing urine during the night (known as micturition syncope)

Consult your doctor
- Only a doctor can measure blood presssure accurately and determine the appropriate treatment for hypotension.

Causes

Hypotension may be brought on by a fall in the blood pressure of the lower limbs (perhaps due to varicose veins). It often occurs on rising, following a prolonged spell of sitting or lying down; this is known as postural hypotension.

The drop in pressure on changing position is common among the elderly. More rarely, hypotension can be caused by cardiac or kidney problems, or sometimes by dehydration due to medication, especially diuretics.

WHICH PLANTS?
WARNING Use only one of the following at any given time

The following plants may be recommended as a complementary treatment to conventional medicine:

Low blood pressure contd

As directed by a medical herbalist

- Winter savory, Ginger, Rosemary

Other measures

- Wear support stockings to avoid varicose veins, which cause circulation problems.
- Get up slowly, gently moving to a sitting position first to avoid sudden falls in blood pressure; be sure to have some support while standing or walking.

Lymphoedema

In this chronic condition a limb may swell excessively due to an accumulation of lymph in the tissues. Lymph is a clear fluid that bathes all the body's cells, removing waste products and fighting infection. It circulates around the body via a network of lymphatic vessels. A malfunction anywhere in this network causes characteristic swelling in one or several limbs.

Symptoms

- Swelling
- Pains, cramp
- Swollen arm (following radical surgery such as a mastectomy, for example
- Permanent, whitish swelling of the leg
- Tension and feeling of tiredness in the limbs

Consult your doctor or medical herbalist

- Lymphoedema requires medical treatment in which plants can play a helpful part. Medical intervention should be sought as soon as lymphoedema strikes any part of the body.

Causes

Lymphoedema is the result of a breakdown in the drainage of lymph. The problem may be caused by poor blood circulation, vein disorders, complications following surgical removal of a vein, or when blood flow is obstructed in some way, as in arthritis of the knee or if cancer spreads through the lymphatic system. It may also occur after surgical removal of lymph nodes or following radiotherapy.

WHICH PLANTS?

WARNING Use only one of the following at any given time

External application

For use in massage
Witch hazel Apply witch hazel-based cream always working towards the heart. Use the cream as directed on the label.

In the bath
Cypress Add up to 8 drops of essential oil to running bath water. Bathe for 10-20 minutes.
Rosemary Add up to 8 drops of essential oil to running bath water. Bathe for 10-20 minutes.

Other measures

- To dissipate the swelling, consult a physiotherapist who can give the appropriate advice and suggest suitable exercises.
- Manual drainage (gentle massages) by a physiotherapist may help.
- Moderate exercise, such as using an exercise bicycle, gentle walking or swimming.
- Support bandages, in layers or spread out, are often a relief, but best applied by a nurse.

Phlebitis

When the wall of a vein becomes inflamed the condition is termed phlebitis. Phlebitis can affect a superficial vein or a more deeply situated blood vessel. The latter is serious and should be treated urgently as there is a risk of the formation of blood clots that may lead to a partial or total blockage of an artery (embolism).

Symptoms

- Swelling and pain over the inflamed vein (shooting pains when you touch it)
- Redness and heat in the skin overlying the affected vein
- Slight fever

Consult your doctor

- Always consult your doctor if phlebitis is suspected so that a correct diagnosis of its seriousness can be made.

DID YOU KNOW?
Phlebitis

Wearing support stockings can be a useful preventative measure, but they should not be worn in existing cases of phlebitis affecting a superficial vein. In such cases the compression only aggravates the condition.

Causes

Long periods of immobility, varicose veins, minor injury to a vein (for example, after an injection or intravenous infusion) and restrictive clothing that hinders blood circulation are among the causes of phlebitis. Smoking, obesity and genetic factors are also associated with the condition.

WHICH PLANTS?

WARNING Use only one of the following at any given time

Medicinal plants can help to relieve problems associated with excessive coagulation, circulation and lesions on the wall of the vein.

As directed by a medical herbalist

- Willow, Meadowsweet, Garlic, Sweet clover, Horse chestnut, Butcher's broom, Grape seed, Witch hazel, Gotu kola

Other measures

- Avoid prolonged periods of inactivity or standing.
- Walk regularly.
- Don't wear restrictive clothing.

Raynaud's disease or phenomenon

This circulatory disorder affects the fingers and toes. On exposure to cold the blood vessels that supply the fingers and toes contract suddenly, cutting off the blood supply. This leads to pallor and then cyanosis (blueness from lack of oxygen) in the extremities for a few minutes. The phenomenon is sometimes limited to two or three fingers or toes.

Symptoms

- First stage: the fingertips (or toes) become pale, then blue. This is accompanied by intense, almost unbearable pain
- Second stage: the fingertips turn red (cyanotic), swell, and become painful again
- Tingling and numbness in the skin

Consult your doctor

- Medical advice is essential for this sometimes severe disorder, which can mask more serious conditions, such as scleroderma and rheumatoid arthritis.

Causes

Raynaud's disease or phenomenon is caused either by the effects of cold followed by sudden warming, or by some form of strong emotion, such as anxiety. It can be a sign of atherosclerosis of the extremities, blood-clotting disorders or a hormonal imbalance (thyroid). It is sometimes caused by certain medications and treatments such as beta-blockers, adrenaline or chemotherapy.

It mainly affects people between 20 and 40 years old, smokers, and is five times more common in women than men. There also seems to be a higher incidence among people who handle vibratory tools such as pneumatic drills.

WHICH PLANTS?

WARNING Use only one of the following at any given time

Internal usage

To improve circulation
Ginkgo (tincture) Take 15 drops in water, three times a day before meals.
Garlic (tincture) Take 40-50 drops three times a day.
Sweet clover (tincture) Take 35 drops in a glass of water twice a day, before meals.

Other measures

- Stop smoking.
- Avoid getting cold – wear double pairs of gloves or socks.
- Warm hands and feet gently.

Vein disorders

Varicose veins are the most common vein disorder. Others include haemorrhoids, phlebitis, and deep vein thrombosis. All are associated with impaired blood circulation.

Symptoms

- Heaviness in the legs, which diminishes during the night or while walking
- Pains and cramps in the calves and the legs
- 'Pins and needles' and restless leg syndrome
- Swelling in the thigh and/or calves.
- Swollen, painful veins in the cases of varicose veins and haemorrhoids.

Consult your doctor

- Vein disorders can be serious so it is improtant to consult your doctor to determine appropriate treatment.

Causes

Inadequate flow of blood from the feet towards the heart is generally caused by damage in the veins of the legs and failure of the small valves in the veins that help to keep the blood moving upwards. Many factors can contribute to this problem, including genetic factors, obesity, hormonal treatment, prolonged standing and raised pressure inside the abdomen.

Some people are particularly prone to vein disorders, including those with a family history of varicose veins, women who are pregnant or taking the contraceptive pill and those whose professions involve a great deal of standing or lifting heavy weights.

WHICH PLANTS?

WARNING Use only one of the following at any given time

Vein disorders contd

Internal usage
To improve blood circulation
Ginkgo (tincture) Take 15 drops in a glass of water, three times a day before meals.
Horse chestnut (capsules, 75mg) Take 2-3 capsules a day. This acts as a 'vein tonic', strengthening the veins and exerting an anti-inflammatory action.
Butcher's broom (capsules, 50mg) Take 3 capsules a day with a large glass of water at mealtimes.
Grape seed (capsules, 30mg) Take 1 capsule a day.
Sweet clover (tincture) Take 35 drops in a glass of water three times a day with meals.

External application
Horse chestnut (cream or gel) Apply horse chestnut-based cream or gel two or three times a day as directed on the label.
Cypress Dilute 3 drops of essential oil in 10ml sweet almond oil and massage into affected area.
Witch hazel Gently massage in witch hazel-based gel or ointment once a day as directed on the label.

Other measures
- As far as possible, avoid prolonged standing or sitting.
- Take regular physical exercise and walk for at least 30 minutes a day.
- Watch your diet to prevent obesity.
- Wear support stockings.
- Try not to lift heavy weights.

Water retention

When too much water is stored in the body it causes swelling known medically as oedema – or water retention. It can affect any part of the body, including the lungs and the abdominal cavity. Localised swelling, of the ankles or fingers, for example, is usually temporary and often rights itself.

Symptoms
- Swollen tissues in the area affected: lower legs, abdomen, face, arms and fingers
- Pressing the skin leaves an indentation for a few moments
- Shortness of breath, particularly when lying down

Consult your doctor or medical herbalist
- Anyone with symptoms of water retention – not to be confused with obesity – should consult a doctor to establish the cause.
- The condition is usually treated with diuretic drugs that increase urinary output. When a large amount of fluid has collected, such as in the abdomen, this may need to be drained via a tube under a local anaesthetic.

Causes
Generalised water retention can be caused by conditions that affect protein levels in the blood. These include kidney disease, liver disease and malnutrition. It can also be caused by anything that increases the leakiness of blood capillaries such as an injury or burns. Hormonal imbalances, as in premenstrual syndrome, may also cause water retention.

When a person suffers from heart failure, water retention occurs because the heart is unable to pump blood round fast enough to clear fluid from the tissues. Common, everyday causes of water retention include a sedentary lifestyle and bad posture – for example, prolonged standing or sitting with your legs crossed. Swollen ankles are common in hot weather, or when flying, especially if movement is restricted.

WHICH PLANTS?
WARNING Use only one of the following at any given time

Water retention can be a symptom of a serious medical problem. Seek advice from your doctor. A medical herbalist can advise which of the following herbs is best suited to help alleviate your symptoms.

If caused by a kidney disorder
- Ash, Barberry, Dandelion, Horsetail, Java tea, Maize, Meadowsweet, Mouse-ear hawkweed

If caused by a liver disorder
- Boldo, Globe artichoke, Hemp agrimony, Lime tree, Maize, Milk thistle, Rosemary

If due to poor circulation
- Agrimony, Butcher's broom, Grape vine, Horse chestnut, Sweet clover

If cardiac in origin
- Hawthorn

Other measures
- Reduce salt intake as sodium encourages water retention.
- Eat foods that stimulate the elimination of water such as horseradish, celery, nettle, beetroot and sorrel.
- Put your feet up during the day, with heels higher than your hips.
- Raise the foot of the bed a few centimetres – on a phone book, for example.
- Walk as much as possible to help the muscles to pump fluid back up to the heart more effectively.
- For congested lungs, sleep propped up on pillows. This will ease breathing and help the kidneys to excrete more fluid.

Brain & nervous system

Alzheimer's disease

A disease that attacks the cells, nerves and transmitters in the brain, Alzheimer's is a form of dementia that rarely affects people under the age of 65. The disease is often accompanied by a reduction in the flow of blood to the brain, and as this happens at different rates from one individual to another, so the rate of memory loss varies between individuals.

Symptoms
- Impairment of short-term memory
- Loss of a sense of time
- Depression, anxiety
- Mood swings
- Difficulty in processing information, leading to confusion

Consult your doctor or medical herbalist
- It is vital that you consult a doctor if you experience short-term memory difficulties and if there is a history of Alzheimer's disease within your family.

Causes
The origins of Alzheimer's disease are still little understood: age is the greatest risk factor, followed by a genetic predisposition. Other triggers include repeated strokes, a diet deficient in fatty acids, stress and a lack of the female hormone, oestrogen. People who smoke, and those who have high blood pressure or high cholesterol levels are at increased risk of developing Alzheimer's disease.

WHICH PLANTS?
WARNING Use only one of the following at any given time

Certain herbs have been shown to help to slow down or prevent the onset of Alzheimer's disease. Others improve the circulation, and a third group helps to alleviate the mood swings and anxiety and sleep problems experienced by sufferers of the disease.

Internal usage
As a preventative treatment
Blackcurrant Put 5g dried leaves in 1 litre of boiling water. Leave to infuse for 5 minutes. Strain. Drink 2-3 cups a day.
Green or black tea: Use 1 teaspoon per cup of boiling water and drink 2 cups a day.
Common sage (capsules, 300mg) Take 1 capsule three times a day.

To improve blood circulation and mental well-being
American ginseng (500mg capsules) Take 2 capsules with breakfast and 2 with lunch.
Schisandra (tincture, 1:5 in 25% alcohol) Put 20-40 drops in a glass of water. Take this dose three times a day.

To reduce anxiety
Lemon balm Put 2-3g dried leaves in 1 cup of boiling water. Drink a cup at midday and one in the evening after meals.
Passionflower (tincture,1:8 in 25% alcohol) Take 25-75 drops a day in water.
Californian poppy (tincture, 1:4 in 45% alcohol): Take 10 drops three times a day in a little cold water after meals.

Other measures
- Eat a balanced diet making sure you include plenty of oily fish and cold-pressed vegetable oils, such as extra virgin olive oil, fresh vegetables and fruit.
- Take vitamins A, C, E and zinc and selenium.
- Take regular exercise.
- Exercise your memory: play card games, recite poems, recall events from your past.

Brain: circulation problems

Many conditions can affect the supply of blood to the brain, including cardiac or respiratory arrest, a brain tumour or brain abscess. A stroke occurs when the blood flow to the brain is interrupted by a blood clot. In a brain haemorrhage, which can occur when a cerebral blood vessel ruptures, the brain is flooded with too much blood and brain cells can die. A major warning sign of blood circulation problems in the brain is the sudden onset of any disorder of brain function – from visual disturbances to paralysis.

Symptoms
- Partial or total paralysis of one side of the body (hemiplegia)
- Numbness in one side of the body (hemianaesthesia)
- Changes in vision
- Inability to communicate due to reduced speech and understanding (aphasia)

Consult your doctor
- It is vitally important to consult a doctor at the first sign of any difficulty with vision, hearing, touch, the normal function of muscles and nerves, or numbness or paralysis.
- These may be warning signs of a serious problem, and early treatment could help to prevent irreversible damage.

Causes
Brain circulation problems as a result of blood clots and strokes tend to affect people over 45, afflicting more men than women.

Certain conditions have been identified as risk factors for strokes or brain haemorrhages. These include high blood pressure, heart disease, diabetes, high blood cholesterol levels, alcoholism and smoking.

Brain: circulation problems contd

WHICH PLANTS?

WARNING Use only one of the following at any given time

Medical herbalism can only help to play a preventative role in circulatory problems affecting the brain.

Internal usage

Garlic (tincture) Take 40-50 drops three times a day.
Olive (500mg capsule, dried leaf) Take 1 capsule a day with food.
Ginger (tincture, 1:5 in 60% alcohol) Take 60-100 drops a day in a glass of water. Do not use if you have high blood pressure.
Ginkgo (tincture) Take 15 drops of tincture in water three times a day before meals.
Lesser periwinkle (tincture) Take 15 drops two to three times a day.

Other measures

• Drink lemon juice every morning.
• Do not smoke.
• Avoid excessive alcohol intake.
• Adopt a Mediterranean-style diet based on olive oil.
• Monitor your cholesterol level.
• Do some sporting activity or take a 30-45 minute walk at least twice a week.
• Avoid putting on weight.

Migraine

The main symptom of migraine is a severe headache, often accompanied by nausea or vomiting. A migraine can last from four hours to three days. The disorder generally starts around puberty and diminishes by middle age. Migraines are often related to menstrual periods or to specific foods. The condition affects more women than men.

Symptoms

• Visual disturbances, such as flashes of zigzag light immediately before a migraine (these occur in about one in five cases)
• Sharp, debilitating headache, felt on one side of the head or face, or all over the head
• Nausea and vomiting
• Strong aversion to bright light or loud noise

Consult your doctor

• If you have more than three or four attacks in a month, you may need long-term medical treatment.

Causes

Most migraines occur for no apparent reason. The condition can run in families, and researchers think that the cause may be related to blood flow in the brain. Sufferers can often pinpoint trigger factors. Some foods, for example, can set off a migraine: the four 'Cs' – citrus, cheese, chocolate and coffee – as well as red wine and fried food are all common culprits. Other causes include bright lights, loud noises, a change in the weather, stress, tiredness, and hormonal changes; an attack is more likely just before a period.

WHICH PLANTS?

WARNING Use only one of the following at any given time

Herbs can help to prevent migraines, but once a migraine has begun, it will run its course.

Internal usage

For long-term preventative treatment

As directed by a medical herbalist

• Feverfew, Rosemary

DID YOU KNOW?

Migraine

Analgesics (painkillers) are best taken at the onset of a migraine headache: once the migraine takes hold, it tends to be resistant to all forms of painkilling medication.

For migraines that accompany the onset of periods
Chaste tree (capsules, 250mg dry extract) Take 2 capsules in the morning and 2 in the evening with a glass of water.

For migraines related to diet
Cinnamon Infuse 1g Chinese cinnamon bark in a cup of boiling water for 10 minutes and strain. Drink 3 cups a day.
Peppermint Put 1 dessertspoon of dried leaves in 150ml of boiling water. Leave to infuse for 10-15 minutes and strain. Drink 1 cup after every meal.

Other measures

• Follow a balanced diet, avoiding known trigger foods.
• Practise relaxation exercises.

Multiple sclerosis

A disease of the central nervous system, multiple sclerosis usually starts early in adulthood. The condition gradually destroys the myelin covering or sheath that protects nerve fibres.

The patches of demyelinated nerve tissue prevent the normal circulation of nerve impulses, resulting in a range of physical disabilities. The disease usually develops gradually, in the form of attacks and remissions over many years; sometimes it can have devastating effect within a matter of months. There is no cure.

Symptoms

These vary from case to case.
- Visual disorders such as double vision or involuntary movement of the eyes
- Extreme fatigue
- Mood changes
- Shaking and poor coordination leading to loss of balance
- Numbness and tingling in certain areas of the body
- Incontinence
- Partial or total paralysis of any part of the body

Consult your doctor or medical herbalist
- Multiple sclerosis must always be treated by a doctor but herbs may bring some relief.

Causes

The exact causes of multiple sclerosis are not known. The disease seems to be caused by several factors, the most common of which are a genetic predisposition to the disease and an imbalance of the immune system. It can also occur after a viral infection. Women appear to be more susceptible than men.

WHICH PLANTS?

WARNING Use only one of the following treatments

Used on their own, medicinal plants are not particularly effective but may help to relieve certain symptoms. Sufferers should avoid plants that stimulate the immune system in favour of regulators and anti-inflammatory agents.

Internal usage

Alfalfa (tincture, 1:4 in 25% alcohol) Put 20 drops in a glass of water. Drink three times a day after meals.
Ginkgo (tincture, 1:4 in 25% alcohol) Take 20 drops in water three times a day after meals.

Other measures
- Try to reduce stress.
- Replace saturated fats such as animal fats and dairy products, with unsaturated fats like olive or sunflower oil.
- Ensure a good intake of omega-3 and omega-6 fatty acids found in fish oils, evening primrose oil and borage oil.
- Take fortifying vitamins and minerals as prescribed by your doctor.

Neuralgia

Pain associated with a nerve, whatever the cause, is known as neuralgia. Related conditions include neuritis – the inflammation of a nerve, and polyneuritis – the inflammation of several nerves.

Symptoms

One or more may be experienced.
- Reduced sensitivity and abnormal sensations
- Heightened sensitivity to touch and other stimuli, sometimes to the point of pain
- Paralysis of one or a group of motor nerves
- In cold weather, facial nerve pain

Consult your doctor
- The symptoms of neuralgia or neuritis require immediate medical attention. Treatment is often difficult and needs regular medical supervision.

Causes

The main causes of neuralgia, neuritis and polyneuritis are injury to the nerve, a nerve abnormality or infections, especially by viruses. They can also be exacerbated by toxic substances such as tobacco and alcohol, by certain types of medication (especially those used in the treatment of HIV) and by conditions such as diabetes and uraemia (an accumulation of waste products in the blood).

WHICH PLANTS?

WARNING Use only one of the following at any given time

Internal usage

Sweet woodruff Put 10g dried herb in a litre of boiling water. Leave to infuse for 10 minutes and strain. Drink 2-3 cups a day.
Bitter orange Put 20g dried flowers in 150ml of boiling water. Leave to infuse for 10 minutes and strain. Sweeten with honey if desired. Take at bedtime.

External application

Juniper Make an infusion using 0.5-2g crushed berries in a cup of boiling water. Leave to infuse for 10 minutes, then strain. Pour this into the bath water.
Nutmeg Dilute essential oil, adding 3 drops essential oil to 50ml carrier oil. Apply once to three times a day; or add some diluted oil to a warm bath.
Lavender Tie 20-100g of flowers in a muslin bag and suspend under the taps while you run the bath.
Capsicum Apply ointment as directed on the label.

Parkinson's disease

A distressing neurological disorder, Parkinson's disease affects around one person in 200. The condition causes a wasting of the nervous system. It damages the area of the brain that controls voluntary movement, causing a progressive loss of motor function, shaking and muscular rigidity. It rarely develops before the age of 60 and is more common in men than in women. For reasons as yet unknown, the incidence of Parkinson's disease is lower among smokers than non-smokers.

Symptoms

- Shaking, tremors
- Partial rigidity of the limbs and face
- Stiff posture, with arms motionless beside the body
- Lack of coordination
- Slurred and laboured speech
- A tendency to dribble
- Depression, insomnia, sudden changes of mood

Consult your doctor

- Anyone with symptoms of Parkinson's disease must be diagnosed and treated by a doctor.

Causes

Parkinson's disease is the result of degeneration of, or damage to certain nerve cells in the brain, affecting their ability to produce the neurotransmitter, dopamine. Dopamine is important in sending the nerve messages that control body movement. The disease is more common in men than in women and tends to be inherited.

WHICH PLANTS?

WARNING Use only one of the following at any given time

Medical treatment can be safely complemented by the use of plants with calming and sedative properties that will help to combat the tendency to depression.

Internal usage

To relax and lift depression

St John's wort Infuse 1 teaspoon of dried herb in a cup of boiling water for 5 minutes and strain. Drink 2 cups a day at mealtimes
Passionflower (tincture, 1:8 in 25% alcohol) Take 25 drops a day in a glass of water.
Lavender Put 2-3g flowers in a cup of boiling water. Leave to infuse for 5-10 minutes and strain. Drink 3-4 cups a day between meals.
Valerian (240mg capsules) Take 1-2 capsules a day.

Other measures

- Regular physiotherapy can help to combat lack of coordination.
- Eat a healthy, balanced diet which includes plenty of fresh fruit, rich in antioxidants.
- Take regular high doses of Vitamins B_1, B_6 and folic acid.

Tetany

Uncontrolled muscle twitching characterises a disorder known as tetany. The recurring spasms and muscular contractions, known as tics, tend to affect the hands and feet but may also affect the face.

Symptoms

- Twitching hands and feet
- Other spasms that may affect facial and spinal muscles
- Chronic fatigue
- Breathing difficulties during a spasm

Consult your doctor

- Tetany usually affects nervous, hypersensitive people. It is more commonly found in women than in men. Only a doctor can make an accurate diagnosis.

Causes

The causes of tetany are not known, though research suggests that it may be symptomatic of a chemical imbalance in the body: it is often associated with low levels of calcium in the blood – which tends to happen when a person is short of vitamin D. Sometimes low blood potassium levels can cause the condition. Hyperventilation (overbreathing) during an anxiety attack can also cause tetany.

WHICH PLANTS?

WARNING Use only one of the following at any given time

Internal usage

To supply minerals

Horsetail Take 2g three times a day with food, or 25 drops of liquid extract in a glass of water.
   Alternatively put 2-4g of the dry plant in 200ml of boiling water, leave to infuse for 10-15 minutes and strain. Drink 1 cup a day.

To calm the nervous system

Californian poppy (tincture, 1:4 in 45% alcohol) Take 10 drops of tincture three times a day in a little cold water after meals.

To prevent or ease spasms

Lime tree Put 5g dried flowers in 1 litre of boiling water. Leave to infuse for 5 minutes and strain. Drink 1 cup a day.
Valerian (capsules, 240mg powder) Take 1-2 capsules a day.
Passionflower (tincture, 1:8 in 25% alcohol) Take 25 drops in a glass of water three times a day.
Black horehound Put 15-30g herb in 1 litre of boiling water. Leave to

infuse for 10 minutes and strain. Take 3 cups a day before meals. Anise (tincture, 1:4 in 45% alcohol) Take 5-10 drops three times a day in a little cold water after meals.

Other measures

- Eat wholefood – have one tablespoon of wholegrains or sprouting seeds every morning.
- Eat calcium-rich foods: dairy produce, sesame seeds, sardines in oil, tofu, dried figs, muesli, runner beans. Avoid foods that hinder the absorption of calcium by the intestine (spinach, dried pulses, nuts) or that are very acidic (rhubarb).
- Maintain your intake of vitamin D which facilitates the absorption of calcium. Eat plenty of fresh fish (herring, trout, salmon, tuna), eggs, margarine and hard cheeses.
- Eat magnesium-rich foods such as cocoa, sunflower and pumpkin seeds.
- If you think the cause might be overbreathing during an anxiety attack, try to slow and deepen your breaths. Rebreathing in and out of a paper bag will help to restore the concentration of carbon dioxide in the blood and relieve muscle twitching.

Travel sickness

Road, sea or air travel can all cause travel sickness in susceptible people. The term nausea actually derives from the Greek word for ship, and was originally used to describe seasickness.

Symptoms

- Pallor
- Headache
- Sudden fatigue
- Cold sweats, dizziness
- Nausea and possibly vomiting

Consult your doctor or medical herbalist

- Travel sickness can be largely avoided by taking medications available on prescription or over-the-counter or by using herbal preparations.

Causes

Travel sickness is caused by the effects of movement on the delicate organs of balance in the inner ear. It is made worse by unpleasant fumes, anxiety, or travelling on a full stomach.

WHICH PLANTS?

WARNING Use only one of the following at any given time

The following should ideally be started 12-24 hours before travel to ensure good blood levels at the onset of travel and during the journey if it is long.

Internal usage

Angelica Take 2-5ml leaf tincture (1:5 in 45% alcohol) or 0.5-2ml root/rhizome tincture (1:5 in 50% alcohol) three times a day. Ginger (1:5 in 60% alcohol) Take up to 30 drops tincture three times a day in a glass of water. Lemon balm (capsules, 200mg) Take 3 capsules a day before meals. For children reduce dose to 2 capsules a day.

Liquorice Add 1-2 teaspoons root powder to 1 cup of boiling water. Allow to steep for 10 minutes before drinking. Drink 2 cups a day. Stinging nettle (tincture 1:4 in 25% alcohol) Take 20 drops in water three times a day after meals. Sweet clover (tincture) Put 35 drops in a glass of water. Take three times a day with meals. Sweet marjoram Infuse 1-2 teaspoons of dried herb in a cup of boiling water, for 5-10 minutes and strain. Drink 3 cups a day.

Other measures

- Eat fruits rich in antispasmodic flavonoids, such as bilberries and blackcurrants.
- When travelling avoid leaning forward and closing your eyes.
- Keep your eyes fixed on the horizon if possible.
- Try to move to the centre of the ship, or to the front – rather than the back – of the car, as this lessens movement.

Vertigo

The term 'vertigo' describes the sensation of objects whirling around you horizontally or vertically. It is not the same as dizziness. Vertigo is caused by a problem in the inner ear, which controls balance. Vertigo may clear on its own without treatment, but it can also be symptomatic of other more serious conditions such as multiple sclerosis.

Symptoms

- Unsteadiness, especially on turning the head suddenly, or lifting it from the pillow
- Nausea, vomiting
- Falling to the ground
- Whistling in the ears and impaired hearing

Vertigo contd

Consult your doctor

- If vertigo continues, consult your doctor who will determine the underlying cause, and prescribe an appropriate treatment that will prevent complications such as permanent deafness.

Causes

Vertigo can be triggered by infections such as influenza or ear infections. Diseases including Ménière's disease and atherosclerosis may also cause vertigo. It can be the result of taking certain medications. Or it can simply arise while watching a film with exaggerated special effects, or taking a spinning fairground ride.

WHICH PLANTS?

WARNING Use only one of the following at any given time

Consult a medical herbalist who will be able to advise you as to the best course of treatment for your particular symptoms. Where poor circulation is a contributory factor, these herbs may be useful.

Internal usage

Ginkgo (tincture) Take 15 drops in water three times a day before meals.
Lesser periwinkle (tincture) Take 15 drops two or three times a day.
Blackcurrant Put 5g dried leaves into 1 litre of boiling water. Leave to infuse for 5 minutes and strain. Drink 2-3 cups a day.

Other measures

- If vertigo occurs suddenly, as a result of an infection, it should be treated with bed rest and appropriate medication.
- If it persists for several days, walk as much as you can to allow the body to adjust and cope with the condition.
- See a physiotherapist if your vertigo is position related.

Children's health
Bronchiolitis in babies

A viral disease that mainly affects babies, bronchiolitis causes the smallest airways in the lungs – the bronchioles – to become inflamed. This can cause fever, cough and breathing difficulties. The disease is prevalent in winter, sometimes in epidemic proportions.

Symptoms

- Blocked nose
- A dry cough
- Rapid or difficult breathing
- Wheezing chest
- Fever
- In severe cases, a bluish tinge to the skin due to lack of oxygen

Consult your doctor

- Consult a doctor urgently if you notice any problems with your baby's breathing.
- In severe cases the baby will need to be admitted to hospital for oxygen and physiotherapy.

Causes

Most cases of bronchiolitis are caused by the respiratory syncytial virus, commonly known as RSV. It is transmitted by airborne droplets, usually when an adult or child nearby coughs or sneezes.

WHICH PLANTS?

WARNING Use only one of the following at any given time

Internal usage

For a cough and fever
Common thyme Infuse 1 sachet of dried thyme in a cup of boiling water for 5 minutes and strain. For babies aged 6-12 months, give 20ml three times a day.

Common elder (elderflower tincture, 1:4 in 25% alcohol) For babies aged 6-12 months, 2 drops in a little water three times a day after meals.

Sweet violet (tincture, 1:4 in 25% alcohol) For babies aged 6-12 months, add a little water and administer 2 drops three times a day after feeds.
Alternatively, make a syrup using 100g dried flowers, 500g sugar and 300ml of water. For babies aged 6-12 months, administer 1ml syrup two or three times a day at mealtimes.

External application
Massage preparation
Lavender Dilute 3 drops of essential oil in 10ml carrier oil and massage 1 teaspoon of this mixture into the chest, back and throat.
Eucalyptus As for lavender (see above).

Other measures

- Massage may help to clear mucus from the baby's bronchioles.
- Ensure the baby drinks regularly to avoid dehydration.

DID YOU KNOW?

Infant bronchiolitis and asthma

Bronchiolitis generally clears up in around a week. It is a viral infection and does not respond to antibiotics. In rare cases, the infection can lead to asthma: a persistent cough can be a sign of this.

Common illnesses

Today, most children are vaccinated against measles, mumps and rubella. All the infections listed confer immunity: it is very rare to catch them more than once.

Mumps causes a tender swelling of the parotid glands beneath the jaw. In adolescents, mumps can lead to testicular inflammation.

Measles is a viral illness that causes a rash and a fever. It is potentially dangerous because it can cause complications including ear infections and encephalitis.

Rubella (German measles) is a mild infection that causes a rash and slight fever. If a mother contracts rubella in the first four months of pregnancy, her unborn child is at risk of deformity.

Chickenpox causes a rash of itchy spots that turn into blisters. When the blisters dry, scabs form, disappearing after 12 days or so. Scratching the spots can lead to bacterial infection and scarring.

Consult your doctor

Consult a doctor urgently if:
- the child has a high fever for more than two days
- the child cries constantly
- there is difficulty in breathing
- the child is confused, delirious or excessively sleepy
- the child has a fit
- the child has a stiff neck
- dark red blotches appear on the skin

Causes

All the childhood illnesses listed are viruses, usually spread by airborne droplets. Children at nursery or at school are more likely to be exposed than those at home. Vaccination confers immunity, and breastfeeding helps to protect babies from infection.

WHICH PLANTS?

WARNING Use only one of the following at any given time

Internal usage

To keep the fever down

Sweet violet Add 2-4g dried flowers to a cup of boiling water. Infuse for 10 minutes and strain. Give the following dose three times a day:

Age 6-12 months: 15ml;
1-6 years: 50ml; **7-12 years**: 75ml

Lavender: Put 2-3g flowers in a cup of boiling water. Infuse for 5-10 minutes and strain. Give the following dose twice a day.

Age 6-12 months: 7ml;
1-6 years: 25ml; **7-12 years**: 40ml

Heartsease Put 1.5g of dried herb in a cup of boiling water. Leave to infuse for 10 minutes and strain. Give the following dose three times a day between meals.

Age 6-12 months: 15ml;
1-6 years: 50ml; **7-12 years**: 75ml

To boost the immune system

Blackcurrant Put 5g dried herb in 1 litre of boiling water. Infuse for 5 minutes and strain. Give the following dose two to three times a day.

Age 6-12 months: 15ml;
1-6 years: 50ml; **7-12 years**: 75ml

External application

To dry up chickenpox blisters

Lavender Swab the spots with essential oil before scabs form.

To soothe an itchy rash

Mallow Put 30g of dried flowers or leaves or both in 1 litre of boiling water and leave to infuse for 10 minutes. Apply to the affected area several times a day.

Other measures

- Ensure the child drinks plenty of liquids to prevent dehydration.
- Keep the child lightly covered.
- In the sick child's room, keep the atmosphere humid and the temperature at 18-20°C.

Coughs, colds and throat infections

Infants are largely protected from coughs and colds by their mother's antibodies for the first few months of life. Thereafter, children build up their own defences against disease. Meanwhile, respiratory and throat infections are rife.

Symptoms

- **Common cold** causes a runny nose, cough and a slight fever
- **Tonsillitis** causes a fever, sore throat and pain on swallowing
- **Sinusitis** causes a fever, a headache, especially on bending forward, a runny nose and reduced sense of smell and therefore appetite

Consult your doctor

- If a child's cold does not clear up quickly, consult a doctor; what began as a cold could end up infecting the middle ear, the tonsils, chest or sinuses, and may require antibiotic treatment.

Causes

The common cold is widespread all year round, but especially in winter. Most coughs, colds and throat infections are spread by airborne droplets when an infected person coughs or sneezes.

WHICH PLANTS

WARNING Only use one of the following at any given time

Internal usage

Most of the plants prescribed are taken as tinctures. Dosage is calculated as a third of the adult dose for children from 1-6 years old, and half the adult dose for children from 7-12 years old. Do not give preparations to infants without the advice of a medical herbalist or a doctor.

Coughs, colds and throat infections contd

To boost the immune system

Echinacea (tincture, 1:5 in 45% alcohol) Administer in water three times a day.
6-12 months: 2 drops; **1-6 years**: 5 drops; **7-12 years**: 7 drops.

For a dry cough

Sundew Add 1-2g dried herb to a cup of boiling water. Infuse for 10 minutes and strain. Give three times a day after meals.
For 6-12 months: 15ml; **1-6 years**: 50ml; **7-12 years**: 75ml.

For a cough with phlegm

Aaron's rod Put 1.5-2g dried herb in a cup of boiling water. Infuse for 15 minutes and strain. Give three times a day.
6-12 months: 15ml; **1-6 years**: 50ml; **7-12 years**: 75ml.
Common elder (elderflower tincture, 1:5 in 25% alcohol) Administer in water three times a day after meals.
6-12 months: 2 drops; **1-6 years**: 6 drops; **7-12 years**: 10 drops.
Common thyme Infuse one teaspoon of dried herb in a cup of boiling water and strain. Spread the following through the day.
6-12 months: up to 30ml, divided into two or more doses; **1-6 years**: 1-2 cups; **7-12 years**: 2-3 cups.

Other measures

- Clear a baby's nose with saline nose drops, available from the chemist.
- Put your baby to sleep on his or her back, but raise the head of the cot by placing books under the legs.
- Keep the room humid by boiling an electric kettle with the lid off for a few minutes every hour.
- Keep a sick child at home.

Ear infections

Medically known as *otitis media*, middle ear infection mainly affects young children. The infection causes inflammation of the cavity between the eardrum and the inner ear. It tends to follow a common cold.

Symptoms

- High temperature
- Headache
- Intense pain in the ear
- Pus may discharge from the ear

Consult your doctor

- Recent research has shown that antibiotics do not significantly reduce the pain of an ear infection, nor its duration or longer term consequences.
- Many doctors advise giving paracetamol or ibuprofen to relieve pain, and letting the infection run its course. If there is a discharge, however, antibiotics may need to be prescribed.

Causes

Most ear infections are caused by the bacteria or viruses responsible for upper respiratory tract infections. These spread, via the Eustachean tubes, to infect the middle ear. Less common causes include hayfever and other allergies, passive smoking and poor diet. Research has shown that children who have been breastfed are less at risk of ear infections.

WHICH PLANTS?

WARNING Only use one of the following at any given time

Internal usage

Aaron's rod Put 2g dried flowers into a cup of boiling water. Infuse for 15 minutes and strain. Give the following three times a day.
6-12 months: 15ml; **1-6 years**: 50ml; **7-12 years**: 75ml.

Blackcurrant Put 5g dried leaves in 1 litre of boiling water. Infuse for 5 minutes and strain. Give the following dosages two to three times a day.
6-12 months: 15ml; **1-6 years**: 50ml; **7-12 years**: 75ml.
Eucalyptus Give the following amounts of tincture in water four to six times a day.
6-12 months: 10 drops; **1-6 years**: 16 drops; **7-12 years**: 25 drops.
Dog rose Put 2.5g chopped rose-hips in a cup of boiling water. Infuse for 10 minutes and strain. Give the following three or four times a day.
6-12 months: 15ml; **1-6 years**: 50ml; **7-12 years**: 75ml.
Mallow Put 5g dry herb in 1 litre of water, boil for 5 minutes and strain. Give the following one to three times a day.
6-12 months: 15ml; **1-6 years**: 50ml; **7-12 years**: 75ml.

Other measures

- Unblock the nose. Children need to be taught how to blow their noses effectively; your health visitor can advise you.

Eczema

The most common type of eczema in children is atopic eczema. It causes itchy, red scaly patches and small fluid-filled blisters, that weep when scratched releasing liquid which then dries into crusts. Atopic eczema is usually found in skin folds – at elbow creases, behind the ears and behind the knees. Most children grow out of eczema after three to five years.

Symptoms

- Red, puffy areas of skin
- Raw, scabbed or flaking skin
- Dry skin
- Persistent scratching may cause the skin to thicken

Consult your doctor

- Consult a doctor as soon as symptoms appear to ensure that there is no viral or bacterial infection.

Causes

Eczema tends to run in families, especially where there is a history of other allergies – asthma or hayfever, for example. Other trigger factors include wearing wool next to the skin, and living in a household where people smoke. Breastfed children are less likely to suffer from eczema.

Sometimes, eczema is caused by food allergies such as to milk, eggs or fish. Airborne allergens include cat or dog hair, house dust mites and pollen.

WHICH PLANTS?

WARNING Use only one of the following at any given time

External application

Marigold Put 5g dried flower-heads in 1 litre of boiling water. Infuse for 5 minutes and strain. Soak a cloth in this infusion and apply to the affected area three or four times a day.

Walnut Apply a cream or gel containing walnut extract. Follow maker's directions, or take advice from a medical herbalist.

Other measures

- Air and vacuum the child's room frequently.
- Keep the house warm and the atmosphere humid.
- Do not allow smoking in the house.
- Avoid woollen clothing next to the skin.
- Take your child outdoors whenever possible: sunlight helps to heal the scabs.
- As a preventative measure, try to breastfeed a newborn baby for at least six months before introducing other foods.

Sleeping problems

Almost a third of infants below the age of three have sleeping problems, either when first being put to bed or during the night.

It is important to remember that some babies and children need more sleep than others: anything from 10 to 15 hours in every 24 is 'normal'. You may find that you need to sacrifice a toddler's daytime nap in order to enjoy a good night's sleep yourself.

Symptoms

- The child resists going to bed and, once put down, remains awake
- After sleeping for 1-3 hours, the child awakes disorientated from a deep sleep and may cry, talk or even sleepwalk
- During the second half of the night, the child has nightmares

Consult your doctor

- Persistent sleep disturbance should be investigated by your doctor or health visitor.
- Family history, environment, previous episodes and the child's behaviour can all give clues as to the source of the problem.

Causes

Sleep problems are often related to something that is happening during the child's waking hours – something in the diet, stress or emotional anxiety, for example. Trouble getting to sleep is often simply the result of external stimulus – the room may be too light, too noisy or too hot.

WHICH PLANTS?

WARNING Use only one of the following at any given time

Do not give a child sedative herbs except in cases of minor sleep problems, those of recent origin or to complement medical treatment.

Internal usage

Bitter orange Put 20g of dried flowers into 150ml of boiling water. Infuse for 10 minutes. Strain, and give the following at bedtime:
6-12 months: 15ml; **1-6 years**: 50ml; **7-12 years**: 75ml.

Lemon balm Put 2-3g dried leaves in 1 cup of boiling water. Infuse for 5 minutes. Strain, and give the following dose after lunch and after supper:
6-12 months: 15ml; **1-6 years**: 50ml; **7-12 years**: 75ml.

Passionflower (tincture, 1:8 in 25% alcohol) Suitable only for children older than four years. Give the following dose in the evening:
4-6 years: 15 drops; **7-12 years**: 20 drops.

Other measures

- Keep to a regular timetable for the child's meals.
- Put the child to bed and wake him or her up at fixed times.
- Establish a regular bedtime and a standard routine for settling down for the night. This will help a child to understand what is expected, and provide the security of knowing when things are going to happen.

Dental & gum problems

Teething

The term 'teething' is used to describe the eruption of a baby's teeth. Teething can be very sore and is often accompanied by gum inflammation and a tummy upset.

Symptoms
- Red, swollen gums
- A red cheek on the side the tooth is emerging
- Dribbling
- Pain, causing the child to refuse food and drink
- Fever
- Diarrhoea

Consult your doctor
- If a fever that you suspect is caused by teething lasts longer than two days, see a doctor. The child may have an unrelated bacterial or viral infection.

Causes
Before it erupts, the budlike tooth is encased in a small sac in the jawbone. When the tooth erupts, it pierces the gum which causes inflammation and pain. Teething pain mainly affects children aged between 6 months and 2 years.

WHICH PLANTS?
WARNING Use only one of the following at any given time

External application
Lavender Dilute 3 drops of essential oil in 10ml carrier oil. Apply a little externally to the cheek on the side where the tooth is aching.
Mallow Put 3g dried flowers or leaves or both in 100ml of boiling water. Infuse for 10 minutes and apply on a clean, lint-free cloth to sore gums.

Other measures
- Give children something hard to chew on – a teething ring if they can hold one.
- Gently massage the gum with your finger.

Gum disorders

People who have been unwell, those who have a poor diet, and anyone who does not observe scrupulous oral hygiene may be susceptible to gingivitis, which causes sore, swollen and bleeding gums. Ulcers are painful, raw lesions on the gums or elsewhere in the mouth.

Symptoms
Gingivitis
- Red, swollen gums that may bleed, especially when brushing the teeth
- Pain

Mouth ulcer
- A small white sore edged in red, acutely sensitive to acidic or salty foods

Consult your doctor
- If symptoms persist for more than a week, see a doctor. Gum disease that does not clear up may indicate a more serious underlying condition.

Causes
Gingivitis is often caused by poor dental hygiene; other causes include hormonal imbalances, some prescription drugs, or conditions such as diabetes, epilepsy, anaemia and leukaemia.
 It is difficult to determine the cause of most mouth ulcers – although they seem to occur more often when a person is run down. Possible triggers include minor injuries, a reaction to streptococcus bacteria or allergies.

WHICH PLANTS?
WARNING Use only one of the following at any given time

Internal usage
Gingivitis
Myrtle Make a decoction by boiling 10g of dried leaves in 1 litre of water for 10 minutes. Strain and drink 2 cups a day.

External application
Gingivitis
Clove Chew a clove three or four times a day.
Marigold Put 5g dried flower-heads into 1 litre boiling water. Infuse for 5 minutes and strain. Gargle with the warm infusion two or three times a day.

Mouth ulcers
Echinacea (tincture, 1:5 in 45% alcohol) Apply neat to the ulcer every hour.
Common sage Put 20g dried leaves into 1 litre of boiling water. Infuse for 10 minutes and strain. Use as a mouthwash two or three times a day.

Other measures
- Brush your teeth and gums after every meal.
- Use floss or interdental brushes between the teeth once a day.
- Cut out foods that can promote ulcers, such as certain fatty foods, chocolate, nuts, dried fruit and spices.
- Avoid smoking, especially a pipe.
- Don't chew toothpicks.

Halitosis

Bad breath, known medically as halitosis, is an embarrassing condition. You rarely know that you have bad breath – and friends are usually too polite to tell you.

Symptom
- Unpleasant odour from the mouth

Causes
Halitosis has many causes. The main ones are smoking, and an empty stomach. Other causes include gum infection, dental caries, decayed food caught between the teeth and infection of the stomach or digestive tract.

Tooth decay

Consult your doctor

- If you suffer from persistent bad breath, consult your doctor to determine the underlying cause.

WHICH PLANTS?

WARNING Only use one of the following at any given time

Internal usage

In all cases and as a preventative

Anise (seed tincture, 1:4 in 45% alcohol) Take 5-10 drops three times a day in a little cold water after meals. Wash around the mouth before swallowing.

Coriander Put 10-30g crushed seeds into 1 litre of boiling water. Infuse for 10 minutes and strain. Drink 1 cup after each meal.

Peppermint Put 1 dessertspoon of dried leaves into 150ml of boiling water. Infuse for 10-15 minutes and strain. Allow to cool, wash around the mouth and swallow.

To prevent gum infection

Echinacea (tincture, 1:5 in 45% alcohol) Add 15 drops, to a little water. Wash around the mouth and swallow. Repeat three times a day for up to a week.

German or Roman chamomile infuse a tea bag in a cup of boiling water for 5-10 minutes. Cool, wash around the mouth and swallow.

To cleanse the digestive tract

Star anise Put 1 teaspoon of dried fruit into a cup of boiling water. Infuse for 10 minutes, strain and take 2 cups a day before meals.

Cloves Add 1-3g of cloves to a cup of water and boil for 10 minutes. Strain. Drink this amount each day.

Cinnamon Put 1g cinnamon bark into a cup of boiling water. Infuse for 10 minutes and strain. Drink 3 cups a day.

To settle poor digestion

Turmeric Put 1g of powdered rhizome into a cup of boiling water. Cover and leave to infuse for 5-10 minutes then strain. Drink 2-4 cups a day.

Rosemary Put 2-4g dried herb into 1 cup of boiling water and infuse for 10 minutes. Strain. Drink 3 cups a day after meals.

Lavender Put 2-3g flowers into a cup of boiling water. Infuse for 5-10 minutes. Strain. Drink ½ cup twice a day.

External application

Ginger (tincture, 1:5 in 60% alcohol) Add 60 drops to a glass of water and use as a mouthwash once or twice a day.

Common sage Put 20g dried leaves in 1 litre of boiling water. Infuse for 5 mins, strain and drink.

Basil Boil 2 tablespoons dried leaves in 250ml of water for 10-15 minutes. Strain and cool. Use as a mouthwash and gargle two or three times a day.

Hyssop Put 1-2 teaspoons dried flowers into a cup of boiling water. Infuse for 5-10 minutes, strain and cool. Use as a mouth-wash three times a day.

Other measures

- Try a toothpaste containing tea tree or eucalyptus essential oil.
- Visit the dentist regularly.
- Limit tobacco and coffee intake.

See also Indigestion, Gastritis, Acid reflux

A small cavity in the protective enamel of the tooth can lead rapidly to tooth decay. If left untreated, the tooth beneath the enamel will begin to rot, eventually causing toothache. If the infection spreads to neighbouring tissue, it can cause an abscess.

Symptoms

- Noticeable sensitivity of the affected tooth to cold and heat
- Pain on contact with sugary or acid foods, and in response to pressure
- Throbbing pain – coinciding with the pulse

Consult your dentist

- Consult a dentist at the onset of toothache so as to minimise the risk of infection.

Causes

Tooth decay, known medically as dental caries, is often exacerbated by diet (too much sugar), or by eating predominantly soft food. Poor dental hygiene encourages invasion by the bacteria that cause caries. Other risk factors for tooth decay include too few minerals in the diet, poor general health, stress, and the menopause.

WHICH PLANTS

WARNING Use only one of the following at any given time

External application

To cleanse the naturally occurring bacteria in the mouth

Marigold Put 5g dried flower-heads in 1 litre of boiling water. Infuse for 5 minutes, strain and cool. Use as a gargle and mouthwash two or three times a day.

Common thyme Infuse 1 sachet in a cup of boiling water for 5 minutes. Cool. Use as a mouth-wash two or three times a day.

Tooth decay contd

For toothache

Capsicum Mix a pinch of capsicum powder with 25ml lemon juice, then add hot water and honey to taste. Wash around the mouth twice a day.

Clove Chew a clove three or four times a day. Alternatively, rub 1 drop of neat essential oil onto the painful tooth two to three times a day for three days.

Lavender Put 2-3g dried flowers into a cup of boiling water. Infuse for 5-10 minutes. Allow to cool, strain and use as a mouthwash two or three times a day.

Peppermint Put 1 dessertspoon of dried leaves into 150ml of boiling water. Infuse for 10-15 minutes. Strain and use warm as a mouth-wash two or three times a day.

Other measures

- Brush your teeth after each meal.
- Use dental floss or interdental brushes once a day.
- Eat a balanced diet.
- Cut down on sugary snacks and soft drinks.
- Don't leave the remains of acidic food, such as apples, in the mouth after eating: rinse the mouth with water or brush the teeth afterwards.
- Chew your food well.
- Do not take fluoride supple-ments: too much fluoride can provoke tooth decay. The amount added to fluoridated toothpaste appears to be both safe and effective.

Acid reflux

The regurgitation of acid from the stomach into the oesophagus is termed gastro-oesophageal, or 'acid', reflux. It occurs when the muscular valve that controls the entrance to the stomach is weak or inefficient. Persistent acid reflux causes oesophagitis (inflammation of the oesophagus).

Symptoms

- Painful burning sensation in the oesophagus, sometimes extending into the mouth
- Reflux may occur when lying down, especially after meals
- Cough, chronic inflammation of the pharynx

Consult your doctor

- Your doctor can usually diagnose gastro-oesophageal reflux by carrying out an examination, though sometimes an X-ray or even endoscopy (fibre-optic camera passed down the oesophagus) is required for this.

Causes

Gastro-oesophageal reflux is often associated with a hiatus hernia. However, other factors can be significant, such as the habit of eating excessively large meals, disorders of the gall bladder, anxiety or stress, wearing tight clothing.

WHICH PLANTS?

WARNING Use only one of the following at any given time

Internal usage

Basil Infuse 4-6g of dried leaves in 250ml of boiling water for 10 minutes. Strain. Drink 1 cup without sugar a day.

Sweet marjoram Infuse 1 dessert-spoon of dried plant in a cup of boiling water for 15 minutes. Strain. Drink 3 cups a day.

Hops (tincture, 1:5 in 60% alcohol) Take 20 drops in water three times a day before meals.

German chamomile Infuse 1 sachet of dried flowers in a cup of boiling water for 10 minutes. Drink 3 cups a day before meals.

Bitter fennel Infuse ¼ to ½ teaspoon of crushed seeds in a cup of boiling water for 10 minutes. Drink 1-3 cups a day.

Lemon balm Infuse 2-3g of dried leaves in a cup of boiling water for 5 minutes. Drink 1 cup at midday and 1 in the evening after meals.

Turmeric Infuse 0.5-1g of powder in a cup of boiling water for 5-10 minutes and strain. Drink 2-4 cups a day.

Other measures

- Eat less and more often, taking your time and chewing properly.
- Drink slightly sparkling mineral water.
- Don't lie down or go to bed immediately after a meal.
- Raise the head of the bed a few inches.
- Reduce your alcohol consump-tion and try to stop smoking (which loosens the valve and so increases reflux of acid back up into the oesophagus).

Colon problems

The lowest part of the intestine, leading to the rectum is called the colon. Several conditions can affect the colon causing abdominal pain. These include colitis, irritable bowel syndrome and diverticulosis.

Colitis is an inflammation of the colon, sometimes caused by an infection. Irritable bowel syndrome – or spastic colon – causes intermittent pain. The disorder seems to stem from a lack of coordination of intestinal movements.

Diverticulosis is the development of small pouches in the intestinal wall. If these become infected they cause severe abdominal pain in a condition known as diverticulitis.

Symptoms

- Abdominal pain that is often colicky – it comes in waves
- Bloating and flatulence
- Intestinal gurgling noises
- Pain before passing a stool
- Constipation, diarrhoea or both
- Blood and mucus in diarrhoea
- Sometimes fever

Consult your doctor

- See your doctor if you have persistent abdominal pain or pass blood-stained diarrhoea.

Causes

Most colon problems are related to diet. Diverticulosis, for example, is usually the result of a lifetime of eating a diet low in fibre. But irritable bowel syndrome may be exacerbated by fibre, and appears to be caused by psychological problems such as stress and anxiety rather than any physical disorder.

WHICH PLANTS?

WARNING Only use one of the following at any given time

Medical herbalism can help to ease many problems affecting the digestive tract.

Internal usage

Aaron's rod Put 1.5-2g flowers in a cup of boiling water. Infuse for 15 minutes and strain. Drink 3 cups a day.

Bitter fennel Add ½ teaspoon crushed seeds to a cup of boiling water, infuse for 10 minutes and strain. Drink 1 cup three times a day (infants: 2-3 teaspoons three times a day).

Caraway (tincture, 1:4 in 45% alcohol) Take 10-15 drops in cold water three times a day after food.

Mallow Put 10-15g dried flowers in 1 litre of boiling water. Leave to infuse for 10 minutes and strain. Drink 3-4 cups a day.

Passionflower (tincture, 1:8 in 25% alcohol) Take 25 drops in a glass of water three times a day.

Peppermint Put 1 dessertspoon of dried leaves into 150ml boiling water. Infuse for 10-15 minutes. Drink 1 cup after every meal.

Roman chamomile Infuse 1 sachet in a cup of boiling water for 10 minutes. Drink 1 cup after meals. Or add 1 dessertspoon of flowerheads to a cup of boiling water, infuse for 10 minutes and strain. Drink three to four times a day.

Star anise Put 1 teaspoon of dried fruit into a cup of boiling water. Infuse for 10 minutes and strain. Drink twice a day before meals.

Other measures

- Eat a balanced diet.
- For irritable bowel syndrome, cut down on fibrous vegetables and increase your intake of soluble fibre such as oats and lentils.
- To prevent diverticulosis and other colon disorders, increase your intake of fibre in the form of wholegrains and vegetables.
- Avoid hot spicy foods.
- Take plenty of exercise.

Constipation

When stools are hard and difficult to pass, or are passed rarely, the condition is known as constipation.

Symptoms

- Stools that are dry, hard and infrequent
- Bloating and wind

Consult your doctor

- Constipation is usually harmless, but if you have been unable to pass a motion for a week, then see a doctor.

Causes

Constipation is usually the result of a lack of fibre and fluids in the diet. Other factors include a lack of exercise, stress, or a reluctance to empty the bowels – perhaps because piles or an anal fissure make it painful to do so. Certain drugs, such as those containing codeine, can also cause constipation. Women suffer from constipation at times of hormonal change, especially during pregnancy and the menopause.

WHICH PLANTS?

WARNING Use only one of the following at any given time

Stools can be made softer and bulkier – and therefore easier to pass – by taking plants containing mucilage such as ispaghula.

The laxative plants suggested below can irritate the intestine and are not recommended for repeated or long-term use. Seek the advice of a medical herbalist or a doctor before taking any of these herbal remedies for more than a few days.

Internal usage

Flax (capsules,100mg flax seed oil) Take 1-3 capsules a day.

Ispaghula (capsules, 430mg) Take 2 capsules before each meal with a large glass of water.

Constipation contd

Rhubarb Boil 20g dried or 40g fresh rhubarb with 750ml water and simmer to reduce to 500ml. Take 100ml in the early evening. Senna (capsules containing 7.5mg sennosides) Take 1-2 capsules at nighttime. Do not take more than 2 capsules in a 24-hour period. Tamarind Take 10-50g of fresh pulp, without the seeds, a day: adjust the quantity according to the individual's reaction to the treatment.

Other measures

- Drink plenty of fluids, at least 2 litres of water a day.
- Take regular exercise.
- Eat more dietary fibre in the form of whole grains (brown rice, wholemeal bread), vegetables and fruit.
- Train your bowel: go to the toilet at the same time of day, every day, even if you do not feel any urgency to do so.
- When you feel the need to empty your bowels, always try to go straight away.

Crohn's disease

Affecting the digestive tract, Crohn's disease is a chronic inflammation of the intestine. It usually affects the end of the small intestine (ileum) at its junction with the large intestine.

Crohn's disease can occur at any age, but it mostly afflicts adolescents and young adults. The condition is incurable.

Symptoms

- Painful abdominal spasms
- Diarrhoea, sometimes with the passage of blood or mucus
- Weight loss

Causes

It is not known what causes Crohn's disease. It could be due to an abnormal allergic response to cereals or to milk-based products, or to a bacterium or virus in the intestine. There may be a family history of the illness, although the genetic link is not a strong one.

Consult your doctor

- People with Crohn's disease need medical supervision. Sometimes, surgery is necessary to remove part of the intestine.

WHICH PLANTS?

WARNING Use only one of the following at any given time

Internal usage

As an anti-inflammatory

Marshmallow Put 2-3g dried root into 1 cup of boiling water. Infuse for 10 minutes and strain. Drink 2-3 cups a day.
Common yarrow Infuse 1 teaspoon dried herb in 250ml of boiling water. Infuse for 5 minutes and strain. Drink 3-4 cups a day.
Aaron's rod Put 1.5-2g of dried flowers into a cup of boiling water. Infuse for 15 minutes and strain. Drink 3 cups a day.
German chamomile Put a sachet into a cup of boiling water and leave to infuse for 10 minutes. Take 1 cup three times a day before meals.

For diarrhoea

Bilberry (tablets, 60mg) Take 1-3 tablets a day.

Other measures

- Follow a balanced diet, avoiding foods likely to upset digestion.
- Drink plenty of fluids so as to avoid dehydration as a result of diarrhoea.
- Take fish oil, rich in omega-3 fatty acids, for its anti-inflammatory properties.

Diarrhoea

The frequent passage of loose motions, often accompanied by stomach cramps, is a symptom of an underlying illness. Most people experience diarrhoea at some time and it often clears up without the need for intervention. Chronic diarrhoea, however, can stem from the inefficient absorption of water from the stools by the colon. Severe or prolonged bouts of diarrhoea can lead to dehydration.

Symptoms

- Abdominal cramps, often preceding the passage of loose or liquid stools
- Bloating and flatulence

Consult your doctor or medical herbalist

- In small children and old people, dehydration caused by diarrhoea can be serious and a doctor should be consulted.
- Chronic diarrhoea should also be investigated and herbal preparations can help to treat it.

Causes

Acute diarrhoea can be caused by anxiety, some medicines, bacterial food poisoning and some tropical infections. It can also be part of a general viral infection.

Chronic diarrhoea is usually a symptom of an intestinal disorder, such as irritable bowel syndrome.

WHICH PLANTS?

WARNING Use only one of the following at any given time

Internal usage

To soothe the bowels

Carob Add 20-30g carob flour to lukewarm water or milk a day.
Purple loosestrife Boil 10g of the dried plant in 1 litre of water for 10 minutes, then strain. Drink 2-3 cups a day.

To ease stomach cramps

Angelica Add 1 teaspoon of root to three quarters of a cup of water, bring to the boil and steep for 5 minutes. Take as two doses during the day.

Lemon balm Infuse 2-3g of dried leaves in a cup of boiling water for 5 minutes. Drink 1 cup at midday and 1 in the evening after meals.

Common thyme Infuse 2g of dried plant in a cup of boiling water for 5 minutes, then strain. Drink 3 cups a day.

To ease intestinal gases

Star anise Infuse 1 teaspoon of dried fruit in a cup of boiling water for 10 minutes. Drink 2 cups a day.

Other measures

- Maintain your fluid intake. You may wish to take a rehydration fluid which can be purchased from a pharmacist.
- Avoid foods that may irritate the bowels such as dairy products, wholegrain cereals, too much sugar and raw vegetables.
- Instead, choose grilled lean meat, fish, ham, pasta, rice, dry biscuits and stewed fruit.

Gall bladder, inflammation of

Cholecystitis is the medical term for inflammation of the gall bladder. The gall bladder swells and becomes tender; infection usually follows. The condition can be acute, where the attack is sudden and severe; or it can be chronic, with repeated, milder attacks. Women over the age of 50 are the most commonly affected.

Symptoms

- Pain on the right side of the abdomen, just beneath the rib cage
- A temperature above 38°C, often accompanied by shivering
- Sudden fatigue and loss of appetite
- Painful abdominal contractions

Consult your doctor

- Cholecystitis is a disorder that can become serious and result in a perforation of the gall bladder involving peritonitis. Therefore you should seek prompt medical attention if you suspect you have this condition.

Causes

Cholecystitis is usually caused by the presence of a gallstone, which blocks the bile duct. The bile becomes trapped in the gall bladder, where it becomes more concentrated and irritates the walls of the gall bladder. It may then become infected with bacteria.

WHICH PLANTS?

WARNING Use only one of the following at any given time

Internal usage

Centaury (tincture, 1:4 in 25% alcohol) Take 10-15 drops in a little cold water 30 minutes before eating three times a day.

Cinnamon Take 0.3-1.5g a day with food.

Lavender Infuse 2-3g of the flowers in a cup of boiling water for 5-10 minutes. Drink ½ cup twice a day.

Rosemary Infuse 2-4g of the dried leaves in a cup of boiling water for 10 minutes, then strain. Drink 3 cups a day after meals.

Turmeric Infuse 0.5-1g of powder in a cup of boiling water for 5-10 minutes and strain. Drink 2-4 cups a day.

Other measures

- Follow a diet that reduces cholesterol levels (see lipid disorders) as most gallstones are cholesterol-based.
- Take rest, lying down rather than sitting, during attacks of cholecystitis.

Gallstones

Thickened bile in the gall bladder may solidify into a calcium-packed gallstone (lithiasis). This may block the normal passage of bile into the intestine and lead to inflammation of the gall bladder. The disorder is often symptomless until the stone or stones become large.

Symptoms

- Intermittent pain under the ribs on the right side of the abdomen
- Nausea, sometimes vomiting
- Inability to digest eggs, milk, chocolate and peanuts. (Bile helps the intestine to digest these fatty substances.)
- Stools may be light-coloured and fatty if the stone is completely obstructing the bile duct. The skin and whites of the eyes then become yellow
- Symptoms suggesting inflammation of the gall bladder

Causes

Gallstones are caused by inefficient functioning and emptying of the bile ducts. An excess or thickening of bile leads to the formation of stones; a structural abnormality of the gall bladder can also lead to the formation of gallstones.

Consult your doctor

- Only a doctor can establish a diagnosis and prescribe the necessary treatment, which can be either medical or surgical.

WHICH PLANTS?

WARNING Use only one of the following at any given time

Plants that stimulate the production of bile are called choleretic. Several are also cholagogic – that is, they stimulate the gall bladder to contract and expel bile.

Internal usage

To soothe the gall bladder

Boldo Infuse 1 sachet of dried leaves in 200ml of boiling water for 10 minutes. Drink 1-3 cups a day.

Peppermint Infuse 1 dessertspoon of dried leaves in 150ml of boiling water for 10-15 minutes. Drink 1 cup after every meal.

Rosemary Infuse 2-4g of dried leaves in a cup of boiling water for 10 minutes. Strain. Drink 1 cup after every meal.

Turmeric Infuse 0.5-1g of powder in a cup of boiling water for 5-10 minutes and strain. Drink 2-4 cups a day.

To combat spasms

Lemon balm Infuse 2-3g of dried leaves in a cup of boiling water for 5 minutes. Strain. Drink 1 cup at midday and one in the evening after meals.

German chamomile Infuse 1 sachet in a cup of boiling water for 10 minutes. Drink 3 cups a day before meals.

Lavender Infuse 2-3g of dried flowers in a cup of boiling water for 5-10 minutes. Strain. Drink ½ cup twice a day.

Other measures

- Avoid foods high in fat.
- Reduce your intake of refined carbohydrates (such as white sugar and flour).
- After a suitable interval, follow your meals with some physical activity.
- Acupuncture may help.

Gastritis, oesophagitis

These two conditions affect the stomach and gullet. In gastritis the lining of the stomach becomes inflamed. It can be either acute, occurring suddenly, or chronic, developing slowly over several years. Oesophagitis is the inflammation of the lining of the oesophagus or gullet.

Symptoms

- Burning and discomfort in the chest with oesophageal spasms
- Flow-back of stomach contents into the gullet accompanied by acid regurgitation into the mouth (acid reflux)
- Bad breath during the episodes of discomfort
- Nausea and spasms of the empty stomach
- Inflammation of the tongue and mouth ulcers
- Sputum specked with blood from intestinal bleeding
- Loss of appetite and weight-loss
- Sometimes chronic cough (as a result of throat irritation)

Consult your doctor or medical herbalist

- Gastritis or oesophagitis may be due to a lack of vitamin B_{12} or iron. They can also be associated with disorders such as an ulcer, hiatus hernia, or even cancer. A medical examination will reveal the cause of the inflammation.

Causes

Gastritis can be due to excessive or insufficient gastric acid in the stomach. It is particularly associated with: stress, excessive alcohol consumption, smoking, a diet that is low in vitamins, or a diet that is high in fatty or acidic food. Certain drugs such as aspirin and anti-inflammatories (like ibuprofen) can cause irritation leading to inflammation of the stomach lining. Gastritis is also more common in people who have irregular eating habits.

Oesophagitis is primarily related to acid reflux, but also commonly occurs when people do not wash down certain types of tablets properly (such as aspirin and anti-inflammatories), or go to bed immediately after taking such medication.

WHICH PLANTS?

WARNING Use only one of the following at any given time

Internal usage

Ginger (tincture, 1:5 in 60% alcohol) Take up to 30 drops a day in a glass of water.
Turmeric Infuse 0.5-1g of powder in a cup of boiling water for 5-10 minutes and strain. Drink 2-4 cups a day.
German chamomile Infuse 1 sachet of dried flowers in a cup of boiling water for 10 minutes. Drink 3 cups a day before meals.
Roman chamomile Infuse 1 sachet of dried flowers or 1 dessertspoon of dried flowers in a cup of boiling water for 10 minutes. Drink 1 cup after each main meal.
Lemon balm Infuse 2-3g of dried leaves in a cup of boiling water for 5 minutes. Drink 1 cup at midday and 1 in the evening after meals.
Peppermint Infuse 1 dessertspoon of dried leaves in 150ml of boiling water for 10-15 minutes. Drink 1 cup after every meal.
Rosemary Infuse 2-4g of the dried leaves in a cup of boiling water for 10 minutes. Drink three cups a day after meals.
Basil Infuse 4-6g of dried leaves in 250ml of boiling water for 10 minutes. Drink 1 cup without sugar a day.

Other measures

- Eat slowly, chewing well.
- Avoid tobacco, alcohol, aspirin, and anti-inflammatories, which irritate the stomach.
- Avoid spicy, fatty or 'rich' dishes, and try to eat little and often. Leave at least a couple of hours between eating and going to bed.
- Always take tablets or capsules with plenty of water.

Gastroenteritis

With this condition there is inflammation of the stomach and intestines. Gastroenteritis may occur quite suddenly, often causing violent vomiting and diarrhoea. It is usually accompanied by severe spasmodic abdominal pains. For most people, gastroenteritis is not a serious illness and it clears up within a few days.

Symptoms

- Loss of appetite, intense thirst from dehydration
- Vomiting, spasms, colic and abdominal cramps
- Shivering
- Diarrhoea, sometimes leading to anal irritation and acute rectal pains
- Flatulence
- Weakness

Consult your doctor or medical herbalist

- If a young or elderly person with these symptoms also has a fever or traces of blood in the stools, consult a doctor immediately.
- The same applies for people who have an impaired immune system or those who have recently travelled abroad.

Causes

Gastroenteritis is commonly caused by viruses, bacteria and other micro-organisms, which are transferred via contaminated water or food. Viral gastroenteritis may be passed on from person to person in much the same way as the common cold or flu.

The ailment can also be caused by taking too much alcohol, eating highly spiced dishes or certain drugs (including antibiotics).

WHICH PLANTS?

WARNING Use only one of the following at any given time

Internal usage

To stop vomiting and reduce inflammation
Ginger (tincture, 1:5 in 60% alcohol) Take up to 30 drops a day in a glass of water.
German chamomile Infuse 1 sachet of dried flowers in a cup of boiling water for 10 minutes. Drink 3 cups a day.

For intestinal spasms
Common thyme Put 1 sachet of dried leaves in a cup of boiling water. Infuse for 5 minutes. Drink 3 cups a day.
Lemon balm Infuse 2-3g of dried leaves in a cup of boiling water for 5 minutes. Drink 1 cup at midday and 1 in the evening after meals.

To ease intestinal gas
Anise (tincture, 1:4 in 45% alcohol) Take 5-10 drops three times a day in a little cold water after meals.
Peppermint Infuse 1 dessertspoon of dried leaves in 150ml of boiling water for 10-15 minutes. Drink 1 cup after every meal.

To prevent infection
Garlic (300mg capsules) Take 1-3 capsules a day.
Ginger (tincture, 1:5 in 60% alcohol) Take up to 30 drops a day in a glass of water.

Other measures

- Stay in bed
- Drink plenty of fluids to make up for water lost through vomiting and diarrhoea: add 4 teaspoons of sugar and ½ teaspoon of salt to each litre of water. Sip throughout the day.
- Take vitamins A, C and E.
- Avoid dairy products. Plain white boiled rice is suitable when the appetite first returns.

Hepatitis, cirrhosis

The term hepatitis refers to the inflammation of the liver. It is commonly caused by a virus (hepatitis A, B, C, D or E), but it can also occur after taking certain drugs or poisons. It damages liver cells and can lead to cirrhosis, in which the function of the liver is seriously and irreversibly impaired.

Symptoms

- Asthenia (tiredness unconnected to any effort)
- Loss of appetite, nausea
- General poor health accompanied by weight-loss
- Oedema (swelling) of the lower limbs
- Whites of the eyes and skin and tissue of the eyelids turn yellow (icterus or jaundice)
- Swelling (oedema) of the abdomen

Consult your doctor or medical herbalist

- Consult your doctor immediately if you have one or several of the above symptoms; rapid detection offers the best chance of a cure.
- A full examination should be made in order to eliminate similar conditions requiring different treatment (such as gallstones and cancer of the liver, gall bladder or pancreas).
- Diagnosis can be confirmed by means of a blood test.

Causes

Most cases of hepatitis are caused by viruses, which produce infections that vary in gravity and difficulty of treatment. Certain kinds of hepatitis can lead to cirrhosis of the liver (whereby liver cells are progressively destroyed).

Cirrhosis can also be caused by alcohol as well as certain drugs and chemicals.

WHICH PLANTS?
WARNING Use only one of the following at any given time

These plants should not be taken without consulting the doctor in charge of the case.

Internal usage
To protect and rejuvenate the liver
Globe artichoke (capsules, 300mg dried leaf extract) Take 1 capsule a day.
Milk thistle (tablets, 200mg) Take 1-2 tablets a day.
Rosemary Infuse 2-4g of the dried plant in a cup of boiling water for 10 minutes. Strain. Drink 3 cups a day after meals.
Sweet woodruff Infuse 10g of dried aerial parts in a litre of boiling water for 10 minutes. Drink 2-3 cups a day.

Other measures
- Stop all alcohol consumption.
- Ask your GP or practice nurse about vaccination against hepatitis A and B.
- Make a point of eating dried fruits, grapes, figs, spinach, watercress, potatoes, carrots, artichokes, rice, wholemeal bread, yoghurt, kephir, chicory (in salad), sunflower oil, olive oil, brewer's yeast, sesame seeds.
- If you belong to a risk group for hepatitis B or C (sex with different partners, intravenous drug use, health worker), regular testing for the presence of these viruses increases the chances of successful treatment, and vaccination against hepatitis B is recommended.
- In the acute stages, adopt a protein-free regime.

Indigestion

The medical term for indigestion is dyspepsia, which covers the variety of symptoms associated with difficulties in digesting foods.

Symptoms

- An uncomfortable feeling of heaviness in the stomach
- Nausea
- Belching
- Flatulence (gas)
- White, furry tongue
- Vomiting
- Fever, in cases of digestive poisoning, accompanied by diarrhoea

Consult your doctor

- A doctor should be called if the dyspepsia is frequent, chronic or involves weight loss. If there is repeated vomiting with blood or jaundice (yellowing of the skin), it is imperative to find out the underlying cause.

DID YOU KNOW?
Digestive problems

Mint and **caraway** essential oils can help to relieve chronic dyspepsia. Double blind studies were carried out on patients suffering from various digestive disorders (but not gastroduodenal ulcers) using a commercial preparation containing 90mg of mint and 50mg of caraway essential oils.

After four weeks the pain disappeared in 63.2 per cent of patients, while 94.5 per cent of patients experienced an improvement in symptoms. Both essential oils are anti-spasmodic.

Causes

Dyspepsia is caused by digestive problems of the stomach or the intestines. It is frequently the result of overindulgence in excessively fatty or spicy foods. It may also be related to a problem in the gall bladder or the pancreas.

WHICH PLANTS?

WARNING Use only one of the following at any given time

Internal usage
For simple indigestion
Caraway (tincture, 1:4 in 45% alcohol) Take 10-15 drops in water three times a day after meals.
Centaury (tincture, 1:4 in 25% alcohol) Take 10-15 drops in a little cold water 30 minutes before eating three times a day.
Cinnamon Take 0.3-0.5g of powder a day with food.
German chamomile Infuse 1 sachet of dried flowers in a cup of boiling water for 10 minutes. Take 3 cups a day before meals.
Ginger (tincture, 1:5 in 60% alcohol) Take 10 drops a day in a glass of water.
Peppermint Infuse 1 dessertspoon of dried leaves in 150ml of boiling water for 10-15 minutes. Drink 1 cup after meals.
Star anise Infuse 1 teaspoon of dried fruit in a cup of boiling water for 10 minutes. Strain. Drink 2 cups a day before meals.
Turmeric (tincture,1:5 in 70% alcohol) Put 35 drops into a glass of water. Take after every meal.

Other measures
- Steer clear of fizzy drinks; avoid completely in cases of flatulence.
- Avoid foods that you have trouble digesting.
- Never overload the stomach; eat smaller meals more frequently.
- Take 1 teaspoon of bicarbonate of soda in water to neutralise stomach acids.

Peptic ulcer

A raw area, about 10-25mm across, in the lining of the oesophagus, stomach or duodenum, is known as a peptic ulcer. The ulcer occurs as a result of erosion by the action of acidic gastric juices. Peptic ulcers are less common now that a wider range of antacid medications are available over the counter.

Symptoms
- Epigastric pain below the sternum, in the pit of the stomach, between 30 minutes and an hour after meals
- Heartburn (dull, burning pain in the centre of the chest)
- Nausea and vomiting
- Black stools due to the presence of digested blood

Consult your doctor or medical herbalist
- A consultation with your GP is recommended to correctly diagnose and treat the condition.

Causes

The development of a peptic ulcer is associated with factors including overwork, anxiety, smoking, eating spicy foods and infection by the bacterium *Helicobacter pylori*. Certain types of medication, including non-steroidal anti-inflammatories and cortisone have also been implicated.

WHICH PLANTS?

WARNING Use only one of the following at any given time

Internal usage
German chamomile Infuse 1 sachet of dried leaves in a cup of boiling water for 10 minutes. Drink 3 cups a day before meals.
Lavender Infuse 2-3g of the dried flowers in a cup of boiling water for 5-10 minutes. Drink ½ cup twice a day.
Lemon balm Infuse 2-3g of dried leaves in a cup of boiling water for 5 minutes. Drink 1 cup at midday and 1 in the evening after meals.
Bitter orange Infuse 20g of dried flowers in 150ml of boiling water for 5 minutes. Take in the evening just before going to bed.

Other measures
- Chew food properly, especially if the food is raw, and eat slowly.
- Eat little meals more often – food is the best way to mop up excess acid.
- If you like spicy food, always use powdered rather than fresh spices as they are less of an irritant for the stomach.
- Fatty or acidic food may also worsen the symptoms.
- Try to avoid stressful situations.

DID YOU KNOW?
Peptic ulcers

The discovery that peptic ulcers are associated with the presence of *Helicobacter pylori* marked the beginning of a new phase in treatment.

Research showed that plant-based substances could inhibit the bacterium. This led to the development of non-antibiotic treatments for peptic ulcers. The plants that inhibit *H.pylori* include garlic, cinnamon, chamomile, marigold, and a blend of mint and caraway.

Ulcerative colitis

The chronic inflammation and ulceration of the rectum and colon is termed ulcerative colitis. The disease is characterised by bloody diarrhoea, which may also contain pus and mucus. Its first manifestation is usually the most severe. Thereafter, its development is characterised by remissions and relapses over a period of years.

Colitis usually affects young adults but also occurs in elderly people.

Symptoms

- Diarrhoea containing blood, pus and mucus
- Fever, extreme fatigue
- Abdominal pain, general malaise
- Loss of appetite, weight loss

Consult your doctor

- Colitis may need urgent treatment, especially during the first attack. Generally speaking, it is crucial to seek medical advice if you suffer an attack of diarrhoea in which blood appears in the stools. Once the condition has been diagnosed, regular medical supervision is required to avoid complications.

Causes

The cause of ulcerative colitis is a subject of debate. It may be an inherited autoimmune disorder, whereby the body produces antibodies that attack its own cells in the gut. It is frequently associated with other diseases whose genetic origins have been proven or suspected (rheumatoid arthritis).

It often affects people who have a diet that is low in fibre and too rich in refined sugars, while non-smokers and ex-smokers are more likely to be affected than smokers. Emotional stress, an associated infection, gastroenteritis or a course of antibiotics can cause a flare-up of the disease.

WHICH PLANTS?

WARNING Use only one of the following at any given time

Internal usage

To soothe the gut
Roman chamomile Infuse 1 sachet of dried flowers or 1 dessertspoon of dried flowers in a cup of boiling water for 10 minutes. Drink 1 cup after each main meal.

To reduce inflammation and ease spasms
Milk thistle (tablets, 200mg) Take 1-2 tablets a day as a food supplement.
German chamomile Infuse 1 sachet of dried flowers in a cup of boiling water for 10 minutes. Drink 3 cups a day before meals.

To prevent anxiety
Lime tree Infuse 5g of dried flowers in 1 litre of boiling water for 5 minutes. Drink 1 cup in the evening to help you fall asleep.
Passionflower (tincture, 1:8 in 25% alcohol) Take 25-75 drops in a glass of water.

Other measures

- Prevent stress by practising yoga or relaxation techniques.
- Avoid milk, dairy products, yeast, raw fruit and vegetables.
- A diet high in protein, iron and potassium will help to replace what has been lost through diarrhoea.
- Take a mineral supplement and probiotics to restore the balance of beneficial bacteria in the gut.

Wind, bloating and flatulence

The presence of gas in the stomach or intestines is experienced as belching, bloating and flatulence.

Symptoms

- Bloating: a painful, distended stomach and difficulty in expelling the gas
- Belching and flatulence

Consult your doctor

- Plants can only be used to treat this type of disorder if a doctor decides that the cause is not serious.

Causes

Wind and bloating occur when you eat too quickly and swallow air at the same time as the food or if you have a fizzy drink with a meal. It can also be due to insufficient chewing of food. People who are anxious and swallow their food awkwardly are particularly susceptible.

Certain foods such as garlic, peas, pulses, cabbage, sugary food, or quantities of raw vegetables or fruit, produce more gas than others. Flatulence can also be the result of excessive bacterial activity in the colon. Equally, intestinal infections, bacterial proliferation and the start of gastroenteritis can often be the cause. Flatulence can also follow constipation, and intestinal blockage or paralysis. It is common among people who are anxious or stressed.

WHICH PLANTS?

WARNING Use only one of the following at any given time

Internal usage

Plants that are antispasmodic, carminative (facilitate expulsion of intestinal gas), sedative and that aid digestion are useful for treating these symptoms.

Bitter fennel Infuse ¼ to ½ teaspoon of crushed seeds in a cup of boiling water for 10 minutes. Drink 1 cup up to three times a day (infants: 2-3 teaspoons up to three times a day).

Caraway (tincture, 1:4 in 45% alcohol) Take 10-15 drops in a glass of cold water three times a day after meals.

Centaury (tincture, 1:4 in 25% alcohol) Take 10-15 drops in a little cold water, 30 minutes before eating three times a day.

Coriander Infuse 10-30g of crushed seed in 1 litre of boiling water for 10 minutes. Strain. Drink 1 cup after each meal.

Cumin Infuse 1 teaspoon of seeds in 250ml of boiling water for 2-3 minutes. Drink ½ cup before main meals.

Lemon verbena Infuse 1 sachet of dried leaves in a cup of boiling water for 5 minutes. Drink 2 cups a day after main meals.

Peppermint Infuse 1 dessertspoon of dried leaves in 150ml of boiling water for 10-15 minutes. Drink 1 cup after every meal.

Rosemary Infuse 2-4g of the dried plant in a cup of boiling water for 10 minutes. Drink 3 cups a day after meals.

Sweet marjoram Infuse 1 dessertspoon of dried plant in a cup of boiling water for 5-10 minutes. Drink 3 cups a day.

Other measures

- Eat small quantities of food at a time, slowly, chewing well.
- Avoid chewing gum.
- Reduce consumption of sugary and starchy food.
- Eliminate excess air by taking charcoal tablets.
- Eat less fibre and avoid fizzy drinks.
- Take regular physical exercise, such as walking.

Ear, nose & throat problems

Common cold and allergic rhinitis

The common cold (rhinitis) is an extremely common viral infection. It is an inflammation of the lining of the respiratory tract, in particular the nasal passages. Recovery usually occurs after a few days.

Allergic rhinitis has similar symptoms to the common cold in that it is characterised by sneezing, nasal itching and congestion. However, it is not caused by a virus. It is frequently associated with allergies to dust, house mites or pollen (see Hay fever). It usually starts during adolescence or in early adulthood, and is associated with a family history of allergy (including hay fever, asthma and eczema).

Symptoms

- Blocked nose
- Frequent sneezing
- Nasal discharge, initially runny and clear and then thick and greenish yellow
- Itching in the nasal area

Consult your doctor

- Only a doctor can distinguish between rhinitis and allergic rhinitis and identify any allergens responsible.

Causes

Rhinitis is usually caused by a virus although it can be caused by bacteria. Allergic rhinitis, however, is becoming increasingly common, and is usually due to an allergy to grass pollen, tree pollens, or the spores of moulds or fungi. When the symptoms persist all year round, they are then the result of other more persistent allergens, or even atmospheric pollution.

WHICH PLANTS?

WARNING Use only one of the following at any given time

Common cold
Internal usage
To combat infection
Echinacea (capsules, 325mg) Take 1-3 capsules a day with a glass of water before meals.

To soothe irritation
Blackcurrant Put 5g of dried leaves in 1 litre of boiling water. Infuse for 5 minutes. Strain. Drink 2-3 cups a day.

Common thyme Infuse 1 sachet of dried leaves in a cup of boiling water for 5 minutes. Strain. Drink 3 cups a day.

Eucalyptus Add 3 drops of essential oil to a bowl of boiled water that has been allowed to cool a little; cover head with a towel and place over the bowl. Inhale deeply for 10 minutes.

Rosemary Infuse 2-4g of the dried plant in a cup of boiling water for 10 minutes. Strain. Drink 3 cups a day after meals.

White deadnettle (tincture, 1:4 in 25% alcohol) Take 20 drops in water three times a day.

Allergic rhinitis
Internal usage
German chamomile Add 1 sachet to 1 cup of boiling water. Infuse for 10 minutes. Drink 3 cups a day before meals.

Ginger (tincture, 1:5 in 60% alcohol) Take 30 drops a day in water.

Other measures

- Increase your fluid intake.
- Increase your vitamin C intake.
- For allergic rhinitis, skin testing can be arranged through your GP to try to discover the identity of the allergen that is causing the reaction.

Ear disorders

Infection of the middle ear (otitis media) is the most common type of ear disorder, particularly in children (*see* Ear infections, p236). In adults, another common disorder is otitis externa – which causes inflammation of the outer ear and is also often the result of an infection.

Outer and middle-ear disorders can also be the result of injury, a boil in the ear canal, or a blockage of ear wax. Earache may also be an accompanying symptom of the common cold, tooth decay or other dental problems.

Symptoms
- Mild to severe earache
- Inflammation of the ear
- Discharge of pus from the ear
- Slight hearing loss

Consult your doctor
- If the pain is severe, see your doctor immediately to determine the cause.
- Antibiotics may be prescribed or an antifungal drug if a fungal infection is the cause.

Causes
Otitis externa can be caused by a bacterial, viral or fungal infection. It is quite common among swimmers as moisture in the ear can encourage infection.

Earache can be caused by a blockage of the ear, and is sometimes worsened by attempts to clear the ear using a cotton bud as this may push it deeper into the ear canal. Rarely a herpes infection can cause blisters in the ear with persisting pain.

WHICH PLANTS?
WARNING Use only one of the following at any given time

Internal usage

To fight infection and reduce inflammation

Aaron's rod Put 1.5-2g into a cup of boiling water. Leave to infuse for 15 minutes, then strain. Take 3 cups a day.

Clove Take 1-3 cloves a day in a decoction.

Echinacea (capsules, 325mg) Take 1-3 capsules a day with a glass of water before meals.

Golden seal (capsules, 540mg), Take 1 capsule three times a day. (Do not take if suffering from high blood pressure.)

Rosemary Put 2-4g of dried plant into 1 cup of boiling water, cover and leave to infuse for 10 minutes. Drink 3 cups a day after meals.

Hoarseness, voice loss

When the larynx, which is responsible for voice production, becomes inflamed through irritation or infection, the result is hoarseness (dysphonia) or complete voice loss (aphonia).

Symptoms
- Hoarseness
- Some pain
- Partial or complete voice loss
- Occasionally, a slight cough

Consult your doctor
- In cases of chronic hoarseness, ask for an ear, nose and throat examination by your doctor or a specialist.
- Sudden hoarseness accompanied by breathing difficulties may be a symptom of severe laryngitis requiring urgent medical intervention.

Causes
Inflammation of the larynx may be caused by infection, allergies, irritation by toxic agents such as tobacco smoke or alcohol, or overuse of the vocal cords. Other less obvious causes of hoarseness, which should be checked if the infection resists medical treatment, include secondary effects of acid reflux, psychological problems, or possibly cancer.

WHICH PLANTS?
WARNING Use only one of the following at any given time

Internal usage

Common thyme Infuse 1 sachet in a cup of boiling water for 5 minutes. Drink 3 cups a day.

Greater plantain (capsules, 280mg) Take 1 capsule three times a day before meals.

Heartsease (tincture, 1:4 in 25% alcohol) Take 20 drops in water three times a day after meals.

Hedge mustard Infuse 1 teaspoon or 5g of the dried plant in a cup of boiling water for 10 minutes. Strain, and drink 2-3 cups a day.

Mallow Boil 5g of the dried plant in 1 litre of water for 5 minutes. Strain, and drink 1-3 cups a day.

Marshmallow (root liquid extract, 1:1 in 25% alcohol) Take 2-5ml three times a day.

External application

Agrimony Infuse 1 teaspoon of the dried plant in 250ml of boiling water for 5 minutes. Strain, cool and use as a gargle three times a day.

Blackcurrant Infuse 5g of dried leaves in 1 litre of boiling water for 5 minutes. Strain, and use as a gargle three times a day.

Eucalyptus Dilute 3 drops of essential oil with 10ml of carrier oil and rub 5ml into the throat and chest area twice a day.

Hyssop Infuse 1-2 teaspoons of dried flowers in a cup of boiling water for 5-10 minutes. Strain, and use as a gargle three times a day.

Lavender (essential oil) Follow instructions for eucalyptus (above).

Sweet fennel Infuse 1 teaspoon of seeds in 200ml of boiling water for 10 minutes. Strain, and use as a gargle three times a day.

Other measures

- Talk as little as possible to rest the vocal cords
- Avoid irritants
- Twice a day, add a few drops of menthol or eucalyptus oil to boiling water and inhale for 10 minutes.

Laryngitis

A common affliction of the voicebox, laryngitis can be acute or chronic and can result in hoarseness and voice loss.

Symptoms

- A cough that is initially dry, later producing phlegm
- Coughing on inhalation
- Pain while coughing (rare)
- Altered or hoarse voice, to the point of loss of voice (aphonia)

Consult your doctor or medical herbalist

- Laryngitis often disappears spontaneously or with the help of medical herbalism. But if symptoms persist, see your doctor to exclude any serious underlying condition.

Causes

Laryngitis is very often the result of a viral infection. However, chronic cases may also be caused by persistent irritation from tobacco smoke, alcohol or fumes, or overuse of the voice (see Hoarseness).

WHICH PLANTS?

WARNING Use only one of the following at any given time

Internal usage

For coughs and catarrh

Aaron's rod Infuse 1.5-2g dried flowers in a cup of boiling water for 15 minutes. Strain, and drink 3 cups a day.

Common thyme Infuse 1 sachet or 2g of dried thyme in a cup of boiling water for 5 minutes. Strain, and drink 3 cups a day.

Common elder (elderflower tincture, 1:4 in 25% alcohol) Take 20 drops in water three times a day after meals.

Greater plantain (capsules, 280mg) Take 1 capsule three times a day before meals.

Mallow Boil 5g of dried plant in 1 litre of water for 5 minutes. Strain, and drink 1-3 cups a day.

Sweet fennel Infuse 1 teaspoon of seeds in 200ml of boiling water for 10 minutes. Strain, and drink three times a day.

White horehound (tincture, 1:4 in 25% alcohol) Take 10-20 drops in a glass of water two or three times a day before meals.

For loss of voice

Hedge mustard Infuse 1 teaspoon or 5g of dried plant in a cup of boiling water for 10 minutes. Strain, and drink 2-3 cups a day.

Aaron's rod Infuse 1.5-2g dried flowers in a cup of boiling water for 15 minutes. Strain, and drink 3 cups a day.

To fight infection

Heartsease (tincture, 1:4 in 25% alcohol) Take 20 drops in water three times a day after meals.

Ginger (root tincture, 1:5 in 60% alcohol) Take 10 drops a day in a glass of water.

To boost the immune system

Echinacea (tincture, 1:5 in 45% alcohol) Take 15 drops in water three times a day.

Rosemary Infuse 2-4g of the dried leaves in a cup of boiling water for 10 minutes. Strain, and drink 3 cups a day after meals.

External application

Eucalyptus Dilute 3 drops of essential oil with 10ml of carrier oil and massage 1-2 teaspoons into the throat, chest and back. Repeat two or three times a day.

Scots pine Infuse 20g of buds in 1 litre of boiling water for 10 minutes. Strain and use as a gargle four or five times a day.

Other measures

- Diffuse eucalyptus oil in a room, or put a few drops in boiling water and inhale the steam from a bowl for 10 minutes, two or three times a day.

Sinusitis

The sinuses are hollow cavities in the facial bones, adjoining and linked to the nose. There are four pairs of sinuses: maxillary, frontal, ethmoidal and sphenoidal. Sinusitis is an inflammation of one or more of these sinuses due to a bacterial infection.

The blocked sinuses associated with the common cold are often misdiagnosed as sinusitis, which can lead to the unnecessary prescription of antibiotics.

Symptoms

- Fever (but not necessarily)
- Pain on the affected side when you lean forward or press on the affected sinus(es)
- Discharge and obstruction of the affected nasal passage
- Coughing at night
- Loss of sense of smell (and therefore also of taste to some extent)
- Generalised headache, often worse in the mornings
- Sometimes pain on chewing

Consult your doctor

- Only a doctor can determine the exact cause of sinusitis and prescribe appropriate treatment.

Sinusitis contd

Causes

Sinusitis often follows infections of the ear, nose and throat such as the common cold. It can also be caused by the presence of polyps in the nose or sinuses or dental extractions and fillings. Some forms of sinusitis are the result of allergies linked to atmospheric pollution (smoke, pollen, dust).

WHICH PLANTS?

WARNING Use only one of the following at any given time

Internal usage

Ash Put 10-20g of dried leaves into 1 litre of boiling water. Leave to infuse for 10 minutes and then strain. Drink 0.5-1 litre a day.
Echinacea (tincture, 1:5 in 45% ethanol) Take 2-5ml a day.
Garlic (300mg powder capsules) Take 1-3 capsules a day.
Golden seal (540mg capsules) Take 1 capsule three times a day.

As directed by a medical herbalist

- Meadowsweet, Greater celandine, Radish, Willow

Other measures

- Try to control the quality of the air you breathe: avoid smoky or dusty atmospheres.
- Place an air humidifier in rooms where you spend several hours at a time.

Throat infections

Tonsillitis and pharyngitis are among the most common throat infections. With tonsillitis the tonsils are inflamed while pharyngitis is an infection of the pharynx (between the tonsils and the larynx).

Symptoms

Tonsillitis
- Redness of the throat and tonsils, often with white patches or spots
- Soreness when swallowing
- Sometimes a slight cough
- Swollen, tender lymph nodes under the jaw
- Ulcerations (small sores) on one tonsil (trench mouth)
- Blisters on the throat with a slight fever

Pharyngitis
- Fever
- Pain in the back of the throat
- Soreness when swallowing
- Often a runny or blocked nose (as in the common cold)

Consult your doctor

- Medical advice should be sought if a sore throat lasts for more than two days, becomes very severe, or you have an immune deficiency or a history of heart or kidney infections.
- Tonsillitis is occasionally troublesome, with a very small risk of complications such as otitis media, sinusitis, abscess on the tonsil (quinsy), rheumatic fever and kidney infections. But antibiotics are not very effective at preventing these complications.

Causes

Tonsillitis and pharyngitis are usually caused by the presence of a relatively benign virus, but they are the work of the streptococcus bacteria in about a third of cases. Tonsillitis can be a manifestation of herpes, glandular fever and other rare infections.

WHICH PLANTS?

WARNING Use only one of the following at any given time

Internal usage

Tonsillitis
Aaron's rod Infuse 1.5-2g of dried flowers in a cup of boiling water for 15 minutes. Strain, and drink 3 cups a day.
Echinacea (tincture, 1:5 in 45% alcohol) Take 2-5ml a day in a glass of water.
Hedge mustard Infuse 1 teaspoon or 5g of dried plant in a cup of boiling water for 10 minutes. Strain, and drink 2-3 cups a day.
Mallow Boil 5g of dried plant in 1 litre of water for 5 minutes. Strain, and drink 1-3 cups a day.
Marshmallow Infuse 2-3g of dried root in a cup of boiling water for 10 minutes. Strain, and drink 2-3 cups a day.
Sweet violet (tincture, 1:4 in 25% alcohol) Take 20 drops in a small amount of water three times a day after food.

Pharyngitis
Common sage Put 20g of dried leaves into 1 litre of boiling water. Leave to infuse for 10 minutes. Strain, and drink 1-2 cups a day.
Common thyme Infuse 1 sachet in 1 cup of boiling water for 5 minutes, then strain. Drink 3 cups a day.

During convalescence
Dog rose Infuse 2-2.5g of broken rosehips in a cup of boiling water for 10 minutes and then strain. Drink 3-4 cups a day.

Rosemary Infuse 2-4g of the dried leaves in a cup of boiling water for 10 minutes. Drink 3 cups a day after meals.
Sea buckthorn Take 1-3 dessert-spoons of sea buckthorn juice a day in a glass of water.

External application
Blackberry Boil 10g of dried leaves in 100ml of water for 2-3 minutes and leave to infuse for 15 minutes. Use as a gargle twice a day.
Eucalyptus Dilute 3 drops of essential oil in 10ml of carrier oil. Rub 5ml into the throat area two or three times a day.
Marigold Infuse 5g of dried flowers in 1 litre of boiling water for 5 minutes. Use as a mouthwash two or three times a day.
Roman chamomile Put 1 teaspoon of dried flowers into a cup of boiling water. Infuse for 10 minutes, strain. Use as a gargle two or three times a day.

Other measures
- Drink a lot of fluids, especially elder infusion.
- Take regular lukewarm baths to help to reduce any fever.
- Eat foods containing vitamin C to fight the infection.

Tinnitus

An auditory sensation in the ear that is not caused by any external noise characterises this stressful condition. Subjective tinnitus refers to buzzing, roaring, ringing or whistling in the ear that may be continuous or intermittent, but is perceived only by the sufferer.

Objective tinnitus is caused by vascular sounds in the head and neck or muscular contractions of the middle ear or the soft palate in the mouth. Upon examination, the noise can be heard by the specialist as well as by the patient.

Symptoms
- Intermittent or continuous thudding, felt in the arteries of the neck, the temples and in the rear part of the head
- A whistling sound in the ear
- Reduction in the ability to hear external sounds
- Reduced ability to hear certain sounds (high or low-pitched sounds, for example)

Consult your doctor
- A visit to the doctor is vital in order to identify the origin of the problem. The treatment will vary according to the type of tinnitus diagnosed.

Causes
The causes are often unknown, which can be frustrating for the tinnitus sufferer. However, certain problems of the middle or inner ear can lead to tinnitus, including ear infections, partial deafness, Ménière's disease, or damage of the acoustic nerve or the auditory centres in the brain. A blockage in the external ear canal and vascular problems (hypertension, athero-sclerosis or congested Eustachian tubes) can also result in tinnitus.

WHICH PLANTS?
WARNING Use only one of the following at any given time

Internal usage
For stress
Passionflower Infuse 1 teaspoon of the dried plant in a cup of boiling water for 5-10 minutes and filter. Strain, and drink 1 cup at bedtime.

For circulatory problems
Ginkgo (tincture, 1:4 in 25% alcohol) Take 15 drops in water three times a day before meals.
Bilberry (60mg tablets) Take 1-3 tablets a day with water.

For infections
Echinacea (tincture, 1:5 in 45% alcohol) Take 15 drops a day in water.
Meadowsweet (tincture 1:4 in 25% alcohol) Take 20 drops in water three times a day after or in between meals.

External application
For congestion in the Eustachian tubes and sinuses
Eucalyptus Dilute 2-3 drops of essential oil in a bowl of freshly boiled water. Cover your head with a towel and place head over bowl. Inhale deeply for 10 minutes.
Scots pine Follow instructions for eucalyptus inhalant (above).

Other measures
- If possible, treat the disorder responsible for the tinnitus.
- If a blockage of earwax is the cause, consult your doctor about its removal.
- Protect your hearing from any very high noise levels that you may experience during the course of your day.
- Acupuncture may help.
- Consider relaxation techniques.

Eye problems
Eye disorders

Problems of the eye, affecting parts such as the retina or macula, can produce a variety of sight defects.

Symptoms
- A reduction in vision
- Inability to see in poor light (night blindness)
- Black specks in the field of vision (scotoma)
- Runny or painful eyes after prolonged visual effort

Consult your doctor
- Visual disorders should always be taken seriously. Always see a GP or optician before consulting a medical herbalist.

Causes
Eye disorders can be due to problems affecting the veins and arteries within the eye, or deterioration of the ophthalmic nerve or they may be caused by high blood pressure or diabetes. They are also often part of the ageing process that affects the retina and ocular tissues.

WHICH PLANTS?
WARNING Use only one of the following at any given time

Internal usage
To treat eye problems
Bilberry (tablets, 60mg) Take 1-3 tablets a day with water.
Blackcurrant Put 5g of dried leaves into 1 litre of boiling water. Leave to infuse for 5 minutes. Drink 2-3 cups a day.

External application
To prevent eye fatigue, irritation and soreness
Eyebright Infuse 1 heaped teaspoon of dried flowers in a cup of boiling water for 15 minutes. Soak two clean cotton pads in the infusion and place over each closed eye for 10 minutes.

Tracheitis

Infectious inflammation of the windpipe (trachea) is called tracheitis. It is usually acute but can become chronic.

Symptoms
- An initially dry and then phlegmy cough
- Coughing on inhalation
- Sometimes a reduction of vocal intensity, a change in the tone of the voice, hoarseness and even loss of speech (aphonia)

Consult your doctor or medical herbalist
- Tracheitis often does not need medical treatment and may be relieved with medicinal plants. If symptoms persist, however, seek advice from a doctor who will determine whether or not it is a more serious condition.

Causes
Tracheitis is commonly caused by a viral infection. It is aggravated by fumes and smoke inhalation. It often occurs with laryngitis and bronchitis.

WHICH PLANTS?
WARNING Use only one of the following at any given time

Internal usage
To prevent coughing and catarrh in the respiratory tracts
Aaron's rod Infuse 1.5-2g dried flowers in a cup of boiling water for 15 minutes. Strain, and drink 3 cups a day.
Bitter fennel Put ¼-½ teaspoon of crushed seeds into a cup of boiling water. Infuse for 10 minutes. Strain, and drink 1 cup up to three times a day.
Mallow Boil 5g of the dried plant in 1 litre of water for 5 minutes. Strain, and drink 1-3 cups a day.

To stimulate the immune system
Echinacea (tincture, 1:5 in 45% alcohol) Take 15 drops a day in a glass of water.

To prevent infection
Common thyme Infuse 1 sachet in a cup of boiling water for 5 minutes. Drink 3 cups a day.
Rosemary Infuse 2-4g of the dried plant in a cup of boiling water for 10 minutes. Strain, and drink 3 cups a day after meals.

External application
Eucalyptus Dilute 3 drops of essential oil in a bowl of freshly boiled water, cover head with a towel and lean over bowl. Inhale deeply for 10 minutes. Repeat twice a day.
Scots pine Infuse 20g of buds in 1 litre of boiling water for 10 minutes and strain. Use as a gargle four or five times a day.

Other measures
- Diffuse menthol or eucalyptus oil in your bedroom or put a few drops into a bowl of boiling water and inhale the steam two or three times a day.

German chamomile Make an infusion with 2 sachets of chamomile – one for each eye – and allow to cool. Squeeze out the excess liquid, then place a sachet over each closed eye and leave it in place for 10 minutes. Repeat two or three times a day.

Sweet clover Boil 20g of dried flowers in 100ml of water for 15 minutes. Soak a cloth in the decoction, squeeze out the excess and place over closed eyes for 10 minutes. Repeat two or three times a day.

Witch hazel Infuse 10g of dried bark in 1 litre of water for 5-10 minutes. Soak a cloth in this liquid and then squeeze out the excess and place over closed eyes. Repeat two or three times a day.

Other measures
- Have your eyesight checked and correct any vision problems.
- Protect your eyes from sun and smoke.
- Give up smoking.
- Eat fresh fruit (berries, tomatoes, sea-buckthorn juice) for their circulatory and antioxidant properties.

Eye infections

Infectious conditions of the eye include conjunctivitis, inflammation of the tear sac (dacryocystitis), inflammation of the uvea or middle layer covering the eyeball (uveitis), infection of the eyelids (blepharitis) and styes. Retinal infection (retinitis) can also occur in people with a compromised immune system.

Symptoms
- Bloodshot eyes
- Itching or pain
- Impaired vision (cloudiness or blurring)
- Over-sensitivity to light

- Inflammation or infection along the rim of the eyelid, often with scaling
- Painful red swelling under the eye can herald dacryocystitis

Consult your doctor
- If any of these infections do not respond to anti-inflammatory treatment or if itching or pain persists for more than 24 hours, consult your doctor as soon as possible. If suffering vision loss, go straight to a hospital accident and emergency department.

Causes
Although the causes of eye inflammation may be environmental (wind, cold, dust), they can lead to, or be caused by, a viral or bacterial infection. An inflamed eye can also be due to seborrhoeic dermatitis (see Scalp problems) that usually affects the scalp and eyebrows.

WHICH PLANTS?
WARNING Use only one of the following at any given time

Internal usage
Bilberry (tablets, 60mg) Take 1-3 tablets a day with water.
Echinacea (tincture, 1:5 in 45% alcohol) Take 15 drops in water three times a day.

External application
Barberry (tincture, 1:3 in 25% alcohol) Add 20 drops to a glass of water. Soak a cloth or pad with this and then squeeze out the excess. Apply to affected closed eye for 15 minutes. Repeat two to three times a day.

Eyebright Infuse a heaped teaspoon of dried flowers in a cup of boiling water for 15 minutes. Soak two clean cotton pads in the infusion and place over each closed eye for 10 minutes.

Lavender Infuse 2-3g of the flowers in a cup of boiling water for 15 minutes. Allow to cool, then soak a cloth in the infusion, squeeze out the excess, and apply to closed eyes for 15 minutes. Repeat two or three times a day.

Marigold Infuse 5g of dried flowers in 1 litre of boiling water for 15 minutes. Allow to cool, then soak a cloth in the infusion, squeeze out the excess, and apply to closed eyes for 15 minutes. Repeat three or four times a day.

Sweet clover Boil 20g of dried flowers in 100ml of water for 15 minutes. Allow to cool, then soak a cloth in the decoction. Apply to closed eyes two or three times a day.

Witch hazel Infuse 10g dried bark in 1 litre of boiling water for 5-10 minutes. Allow to cool then soak a cloth in this liquid, squeeze out the excess, and place over closed eyes. Repeat two or three times a day.

Other measures
- Wear dark glasses to protect your eyes from sunlight.
- Have any ear, nose and throat problems treated promptly.
- Blepharitis (infection of the rim of the eyelids) can be relieved by daily washes using cotton buds soaked in sodium bicarbonate solution or baby shampoo wiped repeatedly along the eyelashes.

Hair & nail problems

Hair loss

Hair is continually falling out and regrowing in cycles that last several months. However, the discovery of an excessive amount of hair on the pillow, or hair that comes out in clumps during brushing may be a cause for concern. The appearance of several small bald patches on the scalp indicate a condition known as alopecia.

Symptoms
- Excessive loss of hair, with or without the roots
- General thinning of the hair

Consult your doctor
- Although baldness in men is usually hereditary, seek a doctor's advice if hair loss – particularly in women – is sudden and excessive, as there may be a more serious underlying cause.

Causes

Excessive loss of hair can be due to a deficiency in certain minerals and proteins. It is sometimes connected to anaemia, fatigue or to problems with the endocrine glands. It can also be caused by alcoholism or by certain drugs (notably anticancer medication).

Well defined patches of complete baldness surrounded by normal hair (alopecia) may be related to other autoimmune conditions (such as some thyroid disorders), but usually resolves itself eventually. Sometimes there is a psychological cause behind hair loss, as in trichotillomania (hair loss due to habitual pulling out of hair).

WHICH PLANTS?

WARNING Use only one of the following at any given time

Internal usage
Evening primrose oil (capsules, 500mg) Take 1-2 capsules a day with food.
Ginkgo (capsules, 50-100mg dry extract) Take 1 capsule three times a day before meals.

External application

As a long-term treatment
Peppermint Dilute 3 drops of essential oil with 10ml carrier oil. Massage into scalp once a week. Shampoo out after 10-15 minutes application.
Rosemary Infuse 50g dried herb in 1 litre of boiling water for 30 minutes. Strain, cool and then massage into the scalp. Shampoo out after 10 minutes. Repeat once a week.
Centaury Boil 30-50g of the dried plant in 1 litre of water for 2-3 minutes. Strain, cool and rub into the scalp once or twice a day.
Stinging nettle Boil 20g dried plant in 750ml water until it is reduced to roughly 500ml. Strain, cool and rub into the scalp twice a week, rinsing after 15 minutes. Use twice the amount of fresh herb.

To nourish the scalp
Maize (oil) Rub into the scalp and leave for 15 minutes, then shampoo out. Repeat once a week.
Flax seed (oil) Follow the same instructions as for maize oil.

Other measures
- Ensure you eat a balanced diet.
- Supplements of iron, sulphur, vitamin A, zinc, copper, magnesium, potassium, fluorine can be taken.
- Take a course of vitamin D.
- Do not panic about generalised hair loss – the hair will usually begin to stop falling out and grow back more thickly again after a few months.

DID YOU KNOW?
Hair

The Sioux Indians made a lotion using **nettle** leaves that helped hair to regrow. When scientists analysed this North American hair preparation they found that the irritant substances contained in the stinging part of the leaves stimulated the blood circulation of the scalp. It is the increased blood supply that encourages cells to produce new hair.

Nail disorders

The main disorders affecting the nails are brittleness, due to a weakness in the tissues that form the nails, and fungal infections of nails and the surrounding skin.

Symptoms
- Striated, transparent-looking nails
- Dry, brittle nails
- Soft nails that split in fine layers
- Thickened, yellowing nails and sore, itchy skin surrounding the nails (fungal infections)

Consult your doctor
- Brittle nails and fungal infections can signify more serious underlying conditions that should be treated by a doctor.

Causes

Brittle nails can be the result of a vitamin, dietary or mineral deficiency, a disorder of the digestive tract or endocrine glands, or localised trauma of the nail. Fungal infections of the nails tend to arise when a person's immune system is weakened due to stress or other illness. Psoriasis can mimic fungal infection of the nails.

WHICH PLANTS?

WARNING Use only one of the following at any given time

Internal usage

For fungal infections

Echinacea (tincture, 1:5 in 45% alcohol) Take 15 drops in water three times a day.

As directed by a medical herbalist

• Barberry

For brittle nails

Evening primrose oil (capsules, 500mg) Take 1-2 capsules a day during meals with a glass of water. Horsetail Infuse 2-4g of the dried plant in 200ml of boiling water for 10-15 minutes. Drink 1 cup a day. Alternatively, take 2g of powder three times a day. Maize (capsules, 150mg dry extract) Take 2-4 capsules a day.

External application

For fungal infections

Common thyme Infuse 1 sachet of dried thyme in a cup of boiling water for 15 minutes. Allow to cool and soak affected nails in the liquid for 15 minutes twice a day. Walnut Infuse 10g of dried leaves in 1 litre of boiling water for 15 minutes. Strain and allow to cool slightly. Soak affected nails in the liquid for 15 minutes twice a day.

Other measures

• To strengthen your nails, take a multivitamin supplement.
• Keep the nails cut short, disinfecting the scissors or clippers after cutting infected nails, to avoid infecting the others.

See also Fungal infections.

Scalp problems

The two main problems affecting the scalp are dandruff (the excessive flaking of the skin of the scalp) and seborrhoeic dermatitis of the scalp (an excessive production of sebum).

Symptoms

Dandruff
• Small shiny, white flakes in the hair, all over the head
• Little or no itching

Greasy dandruff
• Large, thick flakes that are yellowish and moist
• Greasy scalp

Seborrhoeic dermatitis
• Lank hair that becomes greasy rapidly
• Itchiness causing lesions
• An unpleasant smell from the scalp
• Redness around the edges of the scalp
• The scalp can become inflamed
• Sometimes dermatitis spreads to the eyebrows and eyelids

Consult your doctor

• Although dandruff is not a serious disorder, a doctor should be consulted if it becomes severe.
• Other conditions that resemble dandruff include: eczema, psoriasis, ichthyosis, ringworm (a fungal infection) or the presence of lice.

Causes

Dandruff results from an accelerated shedding of dead skin cells. It can be caused by a fungus, anxiety, or hair products that contain too much detergent (or which are used too frequently).

Seborrhoeic dermatitis arises from an excessive secretion of sebum and is often accompanied by a widespread fungal infection. The condition may come and go but is usually aggravated during periods of stress.

WHICH PLANTS?

WARNING Use only one of the following at any given time

Internal usage

To treat dandruff

Rosemary Infuse 2-4g of the dried plant in a cup of boiling water for 10 minutes. Strain and drink 3 cups a day after meals.
Common sage Put 20g of dried leaves into 1 litre of boiling water. Infuse for 10 minutes. Strain and drink 1-2 cups a day.

External application

To prevent dandruff

Great burdock Infuse 5g of dried leaves in 1 litre of boiling water for 10 minutes. When tepid, rub into the scalp and rinse off after 15 minutes. Repeat twice a week.
Lavender Infuse 20g dried flowers in 500ml of boiling water, allow to cool, and then rub into the scalp. Rinse off after 15 minutes. Repeat twice a week.
Juniper Dilute 3 drops of essential oil in 10ml carrier oil and massage into the scalp. Leave for 15 minutes and then shampoo out. Repeat once or twice a week.
Stinging nettle Boil 20g dried leaves in 750ml water until it is reduced to roughly 500ml. Cool and rub into the scalp twice a week, rinsing after 15 minutes. Use twice the amount of fresh herb.
Rosemary Dilute 3 drops of essential oil in 10ml carrier oil and massage into the scalp. Leave for 15 minutes and then shampoo out. Repeat once or twice a week.
Silver birch Infuse 50g of dried leaves in 1 litre of boiling water for 15 minutes and rub into the scalp. Rinse after 15 minutes. Repeat twice a week.

To treat seborrhoeic dermatitis

Common sage Infuse 20g of dried leaves in 1 litre of boiling water for 5 minutes and allow to cool. Massage into the scalp. Rinse after 15 minutes. Repeat twice a week.

Scalp problems contd

Heartsease Infuse 20-30g of fresh flowers in 500ml boiling water until the liquid has cooled. Massage into the scalp and rinse out after 15 minutes. Repeat twice a week.

Marshmallow Infuse 20g of dried root in 500ml of boiling water until liquid cools. Rub into the scalp and rinse off after 15 minutes. Repeat twice a week.

Rosemary Dilute 3 drops of essential oil in 10ml carrier oil and massage into the scalp. Leave for 15 minutes and then shampoo out. Repeat twice a week.

Stinging nettle Boil 20g dried leaves in 750ml water until it is reduced to roughly 500ml. Cool and rub into the scalp rinsing after 15 minutes, twice a week. Use twice the amount of fresh herb.

Witch hazel (witch-hazel water) Rub into the scalp and rinse off after 15 minutes. Repeat twice a week.

Roman chamomile Infuse 20g of dried flowers in 500ml of boiling water until liquid cools. Rub into scalp and rinse off after 15 minutes. Repeat twice a week.

Other measures

- Use mild shampoo or shampoo that is suitable for your scalp condition.
- Try avoiding shampoo altogether – after an initial phase of increased greasiness, the scalp will usually settle back to a normal state, requiring only regular washing with warm water.
- Take a multivitamin and mineral supplement.

Infections & malignant disease

Cancer

There are several types of cancer, all arising from the uncontrollable multiplication of cells in an organ or tissue. The affected cells have been damaged so that they no longer function properly yet they divide more rapidly than the normal cells around them. The body's immune system cannot differentiate between the cancerous cells and normal cells and so does not destroy them.

Symptoms

- Symptoms vary according to the part of the body affected. In the breast or testes, lumps may appear; elsewhere the cancer may not be apparent until the function of the affected organ begins to deteriorate
- There may be pain of varying intensity; severe in some cases
- Loss of appetite
- Severe weight loss and visible signs of serious illness (cachexia)

Causes

A cancer starts off when the genetic material inside a cell is damaged by a carcinogenic substance. It may take several years before the cancer is large enough to be noticed. There are various risk factors associated with cancer, including smoking and drinking alcohol, contact with certain plastics or pollutants that mimic oestrogens. Exposure to asbestos, X-rays and ultraviolet radiation are also responsible for certain cancers. The presence of toxic substances produced by fungi (aflatoxins) in food and certain diseases such as hepatitis C can trigger cancer too.

Consult your doctor or medical herbalist

- Medical herbalism can be used to complement medical treatment for cancer, but it cannot be used to treat cancer alone.
- Some complementary herbal treatments may interfere with the metabolism of certain drugs, and should discussed with the doctor dealing with the case.

WHICH PLANTS?

WARNING Use only one of the following at any given time

Internal usage

Ashwagandha (tincture, 1:3 in 45% alcohol) Take 20 drops in a glass of water three times a day.

Echinacea (tincture, 1:5 in 45% alcohol) Take 15 drops in a glass of water three times a day.

Garlic (capsules, 300mg powder) Take 1-3 capsules a day.

Grape seed extract (capsule, 30-100mg) Take 1 capsule a day.

Green tea Put 1 teaspoon of green tea into a cup of boiling water. Infuse for 10 minutes. Drink 2-3 cups a day.

Liquorice Infuse 1-2 teaspoons of root powder in a cup of boiling water for 10 minutes before straining. Drink 2 cups a day.

Siberian ginseng (capsule, 150mg powder) Take 1 capsule three times a day with a large glass of water.

Stinging nettle (tincture, 1:4 in 25% alcohol) Take 20 drops in water three times a day after meals.

Other measures

- Eat a diet that is rich in oily fish.
- Eat plenty of soya, spinach, celery, asparagus, seaweed, capers, curry, peppers and fruit – all rich in antioxidants that may help to protect against cancer.
- Try to stop smoking, and moderate your alcohol intake.

Fever

Although not in itself an illness, a fever may arise from a wide range of medical problems. It can also be the first sign that something is wrong. Any sustained rise in body temperature above 37.5°C should always be taken seriously.

Symptoms

- Severe shivering followed by drenching sweats
- Alternating between these two states
- Lengthy or serious fevers are often accompanied by a rapid pulse, shortness of breath, a dry mouth and feeling faint
- Confusion, especially in the elderly

Consult your doctor or medical herbalist

- Except in cases where the cause is obviously benign (such as with a common cold), a doctor should be consulted if a fever lasts for more than 12 hours.
- If in doubt, do not try to reduce the fever quickly with medication: fever indicates the progress of the illness that provoked it. To lower it can actually impede the immune system's fight against the virus.
- Instead, call your doctor as soon as possible if the temperature rises suddenly and severely (above 41°C). Get help right away if your child has a temperature of 39°C or more. Remove all but a light layer of the child's clothing and ensure the room is well ventilated.

Causes

In general, fevers arise because of a bacterial, viral or parasitic infection, or an inflammatory condition. They can also result from general metabolic problems, such as hyperthyroidism, or from simply being overtired.

WHICH PLANTS?

WARNING Use only one of the following at any given time

Internal usage

Centaury (tincture, 1:4 in 25% alcohol) Put 30 drops in a glass of cold water. Take three times a day.
Chicory Boil 15-30g dried roots, leaves and flowers in 1 litre of water for 5 minutes, then strain. Drink 1 cup at midday and 1 in the evening.
Common elder (tincture, 1:5 in 25% alcohol) Take 20 drops in a little water, three times a day after meals.
Dog rose Infuse 2-2.5g crushed dried rosehips in a cup of boiling water for 10 minutes, then strain. Drink 3-4 cups a day.
Juniper Boil 10g dried berries in 750ml of boiling water for 20 minutes, then strain. Drink 2-3 cups a day.
Liquorice Steep 1-2 teaspoons of root powder in a cup of boiling water for 10 minutes, then strain. Drink 2 cups a day.
Meadowsweet (tincture, 1:4 in 25% alcohol) Take 20 drops in water, three times a day after or in between meals.
Milk thistle (tablets, 200mg) Take 1 tablet, once or twice a day as a food supplement.
Willow (capsules, 200mg) Take 2-4 capsules, three times a day with water.

External application

German chamomile Mix 3 drops essential oil to every 10ml carrier oil. Rub on your forehead and chest two or three times a day.
Juniper Mix 3 drops of essential oil to every 10ml carrier oil. Rub over your forehead and chest two or three times a day.
Lavender Mix 3 drops of essential oil to every 10ml carrier oil. Rub on your temples, behind your ears and behind your neck twice a day.

Fungal infections

The term 'mycosis' describes various types of infection of the skin and mucous membranes caused by microscopic fungi. These include *candidiasis* (thrush) and various *tinea* (such as ringworm and athlete's foot).

They tend to occur in warm, damp folds of skin, such as in the armpit and groin area. They can also affect the scalp or elsewhere on the body, appearing as crusty round patches, gradually enlarging and leaving a healed centre.

Symptoms

- Red or brown patches partially covered with vesicles (tiny blisters) or small scabs, which sometimes gradually enlarge as described above
- Sore, creamy yellow raised patches in the mouth
- White, cracking, itching inflamed areas in the groin
- Thickened, itchy, scaly patches on the scalp

Athlete's foot
- Thickening of the skin on the sides of the toes, followed by cracking and flaking

Consult your doctor

- Do not treat these infections before asking your doctor to confirm that this is a fungal skin infection and not another type of skin problem such as eczema or psoriasis.

Causes

Candidiasis is caused by a group of fungi similar to yeast, the most common of which is *Candida albicans*. Naturally present in the intestinal flora, these fungi sometimes undergo an abnormal development, especially in areas such as in folds of skin, in the mouth, or in the vagina, following a course of antibiotics or due to an immune deficiency.

Fungal infections contd

Diabetics and people with HIV/AIDS are more susceptible to fungal skin infections and indeed all other types of infection.

Athlete's foot, groin infections and ringworm are usually caused by such fungi as Trichophyton and Epidermophyton. As the name suggests, athlete's foot – associated with wearing shoes and sweating – is found widely among sportsmen and women, and spreads easily on floors of showers and locker rooms.

WHICH PLANTS?

WARNING Use only one of the following at any given time

Internal usage

Echinacea (tincture, 1:5 in 45% alcohol) Take 15 drops in water three times a day.
Grapefruit seed (capsules, 125mg) Take 1 capsule twice a day for the first three days, then 1 capsule three times a day for the next seven days, and finally 2 capsules twice or three times a day for the next 18 days.

External application

Walnut (tincture) Mix 3 drops to every 10ml carrier oil and apply to the affected area two or three times a day.
Winter savory Infuse 30g dried flowering tops in 1 litre of boiling water for 10 minutes, then strain. Apply a cloth soaked in the infusion to the affected area twice a day.

To heal the skin

Marigold Infuse 5g dried flowers in 1 litre of boiling water for 5 minutes. Apply a cloth soaked in the infusion to the affected area three or four times a day.

Other measures

- Prevent athlete's foot by wearing sandals, shoes, and cotton socks that allow your feet to breathe, ensuring your feet are clean, drying your feet and toes well after a bath or shower, keeping your toenails short and disinfecting scissors and other instruments used for foot care.
- Similarly, for tineal infections in the groin, dry well, and wear loose clothes.
- Scalp infections may be helped by keeping the hair short and using the treatments described above and under hair problems.

Glandular fever & cytomegalovirus

Glandular fever (infectious mononucleosis) is an infectious viral disease characterised by tiredness combined with fever, swollen glands, pharyngitis (inflammation of the throat) and sometimes jaundice. It mainly affects adolescents and young adults and is transmitted via saliva, which is why it is known as the 'kissing disease'.

Cytomegalovirus (CMV) affects young adults. Like infectious mononucleosis, it is characterised by tiredness and fever but not sore throat. The glands are not as swollen as with glandular fever. In both cases, the illness lasts around three weeks.

Both of these infections often pass unnoticed, or are thought to be simple flu-like illnesses. They are then only detected in subsequent blood tests.

Symptoms

Both illnesses

- General symptoms can be mild or severe: general malaise, loss of appetite, shivering, headaches, muscle pains
- Fever
- Extreme tiredness
- Swollen glands, more pronounced in the case of mononucleosis

Mononucleosis

- Sore throat
- Jaundice (sometimes)
- Rash similar to scarlet fever

Consult your doctor or medical herbalist

- If the above symptoms are severe, seek medical advice to make sure you do not have a more serious illness. A clinical diagnosis can be easily confirmed with a blood test.

Causes

Both illnesses are incontestably viral in origin and both are primarily transmitted by saliva. Adolescents represent 70 per cent of those affected and incidence peaks at between 14 and 16 for girls, and 16 and 18 for boys.

Cytomegalovirus often affects young adults working in close contact with adolescents. In both cases, the extreme tiredness is caused by the virus and the toxins attacking the liver.

WHICH PLANTS?
WARNING Use only one of the following at any given time

Internal usage

To strengthen the body's immune system and resistance to secondary infections

Echinacea (tincture, 1:5 in 45% alcohol) Take 15 drops in water three times a day.
Garlic (capsules, 300mg) Take 1-3 capsules a day.
Grapefruit seed (capsules, 125mg) Take 1 capsule twice a day for the first three days, then 1 capsule three times a day for the next seven days, and finally 2 capsules twice or three times a day for the next 18 days.
Siberian ginseng (capsules, 150mg) Take 1 capsule three times a day with a large glass of water.

Other measures

- Rest as much as possible.
- Go on a alcohol-free diet for a few days to allow your liver to recuperate and function again normally.
- Drink plenty of grape juice.
- Stop all energetic sports and demanding training programmes for a while.
- Take a break of at least one or two weeks from work or study.

Herpes

Herpes is a recurrent and very contagious viral disease. It can infect the mucous membranes, including that of the eye. There are several variants: labial herpes – cold sores being the most common – and genital herpes, a sexually transmitted disease.

Symptoms

- Tiny white 'fever spots' or blisters, filled with yellowish liquid outlined in red, singly or in groups, appearing around the corners of the lips or inside the lower lip, eventually spreading to the cheek or the tongue
- A burning sensation, followed by eruption of the blisters
- A yellowish scab forms, falling off after a few days
- Itching and a burning sensation
- In the case of genital herpes, fever, painful swelling of the lymph glands of the groin
- In labial herpes in children, small ulcerations appear on the lips, palate, inside the cheeks, with painful under-arm swelling

Consult your doctor

- In cases of swelling, fever or recurring symptoms, consult a doctor without delay.
- If herpes reaches the eyes, it is important to consult an ophthalmologist.
- Genital herpes should be reviewed in a sexual health clinic.

Causes

The virus responsible for herpes is *Herpes simplex*, which is very contagious via skin contact until scabs are formed. It affects adults and children, especially those with weakened immune systems.

Influenza, cold, sunlight, overwork, stress or the onset of menstruation can bring on herpes.

WHICH PLANTS?
WARNING Use only one of the following at any given time

Internal usage

Echinacea (tincture, 1:5 in 45% alcohol) Take 15 drops in water three times a day.
Lemon balm (capsules, 200mg) Take 1 capsule three times a day before meals. Children should take 2 capsules a day.
Liquorice Steep 1-2 teaspoons of root powder in a cup of boiling water for 10 minutes. Strain. Drink 2 cups a day for four to six weeks, accompanied by a low salt diet.

External application

Aaron's rod Soak 3 teaspoons of dried plant in 300ml cold water for 30 minutes. Gently bring to the boil, then strain. Apply a cloth soaked in this decoction to the affected area twice a day.
Lemon balm Infuse 20g dried leaves, stems and flowers in 500ml of boiling water for 10 minutes. Apply twice a day to the lesions.
Marigold Infuse 5g dried flowerheads in 1 litre of boiling water for 5 minutes. Strain. Apply a cloth soaked in this infusion to affected areas three or four times a day.

As directed by a medical herbalist

- Cinnamon (essential oil)

Other measures

- During a herpes (cold sore) attack and for several days afterwards, refrain from all physical contact (kissing and sexual relations) to avoid infecting your partner.
- During an attack of genital herpes, avoid sexual activity until the symptoms have disappeared.
- To prevent subsequent attacks, strengthen your immune system with regular courses of immune-enhancing plants.

Influenza

Influenza is a contagious viral infection of the respiratory tract; it can be epidemic and is often mild, but complications due to bacterial secondary infection can be serious, sometimes fatal.

Symptoms

- Muscular aches, shivering, headache
- High temperature (up to 40°C)
- Sore throat, dry cough
- Chest pains
- Tiredness and general debility

Consult your doctor

- It is important to consult a doctor in the case of those most vulnerable (children, the elderly or those whose immune systems are weak) and when symptoms persist for several days.

Causes

Influenza is caused by a virus, influenza A, B or C. The A virus is the most dangerous and has caused the great pandemics; the C virus is the most benign. It occurs more often in winter as the cold lowers the body's resistance to the virus. Stress, tiredness and certain conditions such as diabetes, or corticosteroid treatment or chemotherapy also weaken the immune system.

WHICH PLANTS?

WARNING Use only one of the following at any given time

Internal usage

To soothe a cough

Aaron's rod Infuse 1.5-2g dried plant in a cup of boiling water for 15 minutes, then strain. Drink 3 cups a day.
Common elder (tincture, 1:5 in 25% alcohol) Take 20 drops in a glass of water three times a day after meals.
Common thyme Infuse 2g of dried thyme in a cup of boiling water for 5 minutes, then strain. Drink 3 cups a day.
Mallow Boil 5g of dried plant in 1 litre of water for 5 minutes, then strain. Drink 1-3 cups a day.
Sweet violet (tincture, 1:4 in 25% alcohol) Take 20 drops with a small amount of water three times a day after meals.
Sundew Infuse 1-2g of dried plant in a cup of boiling water for 10 minutes. Strain. Drink 3 cups a day.

To boost the immune system

Echinacea (tincture, 1:5 in 45% alcohol) Take 15 drops in water three times a day.
Common elder (tincture, 1:5 in 25% alcohol) Take 20 drops in water three times a day after meals.

For fever

Dog rose Infuse 2-2.5g crushed dried rosehips in a cup of boiling water for 10 minutes, then strain. Drink 3-4 cups a day.
Willow (capsules, 200mg) Take 2-4 capsules three times a day with water.

See also Fever.

For general debility, fatigue and convalescence

American ginseng (capsules, 500mg) Take 2 capsules twice a day at mealtimes. Use for up to one month followed by a two month break.
Oats (tincture, 1:5 in 45% alcohol) Take 20 drops in a glass of warm water two to three times a day.
Rosemary Infuse 2-4g of dried plant in a cup of boiling water for 10 minutes, then strain. Drink 3 cups a day after meals.
Sea buckthorn Take 1-3 dessertspoons of juice a day in a glass of water.
Siberian ginseng (capsules, 150mg) Take 1 capsule three times a day with a large glass of water.

External application

Lavender Mix 3 drops of essential oil to every 10ml carrier oil. Rub into the chest, back, throat and temples every 2-4 hours.
Eucalyptus Mix 3 drops essential oil to every 10ml carrier oil. Rub into the chest, back, throat and temples every 2-4 hours.

Other measures

- Drink plenty of water or other liquids (fruit juices, vegetable bouillon, etc.).
- Stay indoors and rest in bed as much as possible.
- Ask your doctor about the possibility of having an annual antiflu vaccination.

Shingles

Shingles (herpes zoster) is a viral infection very similar to herpes. It is characterised by a skin eruption in the form of groups of red plaques or blisters that appear along certain nerve segments. It often affects a narrow area over the ribs, or a strip on the neck and arm or on one side of the lower part of the body, or on the face.

Symptoms

- First phase: a dull aching and burning sensation along the nerve segment; sometimes an intense pain and the skin becoming very sensitive
- Second phase: appearance of red plaques interspersed with blisters, accompanied by a slight fever
- Third phase: after two to three days, the blisters dry up to be replaced by scabs that fall off after about ten days, leaving a white scar
- Pain sometimes persisting for several years after first attack; a symptom usually affecting people over the age of 50

Consult your doctor

- Only a doctor can accurately identify the specific painful rash caused by shingles, prevent possible complications. For example, shingles on the face is particularly dangerous when it affects the skin of the eyelids as it may also affect the cornea.

Causes

Shingles is caused by the chickenpox (varicella) virus, which, after an initial attack of chickenpox, remains in the spinal cord but is suppressed by the immune system.

During an attack of shingles, the virus moves out along the nerves that supply the skin, causing the hypersensitivity and subsequent painful rash. Consequently, only people who have previously had chickenpox are at risk of shingles, and people with shingles can only cause chickenpox in people who have not previously encountered the virus.

An attack of shingles can occur when the immune system has been weakened by a serious illness, such as cancer or tuberculosis, or simply by mental or physical fatigue or stress. The area of the attack may also be linked to a weakness in the corresponding internal organ.

WHICH PLANTS?

WARNING Use only one of the following at any given time

Internal usage

To strengthen the body's resistance

Echinacea (tincture, 1:5 in 45% alcohol) Take 15 drops in water three times a day.
Common elder (tincture, 1:5 in 25% alcohol) Take 20 drops in a glass of water three times a day after meals.
Liquorice Infuse 1-2 teaspoons of root powder in a cup of boiling water for 10 minutes, then strain. Drink 2 cups a day for four to six weeks, and follow a low salt diet.

External application

Aaron's rod Soak 3 teaspoons of dried plant in 300ml cold water for 30 minutes. Gently bring to the boil, then strain. Apply a cloth soaked in this decoction to the affected area twice a day.
Lemon balm Infuse 20g dried leaves, stems and flowers in 500ml boiling water for 10 minutes. Apply twice a day to the lesions.
Marigold Infuse 5g of dried flowerheads in 1 litre of boiling water for 5 minutes. Strain. Apply a cloth soaked in this infusion to affected areas three or four times a day.

Other measures

- Eat meat, fish and dairy products – rich in amino acids – and nuts, beans, seeds and oily fish, which contain essential fatty acids, to help repair cells; take vitamin B.
- Due to a high risk of contagion, avoid contact with other people, especially those who have not previously had a clear attack of chickenpox and are likely to have a low resistance.
- Ensure that the infected areas remain clean and dry.
- Although they may itch, do not rub or scratch the plaques as the blisters may burst and become infected.
- Apply a cool, wet flannel or ice cubes to reduce pain and soothe itching.
- Pregnant women are more at risk from the consequences of shingles, and should consult their midwife, GP, or antenatal clinic if they have been in close contact with it.

Thrush

Thrush (vaginal mycosis) is a fungal infection affecting the – internal and external – female genitals. It can extend to the surrounding area and the anus. Vaginal mycosis affects 75 per cent of women at least once in their life and becomes chronic in 45 per cent of cases. The symptoms can be extremely irritating and painful.

Symptoms

- A white discharge rather like odourless curdled milk
- Itching
- Burning of the vulva and vagina
- A cracking and splitting sensation
- Redness and swelling of the vulva
- Dryness and pain making sexual relations impossible
- Frequent burning on urination

Consult your doctor

- Consult a gynaecologist or doctor in the event of excessive discharge, burning, pain or dryness of the vulva and vagina.

Causes

The fungus *Candida albicans* causes 90 per cent of thrush infections. Naturally present in the intestines, it passes into the vagina via the blood, lymph glands or skin when there is an imbalance in the intestinal flora. Once it reaches the mucous membrane of the vagina, it develops rapidly in the favourable conditions – acid pH, moisture, warmth and high levels of glycogen. Antibiotics, corticosteroids and other immunosuppressants, diabetes and HIV may encourage the development of thrush.

It can be contracted through sexual relations, usually by women though occasionally by men. Infection by the candida fungus may also occur in conjunction with nappy rash in infants.

Thrush contd

WHICH PLANTS?
WARNING Use only one of the following at any given time

Medicinal plants can be used in conjunction with the standard treatments for vaginal mycosis prescribed immediately by the doctor.

Internal usage
To reduce the infection
Grapefruit seed extract (capsules, 125mg) Take 1 capsule twice a day for the first three days, then 1 capsule three times a day for the next seven days, and finally 2 capsules twice or three times a day for the next 18 days.

As directed by a medical herbalist
• Barberry

To detoxify the liver and gall bladder
Dandelion (capsules, 300mg) Take 1 capsule three times a day with water.
Globe artichoke (capsules, 300mg) Take 1 capsule a day.
Rosemary Infuse 2-4g dried plant in a cup of boiling water for 10 minutes, then strain. Drink 3 cups a day after meals.

To stimulate the immune system
Echinacea (tincture, 1:5 in 45% alcohol) Take 15 drops in water three times a day.
Siberian ginseng (capsules, 150mg) Take 1 capsule three times a day with a large glass of water.

External application
Clove Boil 20g dried cloves in 750ml water until the volume is reduced to roughly 500ml, then strain. Use to bathe the vagina once or twice a day.
Common thyme Infuse 1 sachet in a cup of boiling water for 5 minutes. Use to bathe the vagina once or twice a day.
German chamomile Infuse 1 sachet of dried plant in a cup of boiling water for 10 minutes. Use the liquid to bathe the vagina once or twice a day.
Lavender Infuse 2-3g of dried flowers in a cup of boiling water for 10 minutes, then strain. Use the liquid to bathe the vagina once or twice a day.
Roman chamomile Infuse 1 dessertspoon dried flowerheads in a cup of boiling water for 10 minutes, then strain. Use to bathe the vagina once or twice a day.

Other measures
• As far as possible, avoid taking antibiotics or corticosteroids. If this is impossible, use a complementary – topical and oral – antifungal treatment.
• Avoid restrictive clothing and wear cotton underwear.
• Avoid perfumed soaps, bubble baths and other bath products and do not use scented vaginal deodorants.
• In the event of chronic mycosis, use a neutral pH soap for personal hygiene.

Viral infections

A virus is a microscopic foreign body that penetrates a cell, infecting it (unlike a bacterium) and forcing the cell DNA to create thousands more viruses which are released to infect neighbouring cells. The body's only defence is a healthy immune system. The majority of the common respiratory, gastrointestinal and hepatic infections are viral in origin.

Symptoms
• Symptoms differ according to the type of virus and the illnesses that they cause.

Consult your doctor
• Obviously benign viral infections such as the common cold or sore throat can be treated at home but in all other cases, it is imperative to seek medical advice in order to identify which virus is present and to treat it. Treatment of viral infections is largely restricted to alleviating the symptoms and boosting the body's immune system.

Causes
Several factors make the body more vulnerable to viruses, notably an immune deficiency, chronic fatigue or permanent stress. A weakened immune system may also be caused by an inadequate or unbalanced diet. Viruses enter the body by a variety of routes, via food and drink, through punctured skin or during sexual intercourse. Some invade cells near the site of entry or pass into the bloodstream, or along nerve fibres to target specific organs.

WHICH PLANTS?
WARNING Use only one of the following at any given time

Internal usage

To strengthen the body's resistance

Common elder (tincture, 1:5 in 25% alcohol) Take 20 drops in a little water, three times a day after meals.

Echinacea (tincture, 1:5 in 45% alcohol) Take 15 drops three times a day.

Liquorice Steep 1-2 teaspoons of root powder in a cup of boiling water for 10 minutes, then strain. Drink 2 cups a day.

Stinging nettle (tincture, 1:4 in 25% alcohol) Take 20 drops in water three times a day after meals.

To aid convalescence

Dog rose Infuse 2-2.5g crushed rosehips in a cup of boiling water for 10 minutes. Drink 3-4 cups a day.

Oats (tincture, 1:5 in 45% alcohol) Take 20 drops in a glass of warm water two to three times a day.

Rosemary Infuse 2-4g dried plant in a cup of boiling water for 10 minutes, then strain. Drink 3 cups a day after meals.

Sea buckthorn Take 1-3 dessertspoons of juice a day in a glass of water.

Siberian ginseng (150mg capsules) Take 1 capsule three times a day with a large glass of water.

Other measures

- To boost immunity, eat a well-balanced diet that is high in foods containing flavonoids, tannins and proanthocyans (coloured fruits and vegetables such as carrots, broccoli, blackcurrants, bilberries, blackberries). Garlic is also particularly beneficial.
- Avoid excessive consumption of caffeine and alcohol, which weakens the body's natural defences.
- Try not to get too tired or stressed.

Mental health
Anxiety

Anxiety is a state of fear usually arising from a particular cause or threat, which may or may not be obvious to the sufferer. It is accompanied by a feeling of unease that can include physical symptoms.

Its intensity varies from slight anxiousness to terror, and can consequently be acute or chronic, depending on the circumstances.

Panic disorder is a state that occurs when anxiety becomes so acute and intense that it paralyses the sufferer. Panic attacks are recurrent unpredictable anxiety attacks that are of short duration but very intense, occurring among people who would otherwise not be feeling as anxious in the same circumstances.

Anxiety also takes the form of phobias, such as agoraphobia and claustrophobia; phobias are an intense fear of, and attempt to avoid certain objects or specific situations. Obsessive-compulsive disorders, withdrawal syndrome, psychoses and mental disorders also accompany anxiety, varying from slight to very intense.

Symptoms

- Sweating, desire to urinate and defecate, feeling of suffocation, palpitations, dry mouth or copious amounts of saliva, feeling hot or cold, pain, dizziness, bloating, tics
- Insomnia and, more rarely, tremor, feeling the need to escape, anxious thoughts
- In the most serious cases, a feeling of utter helplessness and inability to carry out normal everyday activities

Consult your doctor

- If the symptoms are severe or long-term it is essential to consult a doctor to confirm that they are a result of anxiety and to determine its origin.

Causes

Anxiety is frequently linked to a psychological or emotional problem. It can be caused by an emotional conflict, a feeling of insecurity or stress, or can indicate depression. It can also be a sign of serious mental illness.

WHICH PLANTS?

WARNING Use only one of the following at any given time

Medical herbalism can be used to treat moderate anxiety when insomnia, palpitations and slight dizziness are the most common symptoms.

Internal usage

Preparations for a sedative

Bitter orange Infuse 20g dried flowers in 150ml boiling water for 20 minutes, then strain. Take in the evening before going to bed.

Lavender Infuse 2-3g dried flowers in a cup of boiling water for 5-10 minutes. Drink 3-4 cups a day between meals, or 1 cup before bedtime.

Lemon balm (capsules, 200mg) Take 3 capsules a day, before meals.

Lime tree Infuse 5g dried flowers in 1 litre of boiling water for 5 minutes, then strain. Drink 1 cup in the evening to encourage sleep.

Passionflower (tincture, 1:8 in 25% alcohol) Take 25 drops in a glass of water three times a day after meals.

Valerian (capsules, 240mg) Take 1-2 capsules a day.

Other measures

- Talk to your GP about seeing a psychotherapist or clinical psychologist.
- Take regular physical exercise and take up relaxation exercises, such as yoga.
- Consult an acupuncturist.

Depression

Sadness, pessimism, reduced self-esteem and lack of interest are among the symptoms of depression. It is considered a serious mental condition if it persists without an obvious cause or intensifies and affects behaviour, becoming itself a symptom of a psychiatric illness.

Symptoms

- Feeling sad and tired
- Crying at inappropriate times
- Difficulty in concentrating, and in forming and carrying out plans and ideas
- Self-criticism, lack of self-esteem, even self-loathing
- Lack of appetite and spirit and inability to take pleasure in life
- Weight fluctuation
- Insomnia, particularly waking up frequently during the small hours of the night, or alternatively sleeping to excess
- Thoughts of death or suicide

Consult your doctor

- For people with a history of psychological fragility, getting over a disappointment or an emotional setback can lead to depression.
- If prescribed a chemical or herbal antidepressant, do not discontinue it suddenly without medical advice.

Causes

Depression can affect people who experience great emotional loss, such as the death of someone close, a disappointment in love or a social problem. However, there may be no single obvious cause.

Depression can occasionally be triggered by viral illnesses, or disorders such as hypothyroidism or by hormonal changes after childbirth. Some people also suffer from Seasonal Affective Disorder (SAD) triggered by the long darkness of winter.

As an illness it is more common where there is a history of depression within the family.

WHICH PLANTS?

WARNING Use only one of the following at any given time

Internal usage

Californian poppy (tincture, 1:4 in 45% alcohol) Take 10 drops three times a day in a little cold water after meals. Take up to 20 drops at bedtime.

Lavender Infuse 2-3g dried flowers in a cup of boiling water for 5-10 minutes, then strain. Drink 1 cup before bedtime.

St John's wort (liquid extract, 1:1 in 25% alcohol) Take ½-1 teaspoon three times a day.

Sweet marjoram Infuse 1-2 teaspoons dried leaves in a cup of boiling water for 15 minutes, then strain. Drink 1 cup three times a day.

Other measures

- Take some rest, if possible go on holiday.
- Take a trace element treatment: magnesium, potassium.
- Consult your GP, a trained counsellor, clinical psychologist or psychotherapist.

See also Stress.

Insomnia

The term insomnia encompasses a range of problems that affect sleep. Most people experience it at some time in their lives but as sleeping patterns differ from one individual to another, its symptoms vary and tend to be characterised by the discomfort suffered as a result of not being able to fall asleep or stay asleep.

Symptoms

- Difficulty in getting to sleep

- Premature wakening with a feeling of sleep-deprivation
- Night-time wakefulness at the slightest external stimulus, and prolonged nocturnal wakefulness
- Daytime tiredness, possibly accompanied by a strong desire for sleep

Consult your doctor

- If insomnia persists, consult your doctor.

Causes

Insomnia is generally due to a state of stress, psychological tension, anxiety and various fears, including the fear of sleep. It often accompanies the onset of depression, but it can also be caused by ailments such as atherosclerosis, Alzheimer's disease, or digestive or respiratory problems.

Overuse of coffee, tea, tobacco or even vitamin C can also contribute to insomnia.

WHICH PLANTS?

WARNING Use only one of the following at any given time

Internal usage

Bitter orange Infuse 5g dried flowers in 150ml of boiling water for 20 minutes. Strain. Take in the evening just before going to bed.

Californian poppy (tincture, 1:4 in 45% alcohol) Take 10 drops three times a day in a little cold water after meals. Take up to 20 drops at bedtime.

Hops Infuse 10g dried flowers in 1 litre of boiling water for 10 minutes, then strain. Drink 1 cup just before bedtime.

Lavender Infuse 2-3g dried flowers in a cup of boiling water for 5-10 minutes, then strain. Drink 3-4 cups a day between meals, or 1 cup before bedtime.

Lemon balm (capsules, 200mg) Take 3 capsules a day, before meals.

Lime tree Infuse 5g of dried flowers in 1 litre of boiling water for 5 minutes, then strain. Drink 1 cup in the evening to promote sleep.

Passionflower (tincture, 1:8 in 25% alcohol) Take 25-75 drops a day in a glass of water.

Peppermint Infuse 1 tablespoon of dried leaves in 150ml of boiling water for 10-15 minutes, then strain. Drink 1 cup in the evening for a sedative effect.

Sweet marjoram Infuse 1-2 teaspoons of dried plant in a cup of boiling water for 15 minutes, then strain. Drink 1 cup three times a day.

Valerian (capsules, 240mg) Take 1-2 capsules a day.

Other measures

- Try relaxing exercises such as yoga.
- Take trace elements, notably magnesium.
- Make a point of going for a walk every evening, but avoid stimulating physical or mental exercise soon before retiring.
- Try to go to bed and get up at the same time every day including weekends. If you need to be up at a certain time, use an alarm clock (to avoid the anxiety of oversleeping).
- If you cannot get to sleep, get out of bed and sit in a chair to read, returning to bed again only when you feel sleepy – this avoids the brain associating the bed with wakefulness.
- Self-hypnosis can help to break the cycle of rumination: imagine yourself in a room or garden that you know intimately. Walk very slowly around it in your mind, carefully noticing and examining the details of everything in it.
- Try to avoid sleeping during the day to catch up.

Psychosomatic disorders

A psychosomatic disorder – or, to use the medical term, neurovegetative dystonia – is the repeated manifestation of physical symptoms that seem to have been caused, or worsened, by psychological factors, such as anxiety or stress.

Symptoms

- Cephalgia (headache), especially at the top of the skull
- A dry mouth or over-production of saliva
- Visual disorders
- Nausea, belching, bloated stomach
- Meteorism (intestinal gas), abdominal swelling in the region of the hypochondrium (upper abdomen, below the ribs), flatulence
- Tachycardia (palpitations), a throbbing sensation in the carotid arteries that supply blood to the head and neck
- Twinges of pain in the side
- Isolated instances of diarrhoea
- Yawning
- Frequent but sparse urination
- A feeling of feverishness, burning ears
- Sudden hypotension (low blood pressure), accompanied by feelings of malaise (sweating, buzzing in the ears, clouded vision)
- Tearfulness and emotional disorders

Consult your doctor

- If one of these apparently ordinary symptoms is repeated, consult your doctor. He or she will be able to determine whether it is related to neurovegetative dystonia or to a more serious condition.

Causes

Certain minor nervous disorders, some form of annoyance or slight anxiety can trigger a physical disorder.

WHICH PLANTS?

WARNING Use only one of the following at any given time

Internal usage

To improve general health:

American ginseng (tincture, 1:5 in 70% alcohol) Take 20-40 drops obtained from cultivated American ginseng three times a day.

German chamomile (sachets dried flowerheads) Infuse 1 sachet in a cup of boiling water for 10 minutes, then strain. Drink 3 cups a day before meals.

Lavender (dried flowers) Infuse 2-3g dried flowers in a cup of boiling water for 5-10 minutes, then strain. Drink 3-4 cups a day between meals.

Sweet marjoram (dried plant) Infuse 1-2 teaspoons dried plant in a cup of boiling water for 15 minutes, then strain. Drink 1 cup three times a day.

Other measures

- Practise yoga and relaxation exercises.
- Take trace elements, especially magnesium, manganese.
- Discuss with your GP the idea of seeing a clinical psychologist or psychiatrist, to try to establish the cause of the disorder and hence alleviate it.

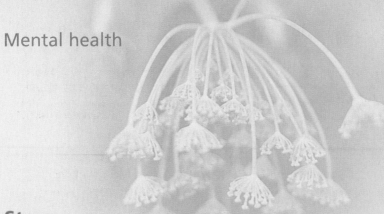

Stress

People experience stress in response to a variety of mental, physical and emotional triggers. Prolonged stress can lead to the development of secondary health problems.

Symptoms

- Extreme fatigue
- Difficulty in sleeping
- Emotional upset, with shaking, vertigo and sudden anxiety
- Poor memory, distraction, difficulty in finding words
- Recurrent infections
- An aggravation of diabetes, premature ageing, arrhythmia and other heart problems

Consult your doctor or medical herbalist

- When stress leads to other mental and physical symptoms, it should be recognised and addressed as soon as possible.
- A person suffering from stress should not take too many stimulants but rather some form of medication that enables the body to adapt to stress.

Causes

There are many different causes of stress: excessive or extended effort without rest almost automatically leads to physical stress, just as family worries, money difficulties or the death of a loved one lead to mental stress.

Prolonged stress weakens the immune system and may be responsible for persistent or recurrent infections.

WHICH PLANTS?

WARNING Use only one of the following at any given time

Internal usage

For fatigue

Cinchona (tincture, 1:5 in 25% alcohol) Take 2-4ml in a glass of water three times a day.

Dog rose Infuse 2-2.5g of fragmented rosehips in a cup of boiling water for 10 minutes, then strain. Drink 3-4 cups a day.

Oats (tincture, 1:5 in 45% alcohol) Take 1-5ml in a glass of warm water two or three times a day.

To fortify without stimulating

Sea buckthorn Take 1-3 dessertspoons of sea buckthorn juice in a glass of water once a day.

To boost the immune system

Echinacea (capsules, 325mg root powder) Take 1-3 capsules a day.

Common elder (tincture, 1:5 in 25% alcohol) Take 20 drops in water three times a day after meals.

Other measures

- Take plenty of rest, interspersed with regular, moderate exercise (such as walking).
- Practise yoga, deep-breathing exercises or t'ai chi.
- Practise relaxation techniques.
- Take a multivitamin and mineral supplement.

See also Insomnia.

Metabolism & Chronic fatigue

Often experienced after a prolonged illness, chronic fatigue (asthenia) can vary in its severity, but should not be trivialised. It is a sign that the body needs rest.

Symptoms

- Weariness that varies in intensity
- An overwhelming need to sleep
- Feeling of muscular numbness with pain of a varying intensity when using limbs
- Difficulty in concentrating
- Reduced resistance to disease

Consult your doctor

- When fatigue is intense and persistent, it is important to consult a doctor to determine its precise nature and also to eliminate other disorders.

Causes

Chronic fatigue can be due to excessive physical or mental activity, stress, depression or other psychiatric illness, infection, anaemia, kidney or liver disorders, cancers, or metabolic disorders such as thyroid insufficiency and diabetes. It is more likely to be experienced during adolescence, pregnancy and in old age.

WHICH PLANTS?

WARNING Use only one of the following at any given time

Internal usage

American ginseng (tincture, 1:5 in 70% alcohol) Take 20-40 drops in water three times a day.

Dog rose (capsules, 50-200mg dry extract) Take 1-2 capsules with a large glass of water three times a day before meals.

Oats (tincture, 1:5 in 45% alcohol) Take 1-5ml in a glass of warm water two or three times a day.

Rosemary Infuse 2-4g of the dried plant in a cup of boiling water for 10 minutes. Strain. Drink 1 cup three times a day after meals.

Sea buckthorn Take 1-3 dessert-spoons of juice in a glass of water once a day.

Siberian ginseng (capsule, 150mg powder) Take 1 capsule three times a day with a large glass of water. Do not use for longer than one month at a time.

Green tea Put 1 teaspoon of green tea into a cup of boiling water. Infuse for 10 minutes. Strain. Drink 2-3 cups a day.

To detoxify the liver

Globe artichoke (capsule, 300mg leaf extract) Take 1 capsule a day.

Dandelion (capsule, 300mg powder) Take 1 capsule three times a day with water.

Milk thistle (tablets, 200mg) Take 1-2 tablets a day with food.

Other measures

- Take relaxation exercises.
- Do some sporting activity.
- Adopt a diet that is rich in fruit but reduced in fat.
- Take a holiday if possible.

Diabetes

This disorder, properly known as diabetes mellitus, is caused by an excess of glucose in the blood (hyperglycaemia) due to the reduced effectiveness or lack of insulin (the hormone that is responsible for the absorption of blood-sugar into the body's cells). There are two types of diabetes mellitus: insulin-dependent (Type 1), which usually occurs in people under the age of 35; and non-insulin dependent (Type 2), which develops mainly in people over 40.

Symptoms

- Feeling thirsty with the need to urinate frequently
- Craving sugary foods
- Weight change (up or down)
- Fatigue

- Slow healing of infections
- Problems with vision
- Poor circulation, pins and needles in the hands and feet, impotence

Consult your doctor

- The disorder can often go unnoticed until it has been present for some time.
- If you have any doubts about the origins of one or several of the symptoms described above, consult your doctor who can recommend a test to detect the presence of sugar in your urine.

Causes

Insulin-dependent diabetes (Type 1) occurs when the insulin-producing cells in the pancreas are destroyed, probably as an immune response during a viral illness, so there is a complete lack of insulin. It tends to occur in children and adolescents, the onset worsening swiftly over several days to a serious illness.

Non-insulin dependent (Type 2) diabetes is effectively the result of exhaustion of the pancreatic cells that produce insulin, or of the inability of the body to use insulin properly. Those most at risk are obese people over the age of 40, with a family history of diabetes but as obesity in younger people increases, it is becoming more common at an earlier age.

Drugs are used to stimulate increased production or effectiveness of insulin, or diet is advised to reduce the need for insulin by the rest of the body. Sometimes, however, non-insulin dependent diabetes becomes so difficult to control with tablets that insulin injections are required.

Diabetes mellitus tends to run in families.

WHICH PLANTS?

WARNING Use only one of the following at any given time

Medical herbalism can only be used to treat mild cases of Type 2 diabetes. It is recommended that you obtain the prior approval of your doctor.

Internal usage

To lower blood sugar levels

Bilberry (60mg tablets) Take 1-3 tablets a day with water.

Dandelion (300mg powder capsules) Take 1 capsule three times a day with water.

Fenugreek Take 2g of powder in a little water three times a day.

Garcinia (400mg powder capsules) Take 1 capsule with a glass of water 30-60 minutes before main meals three times a day.

Olive (500mg powdered leaf tablets) Take 1 tablet a day with food.

Java tea (dried leaves) Infuse 5g in 1 litre of boiling water for 5 minutes. Strain. Drink 1-3 cups a day, the last one several hours before going to bed.

Juniper (tincture, 1:5 in 45% alcohol) Take 10-20 drops in a small glass of sweetened water three times a day.

As directed by a medical herbalist

- **Goat's rue**

Other measures

- Follow a sensible, balanced diet. Reduce your consumption of refined foods (white sugar, flour, bread and rice) and fat.
- Incorporate complex carbohydrates in your diet such wholegrain bread, pasta, rice and oatbran. The body digests these complex carbohydrates slowly, leading to a steady level of sugar in the bloodstream.
- Reduce your weight to a healthy level for your height. This will make your diabetes much easier to control.
- Take regular exercise.

Gout

This painful condition is caused by deposits of uric acid crystals in the joints. The uric acid is a by-product of the breakdown of proteins in the body. The joint in the big toe is commonly the first to be affected with gout. Men are much more likely to suffer from gout than women. There is a family history in about a third of cases.

Symptoms

- Sharp pain in the affected joint (often starting with the big toe)
- The affected joint may be swollen and warm to the touch
- Deformation caused by deposits of uric acid crystals around the affected joint; the crystals may also be deposited in the ear cartilage

Consult your doctor

- Only a doctor can diagnose gout. The doctor must distinguish between gout, arthritis, osteoarthritis, a deep abscess and phlebitis by means of a medical examination, X-ray and blood tests.

Causes

Gout is caused by a combination of two phenomena: excessive breakdown of proteins and the failure of the kidneys to eliminate uric acid. In most cases, there is a genetic disorder in metabolising proteins.

Otherwise the problem may relate to anticancer drugs, some blood pressure drugs and aspirin. It is also associated with psoriasis and some blood cancers.

For those at risk, symptoms can be brought on by over-indulgence in red meat, game, offal, alcohol, protein-rich plants such as peas, lentils and beans, and by drinking too little water.

WHICH PLANTS?

WARNING Use only one of the following at any given time

Internal usage

To treat pain and inflammation

Aaron's rod Infuse 1.5-2g dried flowers in a cup of boiling water for 15 minutes. Drink 3 cups a day.
Devil's claw (capsules, 186mg) Take 1 capsule three times a day before meals.
Gypsy wort (tincture, 1:5 in 45% alcohol) Take 2-6ml in water three times a day.
Java tea Infuse 5g of dried leaves in 1 litre of boiling water for 5 minutes. Strain. Drink 1-3 cups a day, the last one several hours before going to bed.
Oats (tincture, 1:5 in 45% alcohol) Take 1-5ml in a glass of warm water two or three times a day.

To increase urination

Ash Infuse 10-20g of dried leaves in 1 litre of boiling water for 10 minutes and then strain. Drink 0.5-1 litre a day.
Stinging nettle (tincture, 1:4 in 25% alcohol) Take 20 drops in water three times a day after eating.

External application

Lavender Infuse 20-100g of dried flowers in 1 litre of boiling water for 15 minutes and strain. Add the infusion to the bath water and soak for 15 minutes.

Meadowsweet Put 1 tablespoon of dried plant into a cup of freshly boiled water that has cooled slightly. Infuse for 10 minutes, then soak a cloth in the infusion and apply three or four times a day to painful areas.

Other measures

- Drink plenty of water.
- Do not drink alcohol, especially white wine and beer.
- Go on a protein-free diet for at least one week, eliminating even vegetable proteins such as lentils or soya milk.

HIV/AIDS

If left untreated, the virus known as HIV (human immunodeficiency virus) may eventually lead to AIDS (acquired immune deficiency syndrome), which brings about a general collapse of the body's immune system. Multiple infections may follow as well as the development of various types of tumours.

Symptoms

- Extreme fatigue
- The appearance of mouth, chest, eye, brain, or gut infections, herpes, worsening acne, shingles, hepatitis etc
- Infections that recur or become chronic
- The appearance of large purplish blotches on the skin – a possible sign of a vascular skin tumour called Kaposi's Sarcoma (KS)
- Gradual deterioration of the sufferer's general state of health
- When HIV has been contracted it causes a flu-like illness between 10 and 90 days after infection. This often passes unnoticed since its symptoms are similar to a number of common viral illnesses. The symptoms include aching muscles, fatigue, a fine red rash on the trunk and face,

---

DID YOU KNOW?

Gout

A traditional remedy for gout was eating cherries. It has now been discovered that the consumption of 225g of cherries a day (fresh or canned) lowers levels of uric acid in the blood, which may well explain why they can effectively treat the disorder.

---

a dry or ulcerated mouth, and swollen lymph nodes in the neck, groin, and armpits

Consult your doctor

- Consider asking your GP or sexual health clinic about testing if you think you could have picked up the infection. The earlier the presence of the HIV virus is detected, the better the long-term chances of remaining well, and the less the chance of passing it on to someone else.
- Healthy people who are HIV positive may not display symptoms for years. However, they require regular medical supervision to determine when the disease becomes active and requires treatment.

Causes

HIV is one of a group of retroviruses that attack the T-lymphocytes (cells that support the body's immune system). HIV can be transmitted by sexual intercourse, breast milk and via the exchange of infected blood or blood products. AIDS represents the final stage of infection with HIV.

WHICH PLANTS?

WARNING Use only one of the following at any given time

The use of medicinal plants to stimulate the immune system of AIDS patients has not been proven effective or safe as the research is still in the experimental stage. Therefore herbal medicines for this condition should only be taken with the agreement of a doctor or as complementary to medical drugs under the supervision of a medical herbalist. Certain herbs can help to alleviate some of the conditions that affect immuno-deficient patients.

Internal usage

As directed by a medical herbalist

Plants that have shown some potential in fighting HIV
- Hyssop, Mouse-ear hawkweed, Silver birch, Winter savory

To stimulate the immune system
- Echinacea, Liquorice

To treat recurrent infections
- Garlic, Oregano

For fatigue
- Rosemary

Other measures
Whether HIV positive or not:
- Use barrier contraceptives (male and female condoms) for vaginal or anal sex.
- Do not rely on spermicidal gels without the condoms – there's some evidence they may even increase the risk.
- Do not have sex during attacks of other genital infections; you are more at risk of picking up HIV or passing it on.

If already HIV positive:
- Observe all your doctor's prescriptions scrupulously and, above all, take the prescribed antiviral medication regularly. Be honest about any difficulties in taking them because of your daily routine or unpleasant side effects.
- Alternate exercise and rest as much as possible. Regular supervised sessions in the gym can help to build up muscle strength and general vitality.
- If pregnant, talk to your midwife and health visitor about alternatives to breast feeding.
- Eat a varied diet with plenty of fresh fruit and vegetables, especially onions, garlic, pears and the syrup of wild fruits.
- Consider joining a support group with other HIV-positive people.

> **DID YOU KNOW?**
> ## Hyperthyroidism
> Vegetables of the brassica family (including cabbage and turnip) contain glucosinolate, a substance that prevents the synthesis of certain thyroid hormones. Peanuts and soya beans also contain this substance, which means they are all recommended in cases of hyperthyroidism.

Hyperthyroidism

The over-production of thyroid hormones, known as hyperthyroidism, is a malfunction of the thyroid gland. It affects five times more women than men, generally between 30–60 years of age.

Symptoms
- Swelling of the thyroid gland (goitre) at the front of the neck
- Protruding eyeballs (exophthalmia), retraction of the lids, excessive watering, limited vision
- Raised red or purple patches on the shins (pretibial myxoedema)
- Cardiovascular complications: accelerated heart-rate (tachycardia), irregular heartbeats (auricular fibrillation), shortness of breath
- Weight loss despite increased appetite
- Fatigue, muscle weakness
- Thinning hair
- Diarrhoea
- Nervousness, irritability, tremor, anxiety, insomnia, dislike of heat
- Lighter menstruation

Consult your doctor
- If you notice swelling of the neck and any of the other symptoms, consult your doctor.

Hyperthyroidism contd

Causes

In 90 per cent of cases, hyperthyroidism is caused by Grave's disease. This is an autoimmune condition in which the body's own antibodies stimulate the production of thyroid hormones. It can occur at any age, but rarely before puberty and generally between 20–50 years of age. It manifests itself through eye disorders, pretibial myxoedema (see above) and goitre.

In other cases, a tumour of the pituitary gland or thyroid cancer that has developed from secondary growths causes hyperthyroidism.

WHICH PLANTS?

WARNING Use only one of the following at any given time

Internal usage

To relieve anxiety
Lavender Infuse 2-3g of dried flowers in a cup of boiling water for 5-10 minutes. Drink 3-4 cups a day between meals.
Lime tree Infuse 5g of dried flowers in 1 litre of boiling water for 5 minutes. Drink a cup in the evening to help you to get off to sleep.
Valerian (capsules, 240mg powder) Take 1-2 capsules daily.

As directed by a medical herbalist

To regulate heart rhythm
- Hawthorn

To reduce thyroid activity
- Gypsy wort, Lemon balm

Other measures

- Take vitamin C, E and B complex vitamins which are important for maintaining the health of the thyroid gland.

Hypothyroidism

Underactivity of the thyroid gland, known as hypothyroidism is a deficiency of the hormone secreted by the gland. It can be congenital or acquired and affects women six times more than men. There may be a family history of thyroid disease or another autoimmune condition (such as pernicious anaemia, rheumatoid arthritis).

Symptoms

- Tiredness, sleepiness
- Low blood pressure
- Weight gain
- Goitre (swelling in the front of the neck)
- Aversion to the cold
- Hoarseness
- Bradycardia (slow pulse)
- Muscular aches and pains
- Nervous depression, possibly even a type of dementia
- Anaemia
- Dry, scaly skin with vitiligo (white patches ringed by over-pigmented skin)
- Dry, unruly hair
- Irregular or heavier periods
- Sterility, impotence, constipation

Consult your doctor or medical herbalist

- Medical examination is imperative in the case of swelling of the thyroid gland or the appearance of one or more of the above symptoms, in order to diagnose the disorder and to prescribe appropriate medication, and also to eliminate the possibility of cancer.
- Regular monitoring of thyroid hormone levels is also important.

Causes

Hypothyroidism can be congenital, due to spontaneous atrophy of the thyroid gland, or, if there is a goitre, brought on by an inflammatory reaction of the thyroid linked with taking certain drugs, excessive iodine or hormonal under-production. Radiation treatments including radioactive iodine for an overactive gland and several auto-immune diseases can facilitate its development.

WHICH PLANTS?

WARNING Use only one of the following at any given time

Internal usage

To help prevent weight gain
Green tea (capsules, 375mg extract) Take 2 capsules in the morning and 2 at midday.
Java tea Infuse 5g dried leaves in 1 litre of boiling water for 5 minutes. Strain. Drink 1-3 cups a day, the last one several hours before going to bed.

For dry skin
Evening primrose (capsules, 500mg) Take 1-2 capsules a day with a glass of water during meals.

As directed by a medical herbalist

To stimulate thyroid activity
- Bladderwrack

Other measures

- Ask your GP or medical herbalist about mineral supplements, such as zinc and selenium.
- Take vitamin C, E and B complex vitamins which are important for maintaining the health of the thyroid gland.

Immune system deficiency

Immune deficiency occurs when the body is in a state of low resistance to foreign microorganisms such as viruses, bacteria or parasites. The body is incapable of mobilising its immune defences, that is, the innate collection of cells and proteins it normally activates to overpower the invaders.

Symptoms

- Excessive tiredness
- Recurring infections
- Slow recovery from infections
- Infection by generally harmless parasites

Consult your doctor or medical herbalist

- If any of the above symptoms is persistent enough to suggest that the immune system is impaired, it is imperative to seek medical advice.

Causes

A weakened immune system can be a sign of numerous disorders, ranging from allergies to HIV/AIDS. It can be due to toxic products: medications and other synthetic substances. It can also be related to zinc deficiency, Crohn's disease, anorexia nervosa or to a state of depression or anxiety.

WHICH PLANTS?

WARNING Use only one of the following at any given time

As directed by a medical herbalist

To strengthen the body's immune defences

- Ashwagandha, Echinacea, Golden seal, Siberian ginseng

For tiredness and fatigue

- American ginseng, Cinnamon, Dog rose, Oats, Rosemary

Other measures

- Take regular courses of zinc and selenium in trace elements, as well as seaweed extracts.
- Eat plants rich in vitamin C (sea buckthorn).

Low body weight

A person is usually considered underweight if they are well below the weight appropriate for their height and age, as measured by charts such as the Body Mass Index (BMI).

The BMI chart, however, is only appropriate for adults, and has limitations because it cannot distinguish between body fat and muscle, which can make very muscular people appear overweight. Equally the chart may make people who have lost muscle mass, such as the elderly, appear excessively underweight. Some individuals are also genetically disposed to be underweight.

If anyone is more than 20 per cent below the standard weight for their height, the cause may be poor diet or disease. And, if substantial weight loss occurs suddenly or progressively, it is almost certainly symptomatic of a serious disorder.

Medical herbalism can only aid in a limited way by helping to relax, nourish and aid digestion.

Symptoms

- Failing to put on weight while still growing and eating well
- General lack of fatty tissue
- Tiredness, muscular pains, headache and hypotension (low blood pressure)

Causes

Being underweight is often congenital, but may also be due to inadequate diet and a lack of vitamins, poor intestinal absorption, pancreatic dysfunction, stress, overexercising, or a tendency to hyperthyroidism. In young girls, unexplained weight loss may mask Turner's syndrome (a chromosomal abnormality that affects growth in approximately one in 3000 females) or possibly anorexia.

Consult your doctor

- In cases of progressive or sudden weight loss despite following a healthy diet, consult your doctor

WHICH PLANTS?

WARNING Use only one of the following at any given time

Internal usage

To nourish

Fenugreek Take 2g powder in a little water three times a day.
Oats (tincture, 1:5 in 45% alcohol) Take 1-5ml in a glass of warm water 2-3 times a day.
Sea buckthorn Drink 1-3 dessertspoons of pure juice a day in a glass of water.

To aid digestion

Peppermint Infuse 1 dessertspoon of dried leaves in 150ml of boiling water for 10-15 minutes. Strain. Drink 1 cup after every meal.
Yellow gentian (tincture) Take 2-5 drops of tincture with water before eating.

For anxiety

Lavender Infuse 2-3g of dried flowers in a cup of boiling water for 5-10 minutes, then strain. Drink 3-4 cups a day between meals.
Lime tree Infuse 5g of dried flowers in 1 litre of boiling water. for 5 minutes. Strain. Drink 1 cup in the evening to encourage sleep.

For fatigue and tiredness

American ginseng (tincture, 1:5 in 70% alcohol) Take 20-40 drops three times a day.
Dog rose (capsules, 50-200mg dry extract) Take 1-2 capsules with a large glass of water three times a day before meals.

Low body weight contd

Other measures

- Be realistic about your weight loss: it may only be a matter of appearance.
- Do not embark upon any treatment without medical advice.
- Eat dishes you enjoy, in pleasurable circumstances.
- Work towards a balanced diet, and add foods that have a positive medical effect such as dried fruit, rolled oats, rosehip syrup and soya beans.
- Use spices such as ginger and cinnamon, which stimulate digestion.
- Eat chocolate.
- If necessary, try to combat stress and learn relaxation techniques.

Obesity

People are technically obese – rather than simply overweight – when they weigh 20 per cent or more above the normal weight for their height as measured on standard weight charts such as the Body Mass Index (BMI).

Alternatively, it is possible to estimate whether weight could pose a risk of heart problems, diabetes, lipid disorders, or high blood pressure by taking a waist measurement.

For men, a waist measurement of 37in (94cm) or more means increased risk, and of 40in (102cm) or more, suggests substantial risk. For women, a waist size of 32in (80cm) or more, means increased risk, and of 35in (88cm) or more suggests substantial risk.

Obesity is becoming increasingly common in children and young people, and is already leading to serious problems more usually seen at a much later age, such as Type 2 diabetes.

Symptoms

- Excess weight
- Bulky physical appearance
- Abundant fat in the subcutaneous tissues, 'jodhpur thighs' and other physical changes
- Breathlessness when any form of physical effort is involved

Consult your doctor or medical herbalist

- If you are obese, your doctor will be able to determine whether it is due to overeating or the result of a physical dysfunction. You should consult your doctor before undertaking any form of treatment whatsoever.

Causes

Becoming overweight – the first step to obesity – is the result of absorbing more calories than are expended in energy. It can be caused by a wide range of factors, such as lack of physical exercise, an unbalanced diet, heavy drinking, compulsive eating as a result of psychological problems, and physical disorders including diabetes and hypothyroidism.

WHICH PLANTS?

WARNING Use only one of the following at any given time

Internal usage

To help lose weight

Ash (capsules, 300mg powder) Take 2 capsules three times a day with a large glass of water.
Garcinia (capsule, 400mg powder) Take 1 capsule with a glass of water 30-60 minutes before main meals three times a day.
Horsetail Put 2-4g of the dry plant in 200ml of boiling water. Leave to infuse for 10-15 minutes. Strain. Drink 1 cup a day.
Meadowsweet (tincture, 1:4 in 25% alcohol) Take 20 drops in water three times a day after or in between meals.
White horehound (1:4 in 25% alcohol) Put 10-20 drops in a glass of water. Take two or three times a day before meals.

To detoxify the system

Dandelion (capsules, 300mg powder) Take 1 capsule three times a day with water.
Mouse-ear hawkweed Infuse 5-10g of the dried plant in 1 litre of boiling water for 10 minutes and then strain. Drink 1 cup in the morning and 1 at midday.
Maize (tincture, 1:5 in 25% alcohol) Take 5-15ml of the tincture three times a day.
Common elder (tincture, 1:5 in 25% alcohol) Take 20 drops in water three times a day after meals.

Other measures

- Limit your daily calorie intake to 1800kcal.
- Eat balanced meals including plenty of fibre, vegetables and fruit and lean protein foods.
- Cut out sugars and saturated fats.
- Be more energetic: use the stairs instead of taking lifts, and take up physical activities and sports.

Muscles, bones & joints

Back and neck pain

Back and neck pain affects almost two-thirds of the population. In Britain, non-specific back pain is one of the main causes of lost working days. Neither are specific illnesses but rather symptoms that require precise diagnosis, as the causes are many and varied.

Symptoms

- Painful twisting of the neck (torticollis) in which it remains in a fixed tilted position
- Acute painful muscle contraction at the base of the neck, often waking to find the head twisted to one side
- Lumbago (acute muscular contraction in the lower back or lumbar region)
- Intense lumbar pain on one side often associated with a 'blocked' feeling
- Pain in part or along the whole of the sciatic nerve (the main nerve in each leg and the largest nerve in the body). Back pain may be present too, but is often less intense than the leg pain
- Intense, unbearable stabs of sharp pain, aggravated by the slightest effort (coughing, sneezing, defecation)
- A reduction in muscular strength, or in feeling, making walking difficult, sometimes almost impossible

Consult your doctor or medical herbalist

- Back pain generally indicates a minor muscular strain but it can also be a sign of infection, inflammation, tumour, or collapse of the vertebrae, for example, from osteoporosis, that only your doctor can diagnose.

Causes

Back and neck pain can be caused by inefficient functioning of the spinal column or the muscles or ligaments that support it. It can arise from the physical demands of a job, poor posture, housework, gardening or lumbar strain as a result of long and tiring journeys. Sometimes it is stress related.

WHICH PLANTS?

WARNING Use one of the following at any given time

Medical herbalism is effective but takes second place to treatments such as physiotherapy, acupuncture, osteopathy, or chiropractic.

Internal usage

Ash (capsules, 300mg powder) Take 2 capsules in the morning, 2 at midday and 2 in the evening with a large glass of water.
Blackcurrant Put 5g of dried leaves into 1 litre of boiling water. Leave to infuse for 5 minutes. Drink 2-3 cups a day.
Common thyme Add 1 sachet to a cup of boiling water. Leave to infuse for 5 minutes. Drink 3 cups a day.
Devil's claw (capsules) Take a total of 300-750mg a day in three doses before meals.

Maize (tincture, 1:5 in 25% alcohol) Take 5-15ml three times a day.
Meadowsweet (tincture, 1:4 in 25% alcohol) Take 20 drops in water three times daily after or in between meals.
Stinging nettle (tincture, 1:4 in 25% alcohol) Take 20 drops in water three times a day after meals.

External application

Common thyme Infuse 1 sachet in a cup of boiling water for 10 minutes. Soak a cloth in the infusion, then apply to the affected area for 15 minutes. Repeat two or three times a day.
Juniper Add 3 drops of essential oil to 10ml vegetable oil. Rub in two or three times a day. Or, add 2g of crushed berries to 200ml boiling water and infuse for 10 minutes before draining. Add 100-200ml to bath water and bathe for 15-20 minutes.
Rosemary Add 3 drops of essential oil to 10ml carrier oil. Rub in two or three times a day.
Nutmeg Add 3 drops of essential oil to 50ml carrier oil. Apply one to three times a day or use in one bath a day.

Other measures

- Consult a physiotherapist, osteopath or chiropractor and consider acupuncture.
- As a preventative, avoid lifting heavy weights.
- Avoid activities that put too much strain on the back (squash, judo, tennis).
- Try gentle, supervised muscle building in the gym to help to strengthen your back and reduce the severity and frequency of attacks.
- Wear appropriate footwear, possibly with orthopaedic soles.
- Watch your weight and try to avoid being overweight.

DID YOU KNOW?
Backache

Devil's claw is the herb usually prescribed for backache. Medical herbalists consider it a highly effective anti-inflammatory and it has an analgesic effect on non-sciatic, non-inflammatory back pain, as shown in trials conducted in Leipzig, Germany on 117 patients, who were given 480mg of dried extract twice a day. The treatment did not produce any toxic effects in any of the cases studied.

Cramp

An involuntary, painful spasm in a muscle is known as cramp. It is a common occurrence and seldom lasts more than a few moments.

Symptoms

- Muscular pain, usually of the calf muscle or toes, at rest or during the night
- Hardening and contraction of a muscle

Consult your doctor or medical herbalist

- Cramp is usually simply relieved by massage. However, if it occurs regularly at night and interrupts the sleep pattern, a doctor may be able to prescribe a drug to prevent its recurrence.
- If cramp persists for an hour or more, urgent medical attention should be sought.

Causes

Cramp is a muscular spasm that has a variety of causes such as simple muscular fatigue, lying or sitting in an awkward position. It often occurs during or after exercise as a result of the build-up of lactic acid in the muscles. It may also be due to a temporary circulatory problem. Frequently the cause remains unclear.

WHICH PLANTS?

WARNING Use only one of the following at any given time

External application

Common thyme Infuse 1 sachet in a cup of boiling water for 10 minutes. Soak a cloth in the infusion, then apply to the affected area for 15 minutes. Repeat two or three times a day.
Lavender Infuse 20-100g of flowers in 1 litre of boiling water, for 15 minutes before straining. Add the infusion to the bath water and bathe for 15 minutes.
Purslane Put 100g of fresh plant in 100ml of cold water, bring to the boil and allow to simmer for 15-30 minutes. Apply once or twice a day to the painful areas.
Nutmeg Add 3 drops of essential oil to 50ml carrier oil. Apply one to three times a day or use in the bath once a day.
Sweet marjoram Allow 3 drops of essential oil for every 10ml of carrier oil. Massage into affected areas.

Other measures

- Eat sugary foods before physical activity.
- Massage the muscles to relax them. During an attack, get out of the chair or bed and stretch the affected muscle hard.
- Regular stretching of muscles affected can considerably reduce the frequency and severity of subsequent attacks. Stretch the muscle for 10 seconds repeatedly over 3 minutes, three times a day – especially before exercise. For example, to stretch the calf muscles, straighten the knee and use the muscles of the front of the shin to pull your toes up towards you.
- Try raising the head of the bed on a phone book, brick or similarly-sized block of wood.

Fractures

A fracture is a break in a bone. In most cases the two broken ends move apart but in others splintering occurs or bone parts are telescoped into others.

A fracture can be simple (the broken bone does not penetrate the skin surface) or compound (the bone penetrates the skin). The latter is more dangerous, as a wound can lead to infection.

Symptoms

- Sharp pain, easy to locate
- Deformation of a limb
- Inability to move a limb

Consult your doctor

- Compound fractures require urgent medical attention, sometimes followed by surgery and setting in a plaster cast.
- Simple fractures are not always obvious. If you suspect a fracture, ask for an X-ray as even with a mild fracture, the bones can fail to knit in the correct position, causing later problems.

Causes

Most fractures are caused by violent shocks, but elderly people affected by osteoporosis are also at risk, as bones are so fragile that a minor knock or fall can cause a fracture. Athletes are also at risk from injury and may suffer stress fractures – particularly of the shins – caused by excessive exercise.

WHICH PLANTS?

WARNING Use only one of the following at any given time

Internal usage

Alfalfa (tincture, 1:4 in 25% alcohol) Put 20 drops in a glass of water. Drink three times a day after meals.

Horsetail Infuse 2-4g of the dry plant in 200ml of boiling water for 10-15 minutes. Drink 1 cup a day. Alternatively take 2g of powder three times a day with water.

To treat inflammation and pain
Feverfew (capsules, 380mg pure leaf) Take 3 capsules a day with food. Alternatively take one 100mg leaf extract capsule a day with food.

Other measures
- Rest is imperative in the early stages, and the affected bone should be supported; your doctor or nurse will explain what to do about this.
- If possible have physiotherapy to stimulate the muscles in the affected region.
- Increase your calcium intake; eat more dairy foods, nuts and leafy green vegetables.

Fibromyalgia

The symptoms of fibromyalgia, involving painful, stiff joints and muscles, resemble those found in other illnesses. The disorder is chronic and varies in intensity according to the individual. In its most severe forms, it can limit all the activities of those afflicted. Fibromyalgia affects around 2 per cent of the population.

Symptoms
- Pains in all areas of the body
- Joint and muscle stiffness
- Sleeplessness
- Constant tiredness
- Symptoms of depression

Consult your doctor or medical herbalist
- If neglected, fibromyalgia can become a chronic problem. It is therefore essential, if one or several of the symptoms appear, to seek medical advice.

Causes
The precise origin of the syndrome is unknown but it often appears after a traumatic shock. Even if all clinical examinations give normal results, it is important not to assume that fibromyalgia is psychosomatic in origin.

WHICH PLANTS?
WARNING Use only one of the following at any given time

Orthodox medicine may not be particularly helpful. But using plants, treatment can be individually tailored to the symptoms of each particular case.

Internal usage
To improve sleep and reduce anxiety
St John's wort (liquid extract, 1:1 in 25% alcohol) Take 2-4ml three times a day.

For fatigue and tiredness
Ashwagandha (tincture, 1:3 in 45% alcohol) Put 20 drops in a glass of water. Take three times a day.
Oats (tincture, 1:5 in 45% alcohol) Take 1-5ml in a glass of warm water two to three times a day.
Siberian ginseng (capsules, 150mg powder) Take 1 capsule three times a day with a large glass of water. Take for up to one month at a time.

For pain and inflammation
Blackcurrant Put 5g of dried leaves into 1 litre of boiling water. Leave to infuse for 5 minutes. Strain. Drink 2-3 cups a day.
Juniper (tincture, 1:5 in 45% alcohol) Put 10-20 drops in a small glass of sweetened water. Take three times a day.

External application
To relax the muscles
Common thyme Put 1 sachet into a cup of boiling water. Leave to infuse for 10 minutes. Soak a cloth in the infusion, then apply to the affected area for 15 minutes. Repeat two or three times a day.

To treat inflammation
Nutmeg Add 3 drops essential oil to 50ml carrier oil. Apply one to three times a day or use in one bath a day.

Other measures
- Take physical exercise that builds up muscle strength.
- Consider physiotherapy, osteopathy, chiropractic or acupuncture.
- Try to adapt your lifestyle to your state of health.
- Avoid tobacco and excessive alcohol.

Osteoarthritis

Osteoarthritis is a change in the cartilage lining the ends of the joints – especially the hips, knees and spine. Over time – and usually in people aged over 60 – progressive destruction of the cartilage leads to degradation of the bone beneath the cartilage and the membrane containing synovial fluid that lubricates the joint. As a result, joints become painful and swollen and function less well. Severe osteoarthritis affects three times as many women as men.

Symptoms
- Pain in the joints during activity, relieved by rest
- Swelling and stiffness that gets worse over time
- Where pain reduces use of the joint, weakness and shrinkage of surrounding muscles

Consult your doctor or medical herbalist
- A consultation with a doctor is required in order to diagnose osteoarthritis.

Osteoarthritis contd

- Do not use herbal medicines until the diagnosis has been confirmed, as other diseases have similar symptoms but require different treatments.

Causes

The natural wear and tear that occurs with age can lead to the development of osteoarthritis in people over 60. An old joint fracture, a congenital joint deformity and damage to the cartilage may cause it earlier in life.

Overweight people are more at risk, as are sports players and others whose work involves repetitive movement or the use of vibratory machinery.

WHICH PLANTS?

WARNING Only use one of the following at any given time

Internal usage

To treat inflammation and pain
Ash (capsules, 300mg powder) Take 2 capsules in the morning, 2 at midday and 2 in the evening with a large glass of water.
Blackcurrant Put 5g of dried leaves into 1 litre of boiling water, then strain. Leave to infuse for 5 minutes. Drink 2-3 cups a day.
Devil's claw (capsules, 186mg extract) Take 1 capsule three times a day before meals.
Meadowsweet (tincture, 1:4 in 25% alcohol) Take 20 drops in water three times a day after or in between meals.
Siberian ginseng (capsules, 150mg powder) Take 1 capsule three times a day with a large glass of water.
Silver birch (tincture,1:4 in 25% alcohol) Put 15 drops in a glass of water. Take three times a day after meals.

Stinging nettle (tincture, 1:4 in 25% alcohol) Take 20 drops in water three times a day after food.
Willow (capsules, 200mg) Take 2-4 capsules three times a day with water.

To promote healthy bones
Alfalfa (tincture 1:4 in 25% alcohol) Put 20 drops in a glass of water. Drink three times a day after meals.

External application

Capsicum Apply an ointment or capsicum-based cream three or four times a day as directed on the label.
Devil's claw Apply an ointment or devil's claw-based cream twice a day as directed on the label.
Ginger Add 3 drops of essential oil to 10ml of carrier oil and massage into the affected area two or three times a day.
Juniper Add 3 drops of essential oil to 10ml vegetable oil. Rub in two or three times a day.
Lavender Infuse 20-100g of dried flowers in 1 litre of boiling water, for 15 minutes before straining. Add the infusion to the bath water and bathe for 15 minutes.

Other measures

- Take regular gentle exercise that does not strain the joints, such as swimming. It will not worsen the disease, and will gradually reduce pain and stiffness.
- Support painful joints with a special bandage, available from the chemist or a sports shop.

Osteoporosis

The body's bone mass is at its peak at the age of 30. After the age of 45, it starts to decrease, three times faster in women than in men, particularly after the menopause. The term 'osteoporosis' refers to the biological decalcification of the normal bony mass, accompanied by an increased risk of fractures, particularly of the vertebrae, the hip and the wrist, leading to compression of the spinal column and arthritic pain.

Symptoms

- Mainly back pain and occasionally pain in the chest, hip, wrist and pelvic area
- Pain that is mechanical in nature, although it may appear spontaneously, or caused by effort or trauma
- Loss of height (compression of the spinal column)
- Increased risk of fractures from falls

Consult your doctor or medical herbalist

- Although osteoporosis is a natural part of ageing (and may not even become apparent until a fracture occurs), a doctor can advise on preventive measures that will minimise bone loss.
- Do not embark on a course of self-treatment without consulting your doctor.

Causes

The main causes of osteoporosis are the physiological ageing of the bony mass (which reduces the volume of the bones by two-fifths in 20 years), the menopause (because oestrogen protects against osteoporosis and levels fall after the menopause), and long-term immobility of a limb. Cortisone taken over a long period, Cushing's disease, hyperthyroidism, prolonged periods of anorexia or athletic strain in

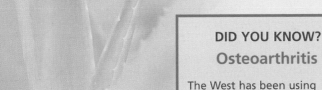

Rheumatoid arthritis

This typical inflammatory disease initially affects a particular joint (hands, knees or feet). It develops in stages with periods of remission and tends to spread to several joints. It affects between 0.5 per cent and 1 per cent of the population, predominately women, who are three times more likely to suffer from the condition than men. Early symptoms can appear around the age of 25 or during the menopause.

Symptoms

- Discomfort or intermittent pain in the joint area
- Stiffness and swelling of the affected joint, particularly after resting
- As it develops, malformation of the joints
- Spread of the disease to other joints
- Increased pain that disturbs sleep
- Ankylosis (fusing of the joints restricting movement)
- Anaemia, fatigue, weight loss, sometimes fever and aching muscles

Consult your doctor or medical herbalist

- Rheumatoid arthritis must be diagnosed by a doctor, who can usually offer treatment.
- If you want to complement this with herbal remedies, consult your doctor or a medical herbalist who will ensure there is no adverse reaction between the prescribed medication and the medicinal plants.

Causes

The disease starts with the inflammation of the synovial membrane lining the joints – this is caused by the body's immune system attacking the lining, believing it

---

The West has been using **devil's claw** (*Harpagophytum procumbens*) against osteoarthritis so successfully that this plant is at risk of disappearing from the Namibian desert. Luckily, it has a cousin, *H. zeyheri*, which has similar properties.

However, despite their overall similarities, only the use of *H. procumbens'* secondary root is authorised by the European pharmacopoeia.

To promote healthy bones
Alfalfa (tincture, 1:4 in 25% alcohol) Put 20 drops into a glass of water. Drink three times a day after meals.

Other measures

- Avoid inactivity: walk regularly, do a work out, go swimming.
- Take vitamin D (but always under medical supervision).
- Ensure a regular intake of calcium-rich foods.
- Reduce alcohol and stop smoking.
- If you feel at risk from osteoporosis, discuss the possibility of bone density (DEXA) scanning with your GP.
- Try to deal with the causes of any amenorrhoea, which increases the risk because it is usually accompanied by reduced oestrogen levels.

---

women (such as marathon runners) causing reduced oestrogen levels, and cancer can also cause osteoporosis. Smoking and heavy drinking increase the risk.

WHICH PLANTS?
WARNING Use only one of the following at any given time

Internal usage
Angelica Take 2-5ml leaf extract (1:1 in 25% alcohol) or 0.5-2ml rhizome/root extract (1:1 in 25% alcohol), three times a day.
Feverfew (capsules, 380mg pure leaf) Take 3 capsules a day with food. Alternatively take one 100mg leaf extract capsule a day with food.
Horsetail Put 2-4g of the dry plant in 200ml of boiling water. Leave to infuse for 10-15 minutes. Drink 1 cup a day. Alternatively take 2g of powder three times a day with water.

Rheumatoid arthritis contd

to be a foreign infection. It can be triggered by a bacterial or viral infection in those who are susceptible. There is often a family history of autoimmune disease.

WHICH PLANTS?

WARNING Use only one of the following at any given time

The treatment of rheumatoid arthritis combines prescribed medicines (often based on corticosteroids) with rest, designed to protect the joints, and physiotherapy, to prevent stiffening. Medicinal plants can complement this treatment.

Internal usage

Devil's claw (capsules, 186mg extract) Take 1 capsule three times a day before meals.
Meadowsweet (tincture, 1:4 in 25% alcohol) Take 20 drops in water three times a day after or between meals.
Turmeric (tincture, 1:5 in 70% alcohol) Take 20 drops in water three times a day after meals.
Stinging nettle (tincture, 1:4 in 25% alcohol) Take 20 drops in a glass of water three times a day after meals.
Willow (capsules, 200mg) Take 2-4 capsules three times a day with water.

External application

Capsicum Apply an ointment or capsicum-based cream three or four times a day as directed.
Ginger Add 3 drops of essential oil to 10ml of carrier oil. Massage into the affected area two or three times a day.
Juniper Add 3 drops of essential oil to 10ml vegetable oil. Rub in two or three times a day.
Lavender Add 20-100g of flowers to 1 litre of boiling water, leave to infuse for 15 minutes, then strain.

Add the infusion to the bath water and bathe for 15 minutes.

Other measures

- Avoid unnecessary fatigue.
- Acupuncture.
- Take vitamin B supplements and trace elements (copper, manganese, sulphur) which are beneficial for bony tissue.
- Eat oily fish from cold regions, which are rich in fatty acids and have a beneficial effect on inflammatory rheumatism.
- Try to maintain your weight within the normal range (see obesity).
- Regular exercise when the joints are not acutely inflamed will help to maintain the strength of the muscles around the joints: swimming is ideal as there is less weight on the joints in water.

Sprains

A sprain is an injury to the ligaments that hold together the bone ends of the joint. In a mild sprain these are stretched; in more severe cases, they are torn. Sprains cause painful swelling around the joint which cannot be moved without considerable discomfort.

Symptoms

- Sharp pain at the moment of trauma, followed by intense pain over at least 24 hours
- Swelling of the joint
- Bruising
- Restricted mobility of the joint

DID YOU KNOW?
Sprains

Arnica has been used in ointments to treat sprains and bruises for hundreds of years. One early proponent was the 12th-century German saint Hildegard of Bingen, who wrote treatises on medicinal plants. Nowadays arnica is sometimes used by plastic surgeons to help reduce post-operative pain and swelling.

Causes

Sprains are usually caused by sudden, excessive force on a joint, such as tripping and twisting an ankle or wrist as the body's full weight falls on the joint. In elderly people, unsteadiness or weakness in the ligaments may lead to this kind of trauma.

Consult your doctor or medical herbalist

- Early attention is important in order to ensure a rapid cure. If joint movement is very painful for more than 18 hours, consult a doctor, who can X-ray the joint to exclude a fracture.
- A benign sprain can be treated simply by rest and topical creams or ointments; in more serious cases the joint may need the support of a splint or plaster.

WHICH PLANTS?

WARNING Use only one of the following at any given time

Arnica, in every form, is excellent for this type of trauma, and other plants can be effective, alone or in combination.

Internal usage

Devil's claw (capsules, 186mg extract) Take 1 capsule three times a day before meals.
Meadowsweet (tincture, 1:4 in 25% alcohol) Take 20 drops in water three times a day after or between meals.
Willow (capsules, 200mg) Take 2-4 capsules three times a day with water.

External application

Arnica Gently massage in an arnica-based cream or gel until it has penetrated completely. Repeat two or three times a day.
Juniper Add 3 drops of essential oil to 10ml vegetable oil. Rub in two or three times a day.
Peppermint Add 3 drops of essential oil to 10ml carrier oil and massage into affected area two or three times a day.
Rosemary Add 3 drops of essential oil to 10ml vegetable oil. Rub in two or three times a day.
Sweet clover Put 20g of dried flowers in 100ml of water. Boil for 15 minutes. Allow to cool a little and then soak a cloth in it. Apply as a hot compress to the sprain two or three times a day.

Other measures

- Rest the affected joint in a supported position while acutely painful, but try to exercise it as soon as possible; this increases the speed and strength of healing.
- If an ankle is affected, wear supportive shoes with laces.
- Apply cold compresses.
- Consider laser treatment or physiotherapy.

Tendinitis

Tendons are the connective tissues that transmit the mechanical effort of the muscles to the bones. Tendinitis is an inflammation of the sheaths of the tendons. It can be traumatic or rheumatic in origin and can last between a week and six months.

Symptoms

- Intense joint pain, usually in the arm or leg
- Limited movement
- Extension of pain to the entire limb
- Waking in pain during the night

Consult your doctor

- Only your doctor can diagnose tendinitis, which can be confused with other conditions with similar symptoms.

Causes

Inflammation of the tendons may occur after overexertion or as a result of a pulled tendon. It can also be linked to muscle fatigue caused by repetitive tasks at work, unaccustomed movement, or intense athletic training.

WHICH PLANTS?

WARNING Use only one of the following at any given time

Internal usage

To treat inflammation and pain
Capsicum (tincture, 1:20 in 60% alcohol) Take 0.3-1.0ml three times a day.

Feverfew (capsules, 380mg pure leaf) Take 3 capsules a day with food. Or, take one 100mg leaf extract capsule a day with food.
Meadowsweet (tincture,1:4 in 25% alcohol) Take 20 drops in water three times a day after or between meals.
Turmeric (tincture, 1:5 in 70% alcohol) Put 20 drops in a glass of water. Take three times a day after meals.

External application

Nutmeg Add 3 drops of essential oil to 50ml carrier oil. Apply one to three times a day or use in one bath a day.
Sweet clover Put 20g of dried flowers in 100ml of water. Leave to boil for 15 minutes. Allow to cool a little and then soak a cloth in it. Apply as a hot compress to the affected area two or three times a day.

Other measures

- At the first sign of tendinitis, stop using the affected limb.
- Place an ice pack on the affected joint.
- Use a strong support bandage on the affected joint.
- Other effective therapies include laser treatment and manipulation.
- After healing, try to strengthen the affected muscles, perhaps at a gym or with physiotherapy.

Reproduction & sexuality

Breast disorders

Breast pain or lumps, known medically as mastopathy, are associated with various anomalies in the structure of the breast – usually benign. Disorders include cysts (tumours which contain fluid), zones of fibrous tissue and glandular nodules.

Breast problems often affect women between the ages of 40–50, and can increase in severity just before the onset of the menopause, following which it lessens. Breast pain is one of the most common symptoms of PMT.

Symptoms
- Breasts swollen, tender, hard, painful, perhaps with nobbly or nodular feel under the skin
- Possibly some discharge from the nipple

Consult your doctor
- It is important to consult a doctor when breast pain becomes too disabling.
- More than half of all breast complaints are related to problems with the cervical and dorsal vertebrae: in such cases, you should consult a physiotherapist or an osteopath.
- Although breast cancer rarely presents with pain as the first symptom, any lump, whether painful or not, should be assessed by your GP.

Causes
Breast pain or lumps can be caused by several factors – they can be hormonal, due to overproduction of oestrogen, circulatory, cancerous or psychological. Hormonal and emotional balances are closely linked, and stress can exacerbate the problem.

WHICH PLANTS?
WARNING Use only one of the following at any given time

Internal usage
Evening primrose oil (soft capsules, 500mg) Take 2 capsules three times a day during the last ten days of the cycle.
See also Premenstrual syndrome.

External application
Marigold Infuse 5g of dried flowerheads in 1 litre of boiling water for 5 minutes. Soak a cloth in the infusion and apply three or four times a day. Alternatively, apply a marigold-based cream three or four times a day.
Marshmallow Infuse 2-3g of dried root in 1 cup of boiling water for 10 minutes and strain. Soak a cloth in the infusion and apply three or four times a day.
Meadowsweet Put 1 tablespoon of aerial parts in 1 cup of water that is barely simmering (above 90°C the salicylates are eliminated). Leave to infuse for 10 minutes. Soak a cloth in the infusion and apply three or four times a day.

Other measures
- Give up smoking.
- If necessary, try relaxation techniques such as yoga, or consider psychotherapy.

DID YOU KNOW?

Mastitis & breast pains

For a woman, her breasts are an important part of how she sees herself and her sexuality. Although pain is a common symptom of a breast disorder, there is often no relation between the intensity of the pain and the gravity of the illness: breast cancer is not very painful. However, fear of breast cancer can give rise to pains in the breasts.

Breastfeeding problems

Problems with breastfeeding can be caused by lack of milk, the appearance of cracks in the nipples, engorgement of the breast, mastitis (inflammation of the lymphatic vessels in the breast) or by an abscess.

Symptoms
- Lack of milk – the baby cries abnormally and does not put on weight
- Lesions on the nipple, ranging from fine to more severe cracks
- Engorged, swollen, hard and painful breasts
- Mastitis – the breast is taut, hot, painful and has a mottled appearance
- Breast abscess – mother's temperature rises, milk and pus leak from the nipple and an abscess forms

Consult your doctor
- It is imperative that a doctor is consulted if you have a temperature, sharp pain or pus from the nipple.
- In the case of mastitis, anti-inflammatory drugs may be prescribed for the first 24 hours, but usually not antibiotics.
- For mastitis or an abscess, antibiotics and anti-inflammatories will often be prescribed.

Causes
Lack of milk can be linked to emotional causes. Cracked nipples can be caused by the baby failing to suck in the correct position, poor hygiene or by nipples that are too short or concave.

Engorgement of the breast usually indicates difficulty with the milk flow rather than an over-full breast. Mastitis is the result of an inflammation of the lymphatic mammary vessels due to the presence of bacteria infecting the breast either via the nipple or the areola, or via blood from another infection in the body.

An abscess develops if inflammation of a milk duct or cracked nipples remain untreated.

WHICH PLANTS?

WARNING Use only one of the following at any given time

Internal usage

It is advisable to seek advise from a professional herbalist or a doctor before starting treatment.

To improve milk flow

Anise (tincture, 1:4 in 45% alcohol) Take 5-10 drops three times a day in a little cold water after meals.

Cumin Infuse a teaspoon of seeds in 250ml of boiling water for 2-3 minutes. Alternatively, use 1-2g of ground seeds and leave to infuse for 10-15 minutes in a cup of boiling water. Strain. Drink ½ cup before main meals.

External application

Marigold Put 5g of dried flowerheads into 1 litre of boiling water. Leave to infuse for 5 minutes. Soak a cloth in this infusion and apply three or four times a day.

Other measures

- To prevent cracked nipples, draw out the nipples during pregnancy to prepare them for breastfeeding. During the ninth month of pregnancy, smear a thick coating of vaseline (40g) and lanolin (40g) on the nipples three times a week.
- For effective feeding, ensure you are comfortable and position the baby so that it takes the entire areola into its mouth.
- Wash the nipples carefully with clean, boiled water.
- Wash your hands before and after each feed, dry the areola with a clean pad or warm air.
- Insert a soft pad in your bra.

Condyloma

A virus known as the human papillomavirus (HPV) is responsible for condyloma – an infection of the skin and genital mucous membrane. Two types of lesion characterise HPV: condyloma acuminatum, in which raised wart-like growths are visible on the external genitalia and less obvious, flatter, condyloma latum affecting the vulva or anus. The latter occurs particularly on the cervix and has been linked to cervical cancer.

Symptoms

- There are frequently no visible signs of the disease
- Sometimes, irritation or itching around the vulva, pain during sex, which may result in frictional burns or bleeding
- In certain types of the virus, abnormal outgrowth from a membrane on the vulva or perineum

Consult your doctor

- You must consult a doctor about any abnormal growth around the genitals.
- A woman who has condyloma latum should have regular smear tests to eliminate to detect abnormal changes in the cervix which can signal cancer.
- Genital warts can be surgically removed, or treated with a laser, or with a cream applied directly to the external genital areas.

Causes

In 95 per cent of cases condylomas are transmitted during sexual activity. The remaining 5 per cent of cases can occur through poor hygiene (dirty hands or underwear). The warts usually take at least three months to appear, but may not become apparent until several years after contact with an infected partner.

WHICH PLANTS?

WARNING Use only one of the following at any given time

Herbal medicine can only complement conventional medical treatment and should be administered over a period of 6-12 months.

Internal usage

Echinacea (tincture, 1:5 in 45% alcohol) Take 15 drops three times a day.

Siberian ginseng (capsules, 150mg powder) Take 1 capsule three times a day with a large glass of water. Take for one month at a time. Do not use if taking oral contraceptives.

External application

Aloe vera Apply the gel two or three times a day until the warts have gone.

Lavender Put 2-3g of the flowers in a cup of boiling water. Infuse for 5-10 minutes, then strain. Soak a cloth in this infusion and apply three or four times a day.

Marigold Put 5g of dried flowerheads in 1 litre of boiling water. Leave to infuse for 5 minutes. Soak a cloth in this infusion and apply three or four times a day.

Other measures

- Ask your partner to see a doctor and take a course of treatment to avoid any reinfection.
- It is recommended that you stop smoking immediately as tobacco encourages the virus to spread.
- Use a condom during all sexual relations to protect against the HPV virus as well as other sexually transmitted diseases.

Endometriosis

The uterus, a hollow muscle, is lined with endometrial tissue, which undergoes changes during the menstrual cycle and is shed during monthly periods. Problems can arise when endometrial tissue is found in an abnormal location. It can, for instance, penetrate to the interior of the muscular wall of the uterus, leading to adeno-myosis or uterine endometriosis. In other cases, it can be found outside the uterine cavity (external endometriosis), on the ovaries, in the Fallopian tubes, on the pelvic colon, the vulva or throughout the pelvic cavity.

This problem often recurs after the cessation of treatment, but diminishes following pregnancy and usually disappears after the menopause. It generally occurs between the ages of 25 and 45, but does not lead to cancer. Both uterine and external endometriosis may be symptomless but can lead to infertility.

Symptoms

Uterine endometriosis
- Heavy menstrual bleeding, with clots
- Lower back pain, pelvic congestion and painful sexual intercourse
- Repeated blood loss between periods leading to severe anaemia

External endometriosis
- Very frequent pain, intensifying around the time of the period: dysmenorrhoea; sharp pain at ovulation, preceded by small bleeds; severe pain during sexual intercourse; abdominal and lower back pain; or pain during defecation
- Urination may be difficult, with bladder pain
- Abnormal bleeding: heavy periods, bleeding between periods

Consult your doctor
- In case of intense pain, severe bleeding or infertility, consult your GP.

Causes

The origin of this complaint is unknown, but it is linked to hormonal problems, in particular to the production of oestrogens. The daughters of women who were prescribed Stilboestrol® (synthetic oestrogen) during pregnancy are predisposed to endometriosis.

WHICH PLANTS?

WARNING Only use one of the following at any given time

Internal usage

For pain and inflammation
Black haw (tincture, 1:3 in 25% alcohol) Take 20 drops in water three times a day after meals.
Common yarrow Put 1 teaspoon of the dried plant into 250ml of boiling water. Infuse for 5 minutes. Strain. Drink 3-4 cups a day.
German chamomile Add 1 sachet to a cup of boiling water. Leave to infuse for 10 minutes. Drink 3 cups a day before meals.
Ginger (tincture, 1:5 in 60% alcohol) Take up to 30 drops a day in a glass of water.

External application

Lavender Dilute 3 drops of essential oil with 10ml carrier oil and massage in enough of this mixture to cover the lower abdomen and lower back. Apply twice a day.

Female infertility

The inability to conceive is known as primary infertility if a woman has never had a baby. It is known as secondary infertility if a woman has already been pregnant, even if the pregnancy was ectopic, terminated or resulted in a miscarriage.

Symptoms
- An inability to become pregnant, despite trying for 1-2 years.

Consult your doctor
- It is important to consult a specialist, who will be able to discover the cause by carrying out various examinations.
- The fertility of a partner may also need to be checked.

Causes

There may be a physical reason for infertility, for example, a malformation of the uterus, Fallopian tubes or ovaries following a genital infection, or endometriosis. It can also be due to a hormonal imbalance or an ovarian or another type of disorder (thyroid, adrenal). It may even be the result of medication. However, there are still cases where there is no apparent cause, in which case doctors may suggest relaxation techniques and the elimination of stress.

DID YOU KNOW?
Fibroids

Avoid plants with an oestrogenic action (such as common sage, ginseng, black cohosh), which may stimulate the production of excess oestrogen and thereby enlarge the fibroids.

WHICH PLANTS?

WARNING Only use one of the following at any given time

Medicinal herbs can help to treat certain contributory factors.

Internal usage

For improving fertility

Chaste tree (tincture, 1:3 in 25% alcohol) Take 30 drops in a little cold water every morning, for up to 6 months. Effects may not be felt until after 3 months.

To reduce stress

Ashwagandha (tincture, 1:3 in 45% alcohol) Take 20 drops in a glass of water, three times a day.
Lime tree Put 5g of dried flowers into 1 litre of boiling water. Leave to infuse for 5 minutes. Strain. Drink 1 cup in the evening.
Passionflower (tincture, 1:6 in 25% alcohol) Take 20 drops with a little cold water after meals, three times a day.

To improve general health

American ginseng (powder, 500mg capsules) Take 2 capsules twice a day, preferably with food. Use for up to 3 months followed by a 6 week break.
Blackcurrant Put 5g of dry leaves into 1 litre of boiling water. Leave to infuse for 5 minutes. Drink 2-3 cups a day.
Grape seed extract (capsules, 30-100mg) Take 1 capsule a day.
Ginkgo (tincture, 1:4 in 25% alcohol) Take 20 drops in water three times a day after meals.

Other measures

- Get your weight up or down to normal (BMI of 18.5 to 30 – see obesity)
- Both partners should stop smoking or drinking heavily.
- Men should wear loose trousers and underwear.

Fibroids

One of the commonest forms of tumour of the uterus, fibroids never become malignant. They vary in size from a pea to a grapefruit and can, in some cases, invade the abdominal cavity. Fibroids cause various kinds of bleeding and tend to grow slowly until the menopause, thereafter decreasing in volume. Sometimes, for unknown reasons, a fibroid may grow rapidly during the reproductive years, resisting all treatment.

While benign in itself, a fibroid may cause infertility and presents a risk of anaemia. A particularly large fibroid may cause pressure on the urinary passage and damage the kidneys. It is a common ailment, affecting 20 per cent of 30-year-old women and 40 per cent of 50-year-olds.

Symptoms

- Abnormally long or heavy periods, with clotting
- Painful periods
- Bleeding between periods
- Discomfort and heaviness, depending upon the size of the fibroid
- Complications due to pressure: urinary complaints, constipation, varicose veins, piles, pelvic inflammation

Consult your doctor

- In cases of infertility, urinary problems, constipation and especially where there is heavy bleeding or serious discomfort, consult your GP.

Causes

A fibroid is caused by hormonal imbalance: insufficient progesterone production and excessive oestrogen production, frequently due to stress, emotional shock, obesity or pre-menopause.

WHICH PLANTS?

WARNING Only use one of the following at any given time

Internal usage

To normalise the menstrual cycle

Evening primrose (capsules, 500mg) Take 2 capsules three times a day during the last ten days of the menstrual cycle.

For pain and inflammation

Black haw (tincture, 1:3 in 25% alcohol) Take 20 drops in a glass of water, three times a day, after meals.
German chamomile Add 1 sachet to a cup of boiling water. Leave to infuse for 10 minutes. Drink 3 cups a day, before meals.
Ginger (tincture, 1:5 in 90% alcohol) Take 10 drops a day in water.
Lavender Put 2-3g of dried flowers into a cup of boiling water. Leave to infuse for 5-10 minutes. Drink 3-4 cups a day, between meals.
Meadowsweet (tincture, 1:4 in 25% alcohol) Take 20 drops in water, three times a day, after or between meals.
Chaste tree (tincture, 1:3 in 25% alcohol) Take 30 drops in a little cold water every morning, for up to 6 months. Effects may not be noticed until after 3 months.

External application

Lavender Dilute the essential oil, allowing 3 drops to 10ml of carrier oil. Massage into the lower abdomen and lower back. Apply twice a day.

Other measures

- Avoid all sporting activities likely to aggravate the pelvis, such as tennis, jogging, skipping, etc.
- Avoid wearing high heels.

Genital infections

There is a difference between lower genital infections (those of the penis, vulva and vagina) and upper genital infections (of the uterus and the Fallopian tubes) which can sometimes be linked to other complications such as peritonitis. Contrary to general opinion, these can afflict anyone, even those who have had sexual relations with just one partner.

Symptoms

As a general rule
- Heavy and unpleasant-smelling discharge
- Itching, burning or pain in the penis, vulva and vagina
- Ulcers, blisters or inflammation
- Pain during sexual intercourse

In cases of lower infection
- Pelvic pain
- Abnormal bleeding (in women)

In cases of upper infection
- Fever

Consult your doctor
- The appearance of any one of the above symptoms means that you should consult a GP or sexual health clinic as soon as possible. Prolonged antibiotic treatment is often prescribed in case of upper genital infection.

Causes

Lower genital infections can be bacterial in origin, springing from intestinal infections (coliform baccili, streptococci B or D, *Staphylococcus aureus*).

Alternatively, they can be caused by skin infection (epidermal staphylococci) or be of vaginal origin, with abnormal proliferation of the infective agents usually present in small quantities (mycoplasmas, corynebacteria).

Most commonly, they can be sexually transmitted (*Gardnerella vaginalis*, *Trichomonas vaginalis*). Lower genital infections of a viral type are due to the human papilloma (wart) virus – which in women presents a risk of cancer of the cervix – or to the recurring herpes virus.

Upper genital infections are principally caused by sexually transmissible microorganisms, such as *Chlamydia trachomatis*, or to gonorrhoea. They can, however, spring from other causes, such as acute appendicitis, after an abortion or, more rarely, following childbirth. *Actinomyces* can cause upper genital infections if women use an IUD for contraception.

Genital infections of every kind can be due to having multiple partners, a careless attitude to sex, ignorance of preventative measures and poor hygiene.

WHICH PLANTS?
WARNING Only use one of the following at any given time

Internal usage

To treat the infection
Echinacea (tincture, 1:5 in 45% alcohol) Take 2-5ml three times a day. Take ten days a month, as a long-term treatment to prevent recurrence of the infection.

For pain and inflammation
German chamomile Add a sachet to 1 cup of boiling water. Leave to infuse for 10 minutes, then strain. Drink 3 cups a day before meals.
Ginger (tincture, 1:5 in 60% alcohol) Take up to 30 drops in a glass of water, every day.
Lavender Put 2-3g of the flowers into a cup of boiling water. Leave to infuse for 5-10 minutes, then strain. Drink 3-4 cups a day between meals.

External application

To treat vaginal discharge
Lady's mantle Put 1-2g of dried plant into 1 litre of boiling water. Infuse for 10 minutes and strain. Add the infusion to a bath. Bathe twice a day.

Other measures
- Use male or female condoms.
- Avoid using tampons, or alternate tampons with sanitary towels.
- After defecation, wipe the anus backwards, not forwards.

See also Condyloma (for genital warts), *and* Fungal skin infections Herpes.

Impotence

Impotence means both the inability of a man to achieve an erection, and also premature or delayed ejaculation.

Symptoms
- Inability to achieve an erection, with or without libido
- Loss of the erection during sexual intercourse
- Premature ejaculation, that is, before penetration or shortly afterwards
- Delayed ejaculation: erection is achieved but impossible to bring to completion by ejaculation

Consult your doctor
- While often psychological in origin, impotence may be caused by other factors, which only a doctor can determine.

Causes

In many cases, impotence springs from psychological problems. These may include: stress, anxiety, depression, fatigue, lack of desire for a partner, anxiety about the sexual act or uncertainty about sexual orientation. Previous episodes of impotence or bad experiences may reinforce the anxiety of it happening again. Chronic tobacco or alcohol abuse may also be factors.

However, sometimes there may be physiological causes: vascular problems, diabetes, high blood pressure, problems affecting the blood reservoirs of the penis that control erection, neurological disorders, low levels of the male hormone testosterone, or the side effects of medication.

WHICH PLANTS?

WARNING Use only one of the following at any given time

Internal usage

Blackcurrant Put 5g of dried leaves into 1 litre of boiling water. Leave to infuse for 5 minutes. Drink 2-3 cups a day.
Fenugreek (tincture, 1:3 in 25% alcohol) Put 20 drops in a little cold water. Take 3 times a day.
Ginkgo (tincture, 1:4 in 25% alcohol) Take 20 drops in water, three times a day, after meals.
Grape seed extract (capsules, 30-100mg) Take 1 capsule a day.
Walnut Put 10g of dried leaves into 1 litre of boiling water. Leave to infuse for 15 minutes. Drink 3-5 cups a day.

For depression, stress and anxiety

Ashwagandha (tincture, 1:3 in 45% alcohol) Take 20 drops in a glass of water, three times a day.
Lavender Infuse 2-3g of dried flowers in a cup of boiling water for 5-10 minutes. Strain. Drink 3-4 cups a day, between meals.
Passionflower (tincture, 1:8 in 25% alcohol) Take 20 drops with a little cold water, after meals, three times a day.

Other measures

- If there are no apparent physiological causes, talk to your GP or sexual health clinic about psychological help – a health adviser or clinical psychologist is usually available on the NHS.
- Avoid smoking and limit your alcohol intake.
- Take physical exercise to boost energy levels.

Libido (problems)

The libido, or sexual drive, can be disturbed, as easily in women as in men, by psychological or physiological factors.

Symptoms

- Lack of sexual desire
- A feeling of tiredness, migraine or other symptoms of discomfort before sexual relations
- Anxiety at the thought of having sex

Consult your doctor or medical herbalist

- A prolonged decline in the libido can be one of the first signs of nervous depression, of a serious nervous illness, of Alzheimer's disease or of another serious mental affliction. A doctor's advice is essential.

Causes

Lack of interest in one's partner, the focusing of this interest on someone or something else, fatigue, stress and an emotional problem, can all affect the libido.

In 90 per cent of cases, loss of libido is psychological in origin. However, chronic alcohol or tobacco abuse can cause problems, as well as medicines such as beta-blockers or certain antidepressants and immunosuppressants.

WHICH PLANTS?

WARNING Only use one of the following at any given time

The role of plants is limited to complementing psychotherapy by their stimulating action on the nervous system.

Internal usage

For depression, stress and anxiety

Lavender Infuse 2-3g of flowers in a cup of boiling water for 5-10 minutes. Strain. Drink 3-4 cups a day between meals.
Lime tree Put 5g of dried flowers into 1 litre of boiling water. Leave to infuse for 5 minutes. Strain. Drink 1 cup in the evening.
Passionflower (tincture, 1:6 in 25% alcohol) Take 20 drops with a little cold water, after meals, three times a day.

For fatigue

Cinnamon Take 0.3-1g of powder three times a day, with food.
Dog rose Put 2-2.5g of broken rosehips into a cup of boiling water. Leave to infuse for 10 minutes and then filter. Drink 3-4 cups a day.
Oats (tincture,1:5 in 45% alcohol) Take 1-5ml in a glass of warm water, 2-3 times a day.
Sea buckthorn Drink 1-3 dessert-spoons of pure juice or syrup in a glass of water, every day.

Reputed aphrodisiac properties

Ashwagandha (tincture, 1:3 in 45% alcohol) Take 20 drops in a glass of water, three times a day.
American ginseng (powder, 500mg capsules) Take 2 capsules twice a day, preferably with food. Use for up to 3 months, followed by a 6 week break.

Other measures

- Do not try to force desire.
- Avoid stress (go on holiday, if possible).
- Consult a GP or a psychotherapist, or ask at the nearest sexual health clinic if you could talk to their health adviser or clinical psychologist.

See also Impotence.

Menopause, pre-menopause

The ending of a woman's fertile years evolves in stages beginning with the pre-menopause, a phase involving menstrual irregularities. It continues with the menopause, the year following the apparent cessation of periods, followed by the post-menopause.

Although some diseases become more prevalent after the menopause (for example osteoporosis and heart disease), there is still no consensus within the medical profession as to whether it should be 'treated' with hormone-replacement therapy – itself subject to some possible serious short and long-term side effects.

Symptoms

Pre-menopause
- Period problems: cycles irregular, shorter or longer
- Bleeding outside period time periods heavier or less heavy
- The appearance or worsening of premenstrual syndrome or of breast problems

Menopause
- Absence of periods
- Hot flushes
- Mood swings
- Vaginal dryness
- Tiredness

Consult your doctor or medical herbalist
- If you have heavy bleeding or unbearable hot flushes and sweats, consult your GP
- Herbs can help, but ask about any possible contraindications to phytoestrogens (naturally occurring oestrogens in plants).
- Never take oestrogenic essential oils (notably sage or mugwort) without medical advice: they can have a toxic effect on the nervous system.

Causes

The menopause concludes the reproductive phase of a woman's life – she has few eggs left in her ovaries, and blood levels of the naturally occurring sex hormones oestrogen and progesterone start to decline. The end of ovulation causes a lack of oestrogens and progesterone, indicating the menopause.

While not totally replacing the sex hormones, herbal medicines can often lessen the symptoms of the menopause.

WHICH PLANTS?

WARNING Use only one of the following at any given time

Internal usage

Pre-menopause
WARNING At the pre-menopausal stage, do not take phytoestrogens
Lady's mantle (tincture, 1:4 in 25% alcohol) Take 20 drops in a little cold water, three times a day.
Chaste tree (tincture, 1:3 in 25% alcohol) Take 30 drops in a little cold water, every morning, for up to 6 months. Effects may not be apparent for up to 12 weeks.

Menopause
WARNING Do not take oestrogenic plants if there is any history of thromboses, or breast cancer or cancer of the uterus
Alfalfa (tincture, 1:4 in 25% alcohol) Take 20 drops in a glass of water, three times a day, after meals. (oestrogenic)
Hop (tincture, 1:5 in 60% alcohol) Take 20 drops in water three times daily after meals. (oestrogenic)

To treat breast pain
Chaste tree (tincture, 1:3 in 25% alcohol) Take 30 drops in a little cold water, every morning, for up to 6 months. Effects may not be apparent for up to 12 weeks.

External application

To treat breast pain
Aloe vera Apply aloe vera gel to the inflamed breast(s) three to four times a day.
Marigold Infuse 5g of dried flower heads in 1 litre of boiling water for 5 minutes. Soak a cloth in this and apply three to four times a day. Or apply a marigold-based cream three to four times a day.
Marshmallow Put 2-3g of dried root into 1 cup of boiling water. Infuse for 10 minutes, then strain. Soak a cloth in this infusion and apply three to four times a day.
Meadowsweet Put 1 tablespoon of aerial parts into 1 cup of water that is barely simmering (above 90°F the salicylates are eliminated). Infuse for 10 minutes, then strain. Soak a cloth in the infusion and apply three to four times a day.

To treat vaginal dryness
Aloe vera Apply the gel to the vagina at night.

Other measures
- Make sure you eat plenty of fruits and vegetables that are rich in vitamins A, C and E, and high in antioxidants.
- At least three times a week eat fish such as salmon, mackerel, tuna, sardines, halibut, herring and anchovies, that are rich in omega-3 fatty acids.
- If you feel you may be at risk of osteoporosis discuss with your GP the possibility of having a bone-density (DEXA) scan.

DID YOU KNOW?
Menstrual problems

In the Middle Ages, feverfew was widely used for menstrual problems and was known as 'the herb of mothers and the mother of herbs'.

Menstrual problems

Such problems include amenorrhoea (the absence of periods) and dysmenorrhoea (painful periods). Amenorrhoea can occur in a girl who is of an age to have started menstruation but has not yet done so, or in a woman who is already menstruating.

Dysmenorrhoea may appear at an early stage in puberty or as a secondary complaint, occurring after several years of pain-free cycles. The pains can take the form of simple cramps or may be so incapacitating that the sufferer is forced to take to her bed.

Menstrual problems mainly affect young girls, women who are stressed, anxious or nervous, and pre-menopausal women.

Symptoms

Amenorrhoea
- Non-appearance of periods at puberty, known as primary amenorrhoea
- The absence of menstruation for at least 3 months in a woman who is menstruating, known as secondary amenorrhoea

Dysmenorrhoea
- Lower stomach pains during periods, frequently severe, which may start several hours before the onset of a period and may continue for 1-2 days.
- Sometimes accompanied by diarrhoea, nausea, vomiting, fainting.

Consult your doctor
- Whatever the nature of the problem it is best to have a clinical examination before embarking on any form of herbal treatment.
- Amenorrhoea may also require several complementary analyses, including radiological and hormonal assessments. An ultra-sound scan of the uterus and ovaries and sometimes an X-ray of the pituitary gland can detect any possible tumour.
- In cases of severe or persistent pain, consult your GP.

Causes

Primary amenorrhoea can be due simply to the delay of the onset of puberty, particularly if there is a family history of this. Much more rarely, it may be caused by genital malformation. Secondary amenorrhoea can be caused by psychological problems; excessively intensive sporting activity; a tumour on the ovary or on the pituitary gland, or certain drugs.

Dysmenorrhoea may be due to circulatory problems, infection, fibroids, endometriosis or polyps. But hormonal problems are the most common cause – possibly as a result of excessive oestrogen or insufficient progesterone and probably stress-related, although the exact cause is not known.

Period problems may also be caused by infection, an intra-uterine device (IUD), other forms of contraceptive, certain types of medication, systemic diseases such as hypothyroidism and blood disorders.

WHICH PLANTS?

WARNING Only use one of the following at any given time

Internal usage

To treat amenorrhoea
Common yarrow Put 1 teaspoon of the dried plant into 250ml of boiling water. Infuse for 5 minutes, then strain. Drink 3-4 cups a day.
Cumin Put a teaspoon of seeds into 250ml of boiling water and leave to infuse for 2-3 minutes. Alternatively, use 1-2g of ground seeds and infuse for 10-15 minutes in a cup of boiling water. Drink ½ cup before main meals.
Mugwort (liquid extract, 1:1 in 25% alcohol) Take 0.5-2ml three times a day.

For relief from menstrual pain
Black haw (tincture, 1:3 in 25% alcohol) Take 20 drops in a glass of water three times a day after meals.
Common yarrow Put 1 teaspoon of the dried plant into 250ml of boiling water. Infuse for 5 minutes, then strain. Drink 3-4 cups a day.
German chamomile Add 1 sachet to a cup of boiling water. Infuse for 10 minutes, then strain. Drink 3 cups a day before meals.
Ginger (tincture, 1:5 in 60% alcohol) Take up to 30 drops a day in a glass of water.

External application
Lavender Dilute 3 drops of the essential oil with 10ml carrier oil and massage in enough of this mixture to cover the lower abdomen and lower back. Apply twice a day.

To treat blood loss between periods
Golden seal (capsules, 540mg powder) Take 1 capsule three times a day.

Other measures
- If menstrual problems are stress-related, relaxation techniques, breathing exercises, yoga and massage can be useful.
- If appropriate, to help you to control your emotions better, consider psychotherapy.

See also Premenstrual syndrome.

Premenstrual syndrome

The term 'premenstrual syndrome' (PMS), also known as premenstrual tension (PMT), is applied to a group of physical and emotional symptoms linked to the menstrual cycle. These symptoms occur just before the period starts and end once it has begun. They can last for between 2 days and 2 weeks (the latter coinciding with the start of ovulation) and affect 40 per cent of women.

Symptoms

- There are about 150 physical and emotional symptoms that can occur separately or together

Physical symptoms including

- Tender, swollen breasts
- A bloated abdomen that can be merely uncomfortable or extremely painful
- Urinary disorders
- Weight gain
- A general feeling of bloatedness, with swollen hands and feet and vascular disorders

Emotional symptoms including

- Unpredictable moods, irritability, aggression, tearfulness, anxiety, depression, nervousness and headaches
- Insomnia, sleepiness, and hypersomnia (sleeping for unusually long spells)
- Lack of concentration, memory disorders
- Loss of appetite or libido problems

Consult your doctor or medical herbalist

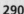

- If the severity of these disorders prevents you from leading a normal life, consult your doctor

Causes

No single cause has yet been identified to explain this wide range of symptoms. However, it appears that PMS is the result of the increased permeability of the capillaries, which causes the swelling of the tissues of the breasts, abdomen and brain.

In some cases, this may be due to the increased production of oestrogen, triggered by a number of factors, including stress and nutritional deficiencies.

WHICH PLANTS?

WARNING Use only one of the following at any given time

Internal usage

Chaste tree (tincture, 1:3 in 25% alcohol) Take 30 drops in a little cold water every morning, for up to 6 months. Effects may not be apparent for up to 12 weeks.
Lady's mantle (tincture, 1:4 in 25% alcohol) Put 20 drops into a little cold water and take three times a day.

For stress, anxiety, depression and sleep problems

Ashwagandha (tincture, 1:3 in 45% alcohol) Take 20 drops in a glass of water, three times a day.
Californian poppy (tincture, 1:4 in 45% alcohol) Take 10 drops in a little cold water, three times a day, after meals. Take up to 20 drops at bedtime.
Lavender Put 2-3g of the flowers into a cup of boiling water. Leave to infuse for 5-10 minutes. Drink 3-4 cups a day between meals.
Lime tree Put 5g of dried flowers into 1 litre of boiling water. Leave to infuse for 5 minutes. Drink 1 cup in the evening.
Passionflower (tincture, 1:8 in 25% alcohol) Take 20 drops with a little cold water, three times a day, after meals.
Valerian (capsules, 240mg powder) Take 1-2 capsules a day.

To relieve breast pains

Evening primrose (capsules, 500mg) Take 2 capsules three times a day, during the last ten days of the menstrual cycle.

Other measures

- Increase your fibre intake (fresh and dried vegetables, fruit, whole cereals). Eat fewer foods with refined sugars and more foods containing slow-release glucose, such as wholemeal bread, Basmati rice and pasta.
- Reduce your intake of animal fats, such as full-fat dairy products, and replace with ones that are monounsaturated or polyunsaturated (sunflower and olive oils).
- Eat less animal protein and more vegetable protein of various types. Cut down on salt.
- Reduce your consumption of stimulants such as cigarettes, coffee and tea.
- Take vitamins B (especially B_6), C (an antioxidant recommended for stress) and E (antioxidant), magnesium, chromium and zinc.

Respiratory problems
Asthma

During an asthma attack, the severity of which can vary, the walls of the airways narrow, become inflamed and produce excessive mucus. The attack may resolve itself spontaneously or may need medical treatment.

Symptoms
- Difficulty breathing in and out
- Spasmodic coughing in children, not accompanied by a fever
- A feeling of suffocating
- Wheezing
- Nocturnal attacks with or without copious production of mucus

Consult your doctor
- Asthma can be severe and is responsible for hundreds of deaths a year. A medical consultation will be needed to distinguish between bronchial asthma, a smoker's cough, a chest infection and other breathing difficulties, such as the simple viral bronchitis that often follows a common cold.
- Cardiac asthma – caused by the water retention in the lungs during heart failure – can mimic bronchial asthma. The doctor will decide upon the treatment with the patient; hospitalisation could be necessary.

Causes
Asthma can be a reaction to allergens such as pollen, perfume and pollution. It can also occur after physical exercise, sudden floods of emotion, or after rapid changes of temperature, such as moving from a warm house to cold street. There may also be an inherited predisposition to asthma.

Smokers, the elderly and those who have already had an allergic reaction such as eczema or allergic rhinitis, are particularly susceptible to asthma. Some medications, such as aspirin, beta-blockers and anti-inflammatories can also trigger asthma in predisposed people.

WHICH PLANTS?
WARNING Use only one of the following at any given time

Internal usage
Aaron's rod Infuse 1.5-2g in a cup of boiling water for 15 minutes. Strain. Drink 3 cups a day.
Angelica (root extract, 1:1 in 25% alcohol) Take 0.5-2ml, three times a day.
Common thyme Add 1 sachet to a cup of boiling water. Leave to infuse for 5 minutes. Strain. Drink 3 cups a day.
Eucalyptus Take 4-10g a day, either in capsule form or as an infusion.
Hyssop Put 1-2 teaspoons of dried flowers into a cup of boiling water. Leave to infuse for 5-10 minutes. Strain. Drink 3 cups a day.
Indian frankincense (tablets, 150mg extract) Take 1-2 tablets, three times a day.
Lavender Put 2-3g of the flowers in a cup of boiling water. Leave to infuse for 5-10 minutes. Drink 3-4 cups a day, between meals.
Liquorice Add 1-2 teaspoons of root powder to a cup of boiling water; allow to infuse for 10 minutes, and then strain. Drink 2 cups a day. Take for four to six weeks at a time, accompanied by a low salt diet.
Turmeric (tincture, 1:5 in 70% alcohol) Take 20 drops with water, three times a day after meals.

As directed by a medical herbalist
- Feverfew, Greater celandine

Other measures
- Take regular exercise unless it provokes an attack. If it does, you could try to prevent the onset of an attack before you start by using some of the treatments above. Get advice from your GP.
- Take minerals such as copper, magnesium, manganese and sulphur.
- Discuss a referral to an allergy clinic, with your GP.
- Try acupuncture treatment.
- Taking breathing lessons from a physiotherapist can sometimes help, too.
- Ask your GP or practice nurse about flu and pneumococcal vaccinations.

Bronchitis, acute and chronic

The disorder known as acute bronchitis is an inflammatory disease of the large bronchi which, in general, follows an infection of the upper respiratory tracts or another illness, such as measles or whooping cough, of which it is one of the symptoms.

With chronic bronchitis there is widespread inflammation of the bronchial tubes with an excessive production of clear or green mucus. The disease is described as chronic when the infection is present for at least three months a year and for more than two years.

Symptoms
Acute bronchitis
- Chesty cough, producing mucus
- Possible fever

Chronic bronchitis
- Persistent chesty cough with clear mucus that turns green if a secondary infection occurs

Consult your doctor or medical herbalist
- The doctor will make a diagnosis by listening to your lungs.
- Plant infusions can be taken to relieve chesty symptoms, but any herbal treatment should be regarded as complementary, and taken only as advised by a qualified herbalist.

Bronchitis, acute and chronic contd

Causes

Acute bronchitis can be due to the presence of both benign and disease-producing bacteria.

Chronic bronchitis tends to affect people who have been weakened by previous infections of the respiratory tract. Tobacco and air pollution are major contributing factors in this disease.

WHICH PLANTS?

WARNING Use only one of the following at any given time

Internal usage

Acute bronchitis

Common thyme Infuse 1 sachet in a cup of boiling water for 5 minutes. Drink 3 cups a day.
Eucalyptus Take 4-10g a day, as a capsule or infusion.
Hedge mustard Infuse 5g of the dried plant in a cup of boiling water for 10 minutes. Strain. Drink 2-3 cups a day.
Hyssop Put 1-2 teaspoons of dried flowers into a cup of boiling water. Leave to infuse for 5-10 minutes. Drink 3 cups a day.
Ivy Put 1 sachet in 200ml of boiling water. Leave to infuse for 5 minutes. Take 1-2 cups a day at mealtimes.
Jujube Put 30-50g of ground fruit into 1 litre of water. Boil for 30 minutes. Strain. Drink 3 cups a day.

Marshmallow (root, liquid extract, 1:1 in 25% alcohol) Take 2-5ml, three times a day.
Oregano Put 20g of the aerial parts in 1 litre of boiling water. Leave to infuse for 10 minutes. Drink 3-4 cups a day.
Senega snakeroot Put 10g of the root into 1 litre of boiling water. Infuse for 10 minutes. Strain. Drink 3-4 cups a day.
Sundew Add 1-2g of the dried plant to a cup of boiling water. Infuse for 10 minutes and strain. Drink 3 cups a day.

Chronic bronchitis

Angelica (root tincture, 1:5 in 50% alcohol) Take 0.5-2ml three times a day.
Buchu Take 350mg powder with a large glass of water, twice daily, at meal times.
Scots pine Put 20g of buds into 1 litre of boiling water. Infuse for 10 minutes and strain. Drink 4-5 cups a day.

To stimulate the immune system

Echinacea (tincture, 1:5 in 45% alcohol) Take 2-5ml, three times a day.

External application

Eucalyptus Dilute 3 drops of essential oil in 10ml carrier oil and rub into the chest and back.
Lavender As for eucalyptus (above).

Other measures

- Stop smoking.
- Do breathing exercises or have respiratory physiotherapy.
- Ask your GP or practice nurse about flu and pneumococcal vaccinations.

Skin problems
Abscess

An abscess is a localised pocket of infection affecting the skin or tissue below. It is most frequently caused by a bacterial infection.

Symptoms

- Sharp pain in the affected area with swelling and intense reddening
- Feeling of a painful build-up under the skin
- Feeling of illness, and fever

Consult your doctor or medical herbalist

- Herbal treatment can only help to bring an abscess to a head. Because a chronic abscess may indicate deep-seated illness, you should always consult a doctor.

Causes

An abscess is caused by an infection being introduced into the skin. This can be the result of a splinter, a bite or a non-sterile injection. An abscess can also form after scraping the skin or having hair removal carried out under unhygienic conditions.

WHICH PLANTS?

WARNING Use only one of the following at any given time

Internal usage

For the infection

Echinacea (tincture, 1:5 in 45% alcohol) Take 2-5ml three times a day.
Garlic (capsules, 300mg powder) Take 1-3 capsules a day.
Siberian ginseng (tincture, 1:3 in 25% alcohol) Take 10-20 drops in a little cold water, three times daily, after meals. Do not take for longer than a month at a time.

External application

To treat inflammation

Aaron's rod Soak 3 teaspoons of the dried plant in 300ml of cold water for 30 minutes. Gently bring to the boil. Strain. Soak a cloth in this liquid and apply twice a day.

Aloe vera Apply the gel two to three times a day.

Fenugreek Add 2g of powder to boiling water and infuse for 10 minutes before straining. Soak a cloth in this infusion and apply for 15 minutes.

German chamomile Infuse 1 sachet for 10 minutes, squeeze out the excess and apply to the abscess for 15 minutes. Repeat two or three times a day.

Lavender Apply 1 drop of pure essential oil to the abscess, once a day.

Stinging nettle Boil 20g of the dried plant in 750ml of water until it reduces by a third, to roughly 500ml. Apply as a poultice for 10 minutes.

Other measures

- Follow the rules of basic hygiene and wash your hands and nails thoroughly before treating the abscess or touching your skin.

Acne

The simplest form of acne affects around 90 per cent of adolescents, appearing as red or white pimples and blackheads that can leave temporary scars on the face, the chest and the back. More serious forms leave the face pockmarked. A rare form is fulminant acne that combines fever with pain in the joints and muscles.

Symptoms

- Greasy look to the face, chest, back and scalp
- Appearance of blackheads
- Presence of whiteheads: the follicle opening is clogged with trapped sebum and sealed by normal coloured skin resulting in inflammation and infection

Consult your doctor

- Unless acne is very mild, a visit to the doctor is recommended, to help prevent any permanent scarring or pigmentation.

Causes

Usually during adolescence, the oil-producing glands in the skin produce excessive amounts of sebum, the oily secretion that protects and lubricates the skin.

Acne occurs when sebum blocks the sebaceous ducts, forming a plug, and bacteria on the surface of or just beneath the skin start to proliferate. The eruption of acne is activated by heat, after exposure to the sun (which may seem to improve the condition of skin but in reality has a negative effect), or before periods in women.

It can also be triggered by some medicines: certain corticosteroids, hormonal treatments, the contraceptive pill, antiepileptic drugs and antidepressants.

WHICH PLANTS?

WARNING Use only one of the following at any given time

Internal usage

Dandelion (capsules, 300mg powder) Take 1 capsule with water, three times a day.

DID YOU KNOW?
Acne

Great burdock is a medicinal plant that has been rather neglected. Yet, its leaves and especially its roots have known antibacterial and antifungal properties. Recent studies have even shown that they contain compounds that remain active after exposure to ultraviolet rays.

Evening primrose oil (capsules, 500mg) Take 2 capsules with a glass of water, three times a day, with meals.

Great burdock (capsules, 350mg root powder) Take 1 capsule with a large glass of water, three times a day, before meals. The dosage can be increased to 5 capsules a day. Not to be administered to children below 15 years of age.

Heartsease (tincture, 1:4 in 25% alcohol) Take 20 drops in water, three times a day, after meals.

External application

Aloe vera Apply an aloe vera-based cream or gel twice a day, as directed on the label.

Basil Dilute 3 drops of essential oil with 10ml carrier oil. Apply to the affected area. Repeat two to three times a week, in the early evening.

Hemp agrimony Add 2-4 teaspoons to 1 litre of boiling water, then cool. Use to wash the face, two to three times a week.

Lavender Dilute 3 drops of the essential oil with 10ml carrier oil. Apply to the affected area, three times a week in the early evening.

Marigold Put 5g of dried flower-heads into 1 litre of boiling water. Leave to infuse for 5 minutes. Soak a cloth in this infusion and apply twice a day. Alternatively, apply a marigold-based cream or ointment twice a day.

Stinging nettle Boil 20g of dried leaves in 750ml water until it reduces by a third, to roughly 500ml. Use to wash the face once a day, three times a week.

Other measures

- Cleanse the skin in the morning and evening with gentle, non-aggressive products. Try to avoid soap; just use plain warm water.
- Never squeeze the pimples.
- Avoid very greasy cosmetics.
- Avoid topical astringents, as they only encourage the skin to produce more oil.

Acne rosacea

Identified by a persistent redness of the skin and a dilation of the blood vessels, and also through the appearance of pimples, acne rosacea afflicts older people. Fair women, with menopausal flushes, are the most susceptible. It can also affect men in middle life, with the nose growing large and warty.

Symptoms
- Redness spread over the face
- Enlargement of the nose
- Appearance of a fine network of tiny red/mauve lines across the cheeks, nose and chin
- Pimples and pustules

Consult your doctor
- It is important to consult a doctor as soon as possible to avoid disfiguring effects on your appearance.

Causes
The cause of rosacea remains unclear, though there is some evidence that it may be caused by a skin infection called Demodex folliculorum and the immune reaction to it. UV light from sunbeds or sunshine may also provoke it.

WHICH PLANTS?
WARNING Use only one of the following at any given time

Internal usage
To relax
Ashwagandha (tincture, 1:3 in 45% alcohol) Take 20 drops in a glass of water, three times a day.
Lime tree Put 5g of dried flowers into 1 litre of boiling water. Leave to infuse for 5 minutes, then strain. Drink 1 cup in the evening.
Passionflower (tincture, 1:8 in 25% alcohol) Take 25 drops with a little cold water, three times a day, after meals.

To fight infection
Echinacea (tincture, 1:5 in 45% alcohol) Take 15 drops in water, three times a day.
Garlic (capsules, 300mg powder) Take 1-3 capsules a day.
Great burdock (capsules, 350mg root powder) Take 1 capsule with a large glass of water, three times a day, before meals. The dose can be increased to 5 capsules per day.

For dilated vessels on the face
Great burdock (capsules, 350mg root powder) Take 1 capsule with a large glass of water, three times a day before meals. The intake can be increased to 5 capsules a day.
Heartsease (tincture, 1:4 in 25% alcohol) Take 20 drops in water, three times a day, after meals.

To improve blood circulation
Blackcurrant Put 5g of dried leaves into 1 litre of boiling water. Leave to infuse for 5 minutes. Drink 2-3 cups a day.
Grape seed extract (capsules, 30-100mg) Take 1 capsule a day.

To detox the liver
Dandelion (capsules, 300mg powder) Take 1 capsule with water, three times a day.
Globe artichoke (capsules, 300mg extract) Take 1 capsule a day.

External application
Aloe vera Apply an aloe vera-based cream or gel twice a day as directed on the label.
Lavender Dilute 3 drops of essential oil with 10ml carrier oil and use to cover the face. Apply three times a week, in the early evening.

Hemp agrimony Put 3g of the dried herb into 100ml of boiling water and infuse for 10 minutes before straining. Use to wash the face three times a week.
Marigold Put 5g of dried flower-heads into 1 litre of boiling water. Leave to infuse for 5 minutes. Soak a cloth in this infusion and apply three to four times a day.
Roman chamomile Dilute 3 drops of essential oil in 10ml carrier oil and apply to the affected area. Apply three times a week, in the early evening.
Witch hazel Massage in a witch hazel-based ointment once or twice a day.

Other measures
- Adopt a diet that is low in animal fats, chocolate and refined sugar.
- Avoid all stimulants (coffee or tea) and spicy food.
- Reduce alcohol consumption.
- Take a course of vitamins A, B, C and E.
- Avoid scented or oily soaps. Use soap-free dermatological cleansers to wash the face, and skin-care products that are suited to your skin type.
- Avoid exposure to bright sunlight and strong winds.

Bedsores

Also known as pressure sores, bedsores are the destruction of the skin and underlying tissues due to a lack of oxygenation allied to poor circulation. They can form very rapidly.

Symptoms
- **First sign**: the skin is discoloured, light or dark red and painful
- The skin then turns black, hardens and becomes dead to the touch
- The dead skin sloughs off, leaving an open sore revealing the underlying tissue

Causes
In general, bedsores are caused by oxygen not getting to the skin, and generally affect those who are bedridden or have reduced mobility and are unable to change position (due to a limb in plaster, for instance). The elderly or diabetics are most at risk, as well as those suffering from circulatory problems in the legs.

Consult your doctor
- Medical or nursing advice is essential in the case of all sores of unknown origin or those showing secondary infection.

WHICH PLANTS?
WARNING Use only one of the following at any given time

Internal usage
To improve the circulation
Ginkgo (tincture, 1:4 in 25% alcohol) Take 15 drops in water, three times a day before meals.
Grape seed extract (capsules, 30-100mg) Take 1 capsule a day.

For healthy skin
Evening primrose oil (capsules, 500mg) Take 2 capsules with a glass of water, three times a day, with meals.

To prevent infection
Echinacea (tincture, 1:5 in 45% ethanol) Take 15 drops in water, three times a day.
Garlic (capsules, 300mg powder) Take 1-3 capsules a day.

External application
Cinchona Put 30g of chopped bark into 1 litre of water. Boil for 5 minutes. Use to wash the bedsore once or twice a day.
Lavender Dilute 3 drops of essential oil with 10ml carrier oil and apply to the affected area once a day, three to four times a week.
Marigold Put 5g of dried flowerheads in 1 litre of boiling water. Infuse for 5 minutes, then strain. Soak a cloth in this infusion and apply three or four times a day.

Other measures
- Change garments and bed linen immediately if damp.
- Help the patient to change position as often as possible – at least every 2 hours.
- Give local massage alternating with hot and cold applications: for instance, apply ice cubes then dry the damp area with a hair dryer, set to warm.

Bruises

A blow to the body with a hard object, or a fall, will result in bruising or contusion. Bruises can range from a small, bluish mark, in the case of minor bruises, to large, black swellings in more severe cases.

Symptoms
- A bump or swelling
- Redness, or a bluish colour, with a burning pain
- Accumulation of blood in pockets beneath the skin

Consult your doctor
- It is recommended that you consult a doctor if you are worried about any bruising or feel that it may be accompanied by a fracture or sprain.
- A doctor should also intervene if the swelling does not go down or if bruising is extensive.

Causes
The underlying tissues or deeper layers of skin, at the site of a bruise become swollen and taut because of the accumulation of blood that has leaked from damaged blood vessels.

WHICH PLANTS?
WARNING Use only one of the following at any given time

Internal usage
Pineapple (capsules, 500mg powder) Take 2 capsules twice a day with a large glass of water.

To aid blood circulation
Ginkgo (tincture, 1:4 in 25% alcohol) Take 15 drops in water, three times a day before meals.
Grape seed extract (30-100mg capsules) Take 1 capsule a day.
Olive (tablet, 500mg leaf powder) Take 1 tablet a day with food.

Antioxidants to protect against free-radical damage
Grape seed extract (capsules, 30-100mg) Take 1 capsule a day.
Green tea (capsules, 375mg green tea extract) Take 2 capsules in the morning and 2 at midday.
Horse chestnut (tablets, 300mg powder) Take 1 tablet a day.
Milk thistle (tablets, 200mg) Take 1-2 tablets a day as a supplement.
Purslane (capsules, 200mg powder) Take 2-3 capsules a day with a large glass of water.
Sea buckthorn Drink 1-3 dessertspoons of pure juice or syrup a day in a glass of water.

Bruises contd

External application

Arnica Gently massage in an arnica-based cream or gel until it has penetrated completely. If necessary, repeat two to three times a day.

Common thyme Add 2g of dried plant to a cup of boiling water. Leave to infuse for 5 minutes, then strain. Soak a cloth in the infusion and apply for 15 minutes. Repeat three times a day.

Dill Put 50-100g of dried dill into 1 litre of boiling water. Leave to infuse for 10 minutes. Apply as a poultice for 15 minutes once a day.

Hyssop Add 3 drops of essential oil to 10ml carrier oil and apply to the bruise twice a day.

Lavender Apply 1 drop of the essential oil, once a day.

Marigold Put 5g of dried flowerheads into 1 litre of boiling water. Infuse for 5 minutes, then strain. Soak a cloth in this infusion and apply three to four times a day.

Sweet clover Simmer 20g of dried flowers in 100ml of water for 15 minutes. Soak a cloth in the warm liquid and apply two to three times a day as a compress.

White deadnettle Put 2 teaspoons of dried flowers into 100ml of boiling water. Leave to infuse for 10 minutes, then strain. Soak a cloth with this infusion and apply two to three times a day.

Other measures

- Place an ice pack on the affected area.
- Take a bath of salt water.

Burns, erythema

Burns are lesions on the skin or the mucous membrane, due to intense heat (or also intense localised cold). They are classified according to their severity. Erythema is the term used for superficial redness of an area of skin.

Symptoms

First degree burn

- Superficial lesions on the outer layer of the skin; localised redness (erythema).

Second degree burn

- More serious damage to the outer layer of skin and tissue below, in the form of blisters; intense pain.

Third degree burn

- Very severe damage, a brown or even burnt look to skin, irreversible lesions and the destruction of nerve endings; the disappearance of pain. State of shock (fainting, pale skin, sweating). This stage always requires urgent medical attention and hospitalisation.

Consult your doctor

- All severe and extensive burns, particularly if they are not painful (indicating third degree burns), require immediate medical attention.

Causes

A burn is caused by exposure to extreme heat or cold. Erythema can have several different causes: irritation, friction, sunburn, infection, viral disease.

WHICH PLANTS?

WARNING Use only one of the following at any given time

Before attempting any treatment to help a wound to heal over, make sure that it is clean and that there is no deep-seated inflammation or infection.

Internal usage

Echinacea (tincture, 1:5 in 45% alcohol) Take 15 drops in water, three times a day.

Gotu kola (capsules, 300mg powder) Take 1-2 capsules with food, up to three times a day.

External application

Aloe vera Apply an aloe vera-based cream or gel two or three times a day.

Eucalyptus Add 3 drops of pure essential oil to 10ml carrier oil and apply to the burn twice a day.

Lavender Apply 1 drop of pure essential oil twice a day.

Marigold Put 5g of dried flowerheads into 1 litre of boiling water. Infuse for 5 minutes, then strain. Soak a cloth in this infusion and apply three or four times a day.

St John's wort Put 1 teaspoon of the dried herb into a cup of boiling water. Infuse for 5 minutes, then strain. Soak a cloth in this infusion and apply twice a day.

Other measures

- Except for severe burns, try to cool the skin and underlying tissue by running cold water over it for some minutes – this may help to limit the damage.

Cellulite

Cellulite is the term given to the dimpled and lumpy appearance of the skin. It affects 90 per cent of women after puberty, afflicting both plump and slim women regardless. It usually appears on the skin of the arms, the thighs, the buttocks and the abdomen.

Symptoms

- 'Orange peel' appearance to the skin, with small dimples
- An increase in fatty mass around the hips and the thighs, down to the knees. It may also affect the upper arms

- If cellulite extends as far as the knees, poor circulation may be the cause

Consult your doctor

- The problem of cellulite is purely cosmetic, but you may wish to consult a your GP or a cosmetic surgeon about treatment.

Causes

The tendency towards cellulite may be hereditary; it is caused by the storage of fat under the skin, complicated by water retention and ageing connective tissue, and can also be provoked by weight gain. Hormonal imbalance may be a factor, particularly at puberty and during the menopause.

WHICH PLANTS?

WARNING Use only one of the following at any given time

Internal usage

For water retention
Dandelion (capsules, 300mg powder) Take 1 capsule with water, three times a day.
Globe artichoke (capsules, 300mg dried leaf extract) Take 1 capsule a day.
Horsetail Put 2-4g of dried stem into 200ml boiling water. Leave to infuse for 10-15 minutes, then strain. Drink 1 cup a day, for no longer than six weeks at a time.

DID YOU KNOW?
Cellulite

Caffeine appears to combat cellulite. A 5 per cent caffeine gel, applied directly to the skin, enhances the beneficial effects of plants such as ivy and horsetail. The gel can stimulate lipolysis – meaning that it helps to eliminate fatty deposits – thus reducing the lumpy appearance of cellulite.

Java tea Put 5g into 1 litre of boiling water. Leave to infuse for 5 minutes. Drink 1-3 cups a day, the last one several hours before going to bed.
Mouse-ear hawkweed Put 5-10g of the dried herb into 1 litre of boiling water. Leave to infuse for 10 minutes. Strain. Drink 1 cup in the morning and 1 at midday.
Stinging nettle (tincture, 1:4 in 25% alcohol) Take 20 drops in water, three times a day, after meals.
Green tea (capsules, 375mg extract) Take 2 capsules in the morning and 2 at lunchtime.

For obesity
Maté Put 2-3g of dried leaves into 1 cup of boiling water. Infuse for 5 minutes and then strain. Drink 1-3 cups a day, preferably before 5pm to avoid difficulty sleeping.
Pineapple (capsules, 500mg powder) Take 2 capsules twice a day, with a large glass of water.

To improve the circulation
Blackcurrant Put 5g of dried leaves into 1 litre of boiling water. Infuse for 5 minutes, then strain. Drink 2-3 cups a day.
Gotu kola (capsules, 300mg powder) Take 1-2 capsules with food, up to three times a day.
Grape seed extract (capsules, 30-100mg) Take 1 capsule a day.
Horse chestnut (tablets, 300mg powder) Take 1 tablet a day.

External application
For obesity and cellulite
Ivy Apply an ivy-based cream or gel, two to three times a day as directed on the label.

Other measures

- Discuss your hormonal balance with your herbalist.
- If you need to lose weight, follow a slimming regime.
- Take regular exercise.

Eczema

A common skin allergy, eczema can occur almost anywhere on the body. There are many variants, and the irritation is often spread by blisters. Eczema generally goes through several stages.

Symptoms

- Redness, inflammation and swelling
- The appearance of very small blisters, at first oozing then dry and cracked
- Itching, which can lead to compulsive scratching, spreading any infection and worsening the condition
- Coarsening or scaling of the skin

Causes

Eczema is often caused by the skin reacting to contact with irritating substances or to certain foodstuffs, as well as overeating, intoxication and extremes of temperature. Some types of eczema run in families, or are triggered by stress or an immune response.

Consult your doctor or medical herbalist

- If the cause of the eczema is not obvious, consult a doctor to get a correct diagnosis and to adapt the treatment.
- Treatment of eczema should not be confined to local therapy, but should address the causes.
- Long-term treatment is often essential in order to avoid relapses, and to prevent the condition becoming chronic.

WHICH PLANTS?

WARNING Use only one of the following at any given time

Internal usage

Great burdock (capsules, 350mg root powder) Take 1 capsule with a large glass of water, three times a day, before meals. The dose can be increased to 5 capsules a day.

Eczema contd

Heartsease (tincture, 1:4 in 25% alcohol) Take 20 drops in water, three times a day, after meals.

For diet-related eczema
Sweet violet (tincture, 1:4 in 25% alcohol) Take 20 drops with a small amount of water, three times a day, after meals.

For stress-induced eczema
Ashwagandha (tincture, 1:3 in 45% alcohol) Take 20 drops in a glass of water, three times a day.
Passionflower (tincture, 1:8 in 25% alcohol) Take 25 drops with a little cold water, three times a day, after meals.
Valerian (capsules, 240mg powder) Take 1-2 capsules daily.

External application
To treat inflammation
Aloe vera Apply an aloe vera-based cream or gel two to three times a day, as directed.
Greater plantain Apply a cream based on greater plantain two to three times a day, as directed.
Marigold Put 5g of dried flower-heads into 1 litre of boiling water. Infuse for 5 minutes, then strain. Soak a cloth in this infusion and apply three to four times a day. Alternatively, apply a marigold-based cream two to three times a day, as directed on the label.
Roman chamomile Apply flower water two to three times a day, as directed on the label.
Sweet violet Add 2-4g of dried flowers to a cup of boiling water. Infuse for 10 minutes, then strain. Soak a cloth in this infusion and apply for 15-20 minutes two or three times a day.
Witch hazel Apply a witch hazel-based ointment or gel, once or twice a day, as directed.

To prevent secondary infection
Marshmallow Put 2-3g of the dried root into 1 cup of boiling water. Leave to Infuse for 10 minutes, then strain. Soak a cloth in this infusion and apply three to four times a day.

For pain relief
Turmeric (tincture, 1:5 in 70% alcohol) Put 20 drops into a glass of water, soak a small cloth in this and apply for 15-20 minutes two or three times a day.

Other measures
- Replace soaps that are harsh, acidic or detergent-based with some that are oil or cream-based.
- Take vitamins (especially vitamin A) to improve skin health and to reduce itching, as well as trace elements such as zinc and sulphur to help prevent scarring.

Itching

Itching is the most common symptom of urticaria, an inflammatory reaction of the skin that is characterised by an eruption resembling the effect of contact with stinging nettles. It can be accompanied by redness and swelling.

Symptoms
- Desire to scratch
- Redness of the skin
- Small spots or blisters

Consult your doctor
- If your face is swollen or you have difficulty in breathing, consult a doctor urgently.

Causes
The body reacts to substances it is allergic to by producing antibodies that release histamine in the skin, which in turn cause redness and itching. The allergenic substance can be external, such as soap or a dye, or internal: certain foods such as strawberries, milk, soya or kiwi fruit. Drugs, notably antibiotics, can cause an allergic reaction.

Stress, dietary excess, ageing or hereditary factors all increase the risk of an allergic reaction.

More rarely, itching is caused by diseases such as scabies or chicken-pox, by systemic disease (such as kidney or liver disease), or is a side effect of chemotherapy.

WHICH PLANTS?
WARNING Use only one of the following at any given time

Internal usage
To soothe itchiness and inflammation
Blackcurrant Put 5g of dried leaves into 1 litre of boiling water. Leave to infuse for 5 minutes, then strain. Drink 2-3 cups a day.
Great burdock (capsules, 350mg root powder) Take 1 capsule with a large glass of water, three times a day, before meals. The dose can be increased to 5 capsules a day.
Greater plantain (capsules, 280mg) Take 1 capsule, three times a day, before meals.
Heartsease (tincture, 1:4 in 25% alcohol) Take 20 drops in water, three times a day, after meals.
Liquorice Add 1-2 teaspoons of root powder to a cup of boiling water. Infuse for 10 minutes, then strain. Drink 2 cups a day. Do not use for longer than four to six weeks at a time and accompany it with a low salt diet.

External application
Aaron's rod Soak 3 teaspoons of the dried plant in 300ml of cold water for 30 minutes. Gently bring to the boil. Strain. Soak a cloth in the liquid and apply twice a day.
Fumitory Put 2 teaspoons of the dried flowers into 150ml of boiling water. Leave to infuse for 10 minutes and then strain. Soak a cloth with the infusion and apply it two or three times a day.
German chamomile Add a sachet to 1 cup of boiling water. Leave to

infuse for 10 minutes. Soak a cloth in this infusion and apply to the affected area for 15 minutes. Repeat two or three times a day.
Lavender Apply a lavender-based cream, ointment or lotion, as directed on the label.
Marigold Put 5g of dried flower-heads into 1 litre of boiling water. Infuse for 5 minutes, then strain. Soak a cloth in this infusion and apply three to four times a day.

Other measures
- Avoid foods that you suspect may give you an allergic reaction.
- Discuss with your GP the possibility of blood and skin tests to identify the substances that are causing the allergies, or a condition that might be causing the itching.
- Do not scratch. This merely worsens the condition and develops into a vicious cycle. Cutting the nails will help to stop them damaging the skin.
- Try to identify any particular clothes or washing materials that aggravate it. Start with wool, soap and biological washing powders. Try using no soap or shampoo at all to wash with – just warm water. This will leave the natural oils undisturbed on the skin.

Perspiration and body odour

Some people have a skin that perspires excessively without the slightest physical exertion. The condition, known as hyperhydrosis, can affect localised areas or the entire body. The skin can also release an unpleasant odour, whether or not it is sweating, in spite of perfectly adequate personal hygiene.

Symptoms
- Excessive perspiration, independent of physical effort
- Sticky perspiration, difficult to eliminate from the armpits
- Unpleasant skin odour

Consult your doctor
- This type of skin disorder can be symptomatic of an internal condition that needs to be diagnosed. Only a doctor can determine whether it is a common disorder or something more serious.

Causes
Certain body odours are defined as idiopathic, which means that their cause is unknown. In some cases, the condition is genetic and several members of the same family are affected. Body odour and excessive perspiration problems also frequently affect people who are obese, anxious, extremely tired or who suffer from digestive, renal and metabolic disorders.

WHICH PLANTS?
WARNING Use only one of the following at any given time

Internal usage
For stress and anxiety
Ashwagandha (tincture, 1:3 in 45% alcohol) Take 20 drops in a glass of water, three times a day.
Lavender Put 2-3g of the flowers into a cup of boiling water. Infuse for 5-10 minutes, then strain. Drink 3-4 cups a day between meals.
Lime tree Put 5g of dried flowers into 1 litre of boiling water. Infuse for 5 minutes, then strain. Drink 1 cup in the evening to help you to fall asleep.

For digestive problems
German chamomile Add 5-8g of dried flowers to a cup of boiling water. Infuse for 10 minutes, then strain. Drink 3 cups a day, before meals.

Passionflower (tincture, 1:8 in 25% alcohol) Take 25 drops with a little cold water three times a day, after meals.
Peppermint Put 1 tablespoon of dried leaves into 150ml of boiling water. Infuse for 10-15 minutes, Strain. Drink 1 cup after meals.

To reduce excessive sweating
Jujube Boil 30-50g of ground fruit in 1 litre of water for 30 minutes, then strain. Drink 3 cups a day.

To detoxify
Dandelion (capsules, 300mg powder) Take 1 capsule with water, three times a day.
Globe artichoke (capsules, 300mg dried leaf extract) Take 1 capsule a day.

External application
Coriander Put 10-30g of crushed seeds in 1 litre of water. Infuse for 10 minutes, then strain. Apply to the affected area twice a day, with a spray.
Heartsease Add 20-30g fresh flowers to 500ml boiling water. Infuse for 15 minutes, then strain. Soak a cloth in this infusion and apply to the affected areas morning and evening.
Marigold Put 5g of dried flower-heads into 1 litre of boiling water. Infuse for 5 minutes, then strain. Soak a cloth in this infusion and apply three or four times a day.
Sandalwood Mix 3 drops of the essential oil with 10ml carrier oil and rub into the affected areas. Leave for 15 minutes before washing off.

Other measures
- Use talc or calendula powder, after taking a shower and drying your skin carefully.
- Try to limit stress; consider relaxation therapy.

Psoriasis

Psoriasis is an extremely common chronic skin disorder associated with severe itching and the presence of well-defined, reddish plaques covered with scales that turn white and flake off, especially when scratched. The condition is often hereditary and tends to affect adolescents and young adults. It usually develops in clearly defined areas of the body such as the elbows, knees and scalp, but it may cover the entire body.

Symptoms

- Reddish plaques covered with whitish scales. They usually occur in the bend of the elbow, at the back of the knee or on the scalp
- Itching, often unbearable
- Scratching and flaking of scales leaves skin red, sometimes causing bleeding
- Erupts and subsides for no apparent reason
- Sometimes plaques occur under the nails, causing them to lift off and become deformed

Consult your doctor

- Psoriasis should be medically diagnosed as, in the initial stages, it can resemble eczema or mycosis (a fungal skin disorder) which are not treated in the same way.

Causes

In 25 per cent of cases, psoriasis is hereditary and several members of the same family are affected. Large numbers of sufferers have been found to have difficulty in the assimilation of fats, or suffer from diabetes.

The condition occurs when the skin cells multiply several times more than normal, causing the thickened plaques and scaling. It is also thought that the disorder can be of nervous origin since its appearance is often triggered by some form of strong emotion.

Alcohol and some medications (especially certain anti-inflammatories and beta blockers) may be culprits too. A particular type of spotty psoriasis (guttate psoriasis) may be triggered by a bacterial infection, especially in the throat. Plaques are more likely to develop over the sites of previous injuries to the skin.

WHICH PLANTS?

WARNING Use only one of the following at any given time

Internal usage

For healthy skin
Evening primrose (soft capsules, 500g oil) Take 3 capsules a day.

For stress and anxiety
Ashwagandha (tincture, 1:3 in 45% alcohol) Take 20 drops in a glass of water, three times a day.
Lavender Put 2-3g of dried flowers into a cup of boiling water. Infuse for 5-10 minutes, then strain. Drink 3-4 cups a day between meals.
Lime tree Put 5g of dried flowers into 1 litre of boiling water. Infuse for 5 minutes, then strain. Drink 1 cup in the evening to help you to fall asleep.

To aid digestion
German chamomile Add 5-8g of dried flowers to 1 cup of boiling water. Infuse for 10 minutes, then strain. Drink 3 cups a day before meals.
Passionflower (tincture, 1:8 in 25% alcohol) Take 25 drops with a little cold water after meals, three times a day.
Peppermint Put 1 tablespoon of dried leaves into 150ml of boiling water. Infuse for 10-15 minutes, then strain. Drink 1 cup three times a day after meals.
Turmeric (tincture, 1:5 in 70% alcohol) Take 20 drops in a glass of water, three times a day, after meals.

To treat infections
Barberry (tincture, 1:3 in 25% alcohol) Take 10 drops in cold water, three times a day, before meals. Do not take for longer than four weeks at a time. Consult a medical herbalist before using.
Golden seal (capsules, 540mg powder) Take 1 capsule, three times a day.

For inflammation
Blackcurrant Put 5g of dried leaves into 1 litre of boiling water. Infuse for 5 minutes, then strain. Drink 2-3 cups a day.
Liquorice Add 1-2 teaspoons of root powder to 1 cup of boiling water. Infuse for 10 minutes, then strain. Drink 2 cups a day. Do not take for longer than four to six weeks at a time and accompany with a low salt diet.
Stinging nettle (tincture, 1:4 in 25% alcohol) Take 20 drops in water, three times a day, after meals.

To detox
Dandelion (capsules, 300mg powder) Take 1 capsule with water, three times a day.
Globe artichoke (capsules, 300mg dried leaf extract) Take 1 capsule a day.

For a healthy liver
Milk thistle (tablets, 200mg) Take 1-2 tablets a day, as a supplement.

External application

For pain and inflammation
Aloe vera Apply a cream or gel to the area two to three times a day, as directed on the label.
Fumitory Put 2 teaspoons of dried flowers into 150ml of boiling water. Infuse for 10 minutes, then strain. Soak a cloth in the infusion and apply it to the affected areas two to three times a day.
Greater celandine Apply fresh sap to affected areas between one to three times a day as directed on the label.

Lavender Add 20-100g of dried flowers to 1 litre of boiling water. Infuse for 15 minutes, then strain. Add the infusion to the bath water and bathe in it for 15 minutes.

Red clover Infuse 2 teaspoons of dried flowers in a cup of boiling water for 10 minutes before straining. Soak a clean cloth in this infusion and apply to affected area for 15 minutes. Repeat two to three times a day.

Roman chamomile Apply flower water two to three times a day, as directed on the label.

Silver birch Put 50g of dried leaves into 1 litre of boiling water. Infuse for 15 minutes, then strain. Wash affected areas with this infusion two to three times a day.

Other measures

- Add a blend of essential oils to your bath: 5 drops of niaouli, 3 drops of chamomile, 2 drops of common thyme, diluted in a quarter of a glass of alcohol (such as vodka or gin).
- Sunbathing can help, but consult your doctor first about the risk of skin cancer.
- PUVA treatment (ultraviolet radiation treatment) may also be beneficial.

Skin conditions

The skin is a major organ in the body, helping to regulate the body's water content. Dry skin is, at best, uncomfortable and, at worst, can lead to flaking and discomfort. It can be exacerbated by climatic conditions or contact with irritants such as detergents or the salt in sea water. Greasy skin may lead to acne and other skin problems.

Symptoms
Dry skin
- A dull, fine-grained appearance
- Extremely fragile, itchy and flaky

- Feelings of tautness
- Rough to the touch

Greasy skin
- Shiny, moist appearance
- Coarseness, with subcutaneous fat
- Blocked or open pores, with blackheads

Consult your doctor
- The more serious skin condition, eczema, can present itself as dry skin, and seborrhoeic dermatitis as greasy skin, so ask your doctor for advice.

Causes
Dry skin is usually caused by the inefficiency of the oil-producing glands in the skin: if they fail to produce enough sebum, the skin is unprotected from outside irritants. Greasy skin is caused by over-production of sebum, and may be due to extreme nervousness, obesity, an over-rich diet or oral contraceptives.

WHICH PLANTS?
WARNING Use only one of the following at any given time

Internal usage
Dry skin
Evening primrose (soft capsules, 500mg oil) Take 1-2 capsules a day, with a glass of water at mealtimes.

Gotu kola (capsules, 300mg powder) Take 2 capsules with food, twice a day.

Grape seed extract (capsules, 30-100mg) Take 1 capsule a day.

Maize Put 1 teaspoon of stamens into 1 cup of water. Bring rapidly to the boil and leave to infuse for 10 minutes, then strain. Drink 3 cups a day.

Greasy skin
Great burdock (capsules, 350mg root powder) Take 1 capsule with a large glass of water, three times a day, before meals. The dose can be increased to 5 capsules a day.

To aid digestion
German chamomile Add 5-8g of dried flowers to 1 cup of boiling water. Leave to infuse for 10 minutes, then strain. Drink 3 cups a day, before meals.

Peppermint Add 1 tablespoon of dried leaves to 150ml of boiling water. Leave to infuse for 10-15 minutes, then strain. Drink 1 cup after meals.

External application
Dry skin
German chamomile Add 3 drops of essential oil to 10ml carrier oil. Apply to the affected area two to three times a day.

Mallow Put 30g of dried flowers or leaves into 1 litre of boiling water. Infuse for 10 minutes, then strain. Apply to the affected area three to four times a day.

Marigold Put 5g of dried flower-heads into 1 litre of boiling water. Infuse for 5 minutes, then strain. Soak a cloth in this infusion and apply three to four times a day. Alternatively, apply a marigold ointment or cream, as directed on the label.

Oats Boil 20g of dried plant in 1 litre of water for 3 minutes, then leave to soak for 10-20 minutes. Strain, add to bath water and bathe for 15-20 minutes.

Greasy skin
Lavender Put 2-3g of dried flowers into a cup of boiling water. Infuse for 10 minutes, then strain. Use to wash the skin two to three times a day.

Stinging nettle Boil 20g of the dried plant in 750ml water until it reduces to about 500ml. Use cotton wool to wipe the face with this liquid. Leave on for 15 minutes, then rinse off. Repeat two to three times a week.

Witch hazel Apply witch hazel water once or twice a day, as directed on the label.

Skin problems

Skin conditions contd

Other measures
- Protect your skin from natural damage: cold, heat (including saunas), sun, sea water and atmospheric pollution.
- Keep your skin moist with a pure-water spray.
- Take low doses of zinc, vitamin A and also vitamin E (100mg).

Skin infections

Some skin infections are viral in origin (herpes, warts, molluscum contagiosum, chickenpox and shingles), some are bacterial (boils, cellulitis, erysipelas and impetigo) and others are fungal (athlete's foot and ringworm). They can have serious complications: in the case of impetigo, they can lead to kidney disease or to a general organic infection (septicaemia). In boils, the spread of infection can lead to a type of carbuncle.

Symptoms
Impetigo
- Reddened skin
- Fluid-filled blisters, which burst leaving yellowish scabs
- Fever and swellings (lymph nodes) in serious cases

Boils and carbuncles
- Rounded nodules appear
- Inflammation (redness, heat and swelling) with pain on contact
- Swelling of the nodules, which fill with pus
- A white spot appears in the centre (the head of the boil)

Consult your doctor
- In case of complications such as swollen lymph nodes, fever or general poor health, it is important to consult your doctor.

Causes
Impetigo is a bacterial infection. It is a common and very contagious ailment that frequently attacks children. Boils develop when hair follicles become infected. The infection spreads to surrounding tissues which fill up with puss. Diabetes can also cause boils.

Skin infections are spread by scratching the infected areas and by poor personal hygiene. Those susceptible are primarily infants in crèches and schools, and those already suffering from dermatitis, whose immunity is low.

WHICH PLANTS?
WARNING Use only one of the following at any given time

Internal usage
For infection
Echinacea (tincture, 1:5 in 45% alcohol) Take 15 drops in water, three times a day.
Garlic (capsules, 300mg powder) Take 1-3 capsules a day.
Siberian ginseng (tincture, 1:3 in 25% alcohol) Take 10-20 drops in a little cold water, three times a day, after meals. Do not take for more than a month at a time.

To detoxify the liver and kidneys
Dandelion (capsules, 300mg powder) Take 1 capsule with water, three times a day.
Globe artichoke (capsules, 300mg leaf extract) Take 1 capsule a day.
Great burdock (capsules, 350mg, root powder) Take 1 capsule with a large glass of water, three times a day, before meals. The dose can be increased to 5 capsules a day.

External application
Common thyme Add 2g of dried plant to a cup of boiling water. Infuse for 15 minutes, then strain. Soak a cloth in this infusion and apply to the affected area for 15 minutes, three to four times a day.
Juniper Add 2g of crushed berries to 200ml boiling water and infuse for 10 minutes, then strain. Add 100-200ml to your bath water and bathe in it for 15-20 minutes. Alternatively, add 3 drops of essential oil to 10ml vegetable oil. Rub in two or three times a day.
Lavender Dilute 3 drops of the essential oil in 10ml carrier oil and cover the affected area. Repeat two or three times a day.
Winter savory Put 20g of dried flowering tops into 1 litre of boiling water. Infuse for 10 minutes, then strain. Soak a cloth in this infusion and apply to the affected areas two to three times a day.

Other measures
- Avoid spreading the infection by scratching affected areas.
- Never squeeze a boil to remove the pus; it should be left to clear up, untouched.
- Avoid sausages and fatty meats (to spare the liver, intestines and kidneys from overload), as well as desserts.

Stretch marks

When there is a significant increase in weight, often as a result of pregnancy, the skin is distended and tissues may rupture. This may occur on the breasts, stomach and buttocks and take the form of fine stretch marks of unequal lengths, of up to 20cm.

Symptoms
- Pink or purplish red raised lines that after a few months usually become pale and flatten

Consult your doctor or medical herbalist
- Herbal treatments are only complementary and should not replace regular medical supervision, especially in cases of extreme weight variation.

Causes

Stretch marks are usually caused by thinning and lack of elasticity in the skin, at a time of weight increase. They can sometimes be linked to an endocrine disorder such as hyperthyroidism. Body-builders may also develop them, because of the extra muscle bulk, the stretching of the skin during exercising or even the alteration of adrenal or testicular hormones.

WHICH PLANTS?

WARNING Use only one of the following at any given time

It is difficult to treat stretch marks. However, medicinal plants can help by stimulating the rebuilding of the elasticity of the skin, and by improving both the quality of the collagen in the connective tissue, and blood circulation.

Internal usage

For healthy skin
Evening primrose oil (capsules, 500mg) Take 2 capsules, three times a day, during the last ten days of the menstrual cycle.
To improve blood circulation
Ginkgo (tincture, 1:4 in 25% alcohol) Take 15 drops in water, three times a day, before meals.
Golden seal (capsules, 540mg powder) Take 1 capsule, three times a day.
Grape seed extract (capsules, 30-100mg) Take 1 capsule a day.

External application

Bladderwrack Massage in a cream, oil, lotion or ointment based on bladderwrack, as directed on the label.
Gotu kola Massage in cream, ointment or lotion based on gotu kola, once or twice a day, as directed on the label.
Lady's mantle Boil 40g of dried leaves in 1 litre of water. Leave to infuse for 10 minutes. Soak a cloth in the liquid and apply three times a day.

Maize Massage in maize oil as directed on the label.

Other measures

- Immerse the lower part of your body in cold and then hot baths.
- Have massages.
- Take small doses of vitamin A or, after consulting your doctor or pharmacist, vitamins D and E.
- Take trace elements: special preparations of zinc, iron and silicon.

Sunburn

Depending on its severity, sunburn can cause anything from an acute inflammation of the skin to severe blistering.

Symptoms

- Redness of the skin with a sharp burning sensation
- Blisters, then peeling of the skin
- In severe cases, fever, nausea and headaches

Consult your doctor or medical herbalist

- If you have several or all of the above symptoms, you should consult a doctor: all serious sunburn needs rapid medical attention.

Causes

Exposing fair or delicate skin to the sun and to reflection of the sun's rays from snow or the sea, without protection, are the principal causes of sunburn.

Certain drugs can also make you more susceptible to sunburn (some antibiotics and acne treatments in particular) as can creams that are said to be photosensitive. PUVA therapy (the technique of using the sun's rays to treat certain skin complaints, such as psoriasis) can also have the same effect.

WHICH PLANTS?

WARNING Use only one of the following at any given time

Internal usage

Gotu kola (capsules, 300mg powder) Take 1-2 capsules with food, up to three times a day.
Grape seed extract (capsules, 30-100mg) Take 1 capsule a day.
Pineapple (capsules, 500mg powder) Take 2 capsules in the morning and 2 in the evening with a large glass of water.

External application

Aloe vera Apply gel two to three times a day, as directed on the label.
Lavender Dilute 3 drops of essential oil with 10ml carrier oil and apply to the affected area two to three times a day.
Marigold Put 5g of dried flowerheads into 1 litre of boiling water. Leave to infuse for 5 minutes. Soak a cloth in this infusion and apply three to four times a day.
Sea buckthorn Apply buckthorn oil, or a preparation with a base of buckthorn oil, once or twice a day, as directed on the label.
St John's wort Infuse 1 teaspoon of dried plant in a cup of boiling water for 5 minutes. Strain. Apply to the affected skin twice a day.
Witch hazel Apply witch hazel water to the affected skin once or twice a day as directed on the label.

Other measures

- Protect your skin before any exposure to the sun and do not tan to excess. Prolonged sunbathing can lead to skin cancer. Do not use a sun block simply to allow you longer in the sun – the risk is as great.
- Avoid the sun from noon to 3pm.
- In the case of delicate or fair skin it is imperative that you use a total sun block.

Warts

Warts are a common but unpleasant skin condition. They are small, benign skin tumours that appear in the form of growths of varying shape. They tend to develop slowly and haphazardly, can disappear for no apparent reason and may be slightly contagious.

Symptoms
- Discoloration of the skin, in raised patches
- Appearance of one or more small, rough growths
- In some cases, itching

Causes
Warts are caused by viruses, including the Papilloma virus, which provoke an abnormal growth of cells in a given place. The Papilloma virus can cause different types of wart: common warts (on the hands), plantar warts or verrucas (on the feet), plane warts and laryngeal warts. Genital warts (condyloma acuminata) are caused by a different type of virus, as is Molluscum contagiosum, a harmless but highly contagious infection, often found among children and characterised by shiny papules on the skin's surface.

Scratching, warm, damp feet and fungal skin infections encourage the development of warts as the virus enters the skin via small cuts or scratches. Fatigue and stress can increase susceptibility to warts.

WHICH PLANTS?
WARNING Use only one of the following at any given time

The following plants are particularly effective for common and plantar warts, occasionally for plane warts and Molluscum contagiosum, but not for genital warts.

Internal usage
For infection
Common elder (tincture, 1:4 in 25% alcohol) Take 20 drops in a glass of water, three times a day, after meals.
Echinacea (tincture, 1:5 in 45% alcohol) Take 15 drops three times a day.
Garlic (capsules, 300mg powder) Take 1-3 capsules a day.
Liquorice Add 1-2 teaspoons of root powder to a cup of boiling water, allow to infuse for 10 minutes before straining. Drink 2 cups a day. Do not use for longer than four to six weeks, and accompany with a low salt diet.
Siberian ginseng (tincture, 1:3 in 25% alcohol) Take 10-20 drops in a little cold water, three times a day, after meals. Do not take for more than a month at a time.
Stinging nettle (tincture, 1:4 in 25% alcohol) Take 20 drops in water three times a day after meals.

External application
For their antiviral properties
Aaron's rod Soak 3 teaspoons of the dried plant in 300ml of cold water for 30 minutes. Gently bring to the boil. Strain. Soak a cloth in the liquid and apply twice a day.
Greater celandine Apply juice to affected area one to three times a day, as directed on the label.
Cinnamon Add 3 drops of essential oil to 10ml of carrier oil and apply twice a day.
Lemon balm Add 20g of dried parts to 500ml of boiling water. Infuse for 10 minutes and apply twice daily to the lesions.
Marigold Put 5g of dried flowerheads into 1 litre of boiling water. Leave to infuse for 5 minutes. Soak a cloth in this infusion and apply three to four times a day.

Other measures
- Avoid walking barefoot in public places (especially swimming pools).
- Try not to touch the infected area(s) and avoid contact with anyone who has warts.

Whitlow

Often confused with the less painful paronychia, whitlows are pus-filled inflammations of the top of a finger or thumb. Paronychia is inflammation of the fold of skin at the side of a fingernail or toenail and is often a more chronic fungal infection, or occasionally acute.

Symptoms
Whitlow
- Tenderness and pain in a finger pad, which becomes tense but does not swell
- Pain reaches a peak after a day or two
- Fever, shivering; crying and sleeplessness in children

DID YOU KNOW?
Warts

Our ancestors were familiar with the properties of the greater celandine, a wild flower that is still common today. The latex it contains has traditionally been used to cure warts (though it must be applied carefully as it stains clothing).

Now modern phytochemical research has discovered that the constituents of the latex include certain antimitotic alkaloids, that is, alkaloids that prevent cell division. This may explain why it was such an effective cure for warts, which are benign tumours that cause rapid skin growth.

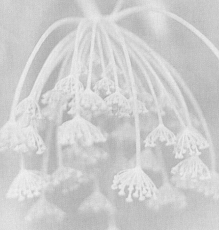

Paronychia

- Swelling and reddening of the finger, with sudden, shooting pains
- Pus develops and is visible under or alongside the nail

Consult your doctor

- It is crucial to seek medical advice if the fever has not subsided after 48 hours.
- Whitlows can have complications which, although rare, can be severe: osteomyelitis (the infection of the bone tissue of the finger or toe joints, especially in children and adolescents) or septicaemia (a general infection of the blood).

Causes

Whitlows are usually the result of a staphylococcal infection. The pain is caused by the accumulation of pus which cannot form a boil and come to a head, because the skin is too thick.

DID YOU KNOW?
Paronychia

Marseilles soap applied to an affected finger or toe and left overnight will draw the pus from paronychia. The soap, a natural product made from olive and other vegetable oils, is available from health shops.

Paronychia is caused when infection enters the skin beside a nail, through a small cut or wound; biting nails, and pulling 'hangnails' can be causes. The condition is painful, but subsides as soon as the pus is released.

WHICH PLANTS?
WARNING Use only one of the following at any given time

Internal usage
To treat inflammation and pain

Echinacea (tincture, 1:5 in 45% alcohol) Take 15 drops three times a day.
Feverfew (tincture, 2:5 in 25% alcohol) Take 20 drops in water twice a day after meals. The supervision of a professional herbalist or doctor is strongly recommended.
Ginger (tincture, 1:5 in 60% alcohol) Take up to 30 drops in a glass of water, every day.
Lavender Put 2-3g of dried flowers into a cup of boiling water. Leave to infuse for 5-10 minutes. Drink 3-4 cups a day, between meals.

External application
German chamomile Dilute 3 drops of essential oil with 10ml carrier oil and apply to the affected area. Repeat two to three times a day.
Lavender Dilute 3 drops of essential oil with 10ml carrier oil and apply to the affected area. Repeat two to three times a day.
Marigold Put 5g of dried flowerheads into 1 litre of boiling water. Leave to infuse for 5 minutes. Soak a cloth in this infusion and apply three to four times a day.

Other measures
- Disinfect all manicure instruments; do not pick at hangnails.
- Ensure that your tetanus injections are up to date: they should be boosted every ten years.

Wounds and grazes

Wounds are cuts, punctures or tears in the skin or other tissues. They vary in depth and are more or less clearly defined. Grazes are wounds that only affect the superficial skin tissues.

Symptoms
Wounds
- A cut or tear with either 'clean' or irregular edges
- Bleeding, often profuse

Grazes
- An abrasion or scratch on the outer layer of the epidermis
- Short-lived bleeding

Consult your doctor
- You can treat simple grazes yourself, provided they are not infected or inflamed.
- For wounds, see your doctor or go to the emergency department at the local hospital, especially if they contain foreign bodies such as pieces of glass or gravel, are infected or inflamed.
- A wound with irregular edges can not be stitched or drawn together and usually has to be dressed. Ensure that your tetanus injections are up to date and, if necessary, ask for an injection or booster.

Causes
Like bruises, wounds and grazes are localised damage caused by some form of violent contact with a sharp or heavy object. Cuts usually create wounds with clean edges, unlike contusions and tears, which can be external or internal.

WHICH PLANTS?
WARNING Use only one of the following at any given time

Only use medicinal plants if your injections are up to date and if the wound is not serious.

Wounds and grazes contd

Internal usage

To prevent infection

Echinacea (tincture, 1:5 in 45% alcohol) Take 15 drops three times a day.

Garlic (capsules, 300mg powder) Take 1-3 capsules a day.

External application

To disinfect the affected area

Echinacea (tincture, 1:5 in 45% alcohol) Add 2-5ml to a little cold water. Soak cotton wool in this and apply to the affected area.

To cover an infected wound

Lavender Pour 1-2 drops of essential oil onto the compress used to dress the wound.

For inflammation

Aloe vera Apply gel to affected areas two to three times a day.

Lavender Pour 1 drop of essential oil onto the affected area. Alternatively, add 20g dried flowers to 500ml boiling water and infuse for 15 minutes before straining. Soak a cloth in the infusion and apply to the affected area for 15 minutes. Repeat two or three times a day.

Marigold Put 5g of dried flower-heads into 1 litre of boiling water. Leave to infuse for 5 minutes. Soak a cloth in the infusion and apply three to four times a day.

To aid healing

Cinchona Put 30g of chopped bark into 1 litre of water. Boil for 5 minutes. Wash the affected areas once or twice a day.

Other measures

- Always clean grazes and wounds with a disinfectant.
- Use a sticking plaster to draw the edges of a wound together, put a light dressing on a graze to keep out infection.

Urinary tract & kidney problems
Cystitis, urethritis

Cystitis is an inflammation of the bladder, and urethritis is an inflammation of the urethra or passage through which the bladder is emptied. Attacks can be sudden and acute, or chronic and long term. Occurring only rarely among men, cystitis is very common among women.

Symptoms

- Burning pain when urinating, more intense in the case of urethritis
- Frequent urge to urinate, often without a real need to do so
- Urine is dark, and blood or pus may be present
- Often shivering and fever

Causes

Cystitis and urethritis are caused by a bacterial infection of the bladder, which can be linked to constipation, diarrhoea, or sexual relations. In women, poor personal hygiene can sometimes be a cause of cystitis.

Consult your doctor or medical herbalist

- Despite the fact that most women are able to identify cystitis themselves, a doctor's diagnosis should still be sought to ensure that there is no other disease present.
- A simple examination of the urine is usually sufficient. Cystitis may not appear to be a serious complaint, but without correct treatment even a benign inflammation is at risk of becoming more serious.

WHICH PLANTS?

WARNING Use only one of the following at any given time

Internal usage

Buchu (powder, 350mg capsules) take one with a large glass of water, twice a day, at meal times.

Cranberry (capsules, 400mg dry extract) Take 1 capsule twice a day with plenty of water. Or drink 500ml of fresh juice twice a day.

Dandelion (capsules, 300mg powder) Take 1 capsule with water, three times a day.

Garlic (capsules, 300mg powder) Take 1-3 a day.

Goldenrod Put 1.5-3g of the parts that grow above ground into a cup of boiling water. Leave to infuse for 10-15 minutes and strain. Drink 3-5 cups a day.

Java tea Put 5g into 1 litre of boiling water. Leave to infuse for 5 minutes. Drink 1-3 cups a day, the last one several hours before bed.

Maize (tincture, 1:5 in 25% alcohol) Take 5-15ml three times a day.

Silver birch (tincture, 1:4 in 25% alcohol) Take 15 drops in a glass of water, three times a day, after meals.

Uva ursi (tincture, 1:1 in 25% alcohol) Take 2-4ml three times a day.

DID YOU KNOW?
Urinary infection

Goldenrod, which was used in urology in ancient times, is enjoying a revival and appears to be particularly effective for treating urinary infections. It is an anti-inflammatory, a diuretic, a urinary antiseptic and it stimulates the immune system, as has been recently discovered. Its action is both local (on the urinary passages) and general, thanks to its effect on the pituitary gland, which influences the working of the adrenal glands. It can be employed to treat practically all urinary problems.

As directed by a medical herbalist

- Barberry (tincture)

Other measures

- Drink plenty of fluids: 1.5-2 litres a day (water, infusions, juice).
- Ensure you urinate regularly, at least four or five times a day, emptying the bladder completely, each time.
- If you are constipated, eat fresh fruit and green vegetables, take meals at regular times and drink plenty of fluids with them.
- Avoid wearing tight clothes.
- After urinating, or a bowel movement, wipe yourself from front to back and not vice versa.
- If bouts of cystitis occur after sexual activity, get into the habit of urinating after sex.
- Avoid substances that can be irritants, such as tea, coffee, spices and alcohol.
- Avoid vaginal deodorants, douches, or underwear made of artificial fibres.

Kidney failure

When functioning normally, the kidneys filter 125ml of blood a minute, excreting waste products in the form of urine. Kidney or renal failure leads to the accumu-lation of toxic elements in the blood, which, without medical treatment, can prove fatal. Renal failure may be acute or chronic.

Symptoms

- Swelling of the lower limbs together with retention of fluid in the abdomen and the lungs
- Normal or greatly reduced volume of urine, with blood
- High blood pressure
- Symptoms of advanced renal failure can include serious difficulty in breathing, tiredness, nausea, vomiting and skin irritation

Causes

Acute kidney failure can be the result of an injury or major illness. Renal tissue breaks down after an infection, inflammation or kidney disease. Chronic failure can be caused by high blood pressure, diabetes or the formation of renal cysts (polycystic kidneys). It can also follow the removal of a kidney or a narrowing of the renal artery.

Consult your doctor

- Kidney failure, with or without uraemia, must not be ignored. Your doctor should look for renal or external causes, for example, narrowing of the renal arteries or heart problems.

WHICH PLANTS?

WARNING Use only one of the following at any given time

To promote healthy kidneys
Globe artichoke (capsules, 300mg dried leaf extract) Take 1 capsule a day.

To treat inflammation
Mouse-ear hawkweed Put 5-10g of the dried plant into 1 litre of boiling water. Infuse for 10 minutes, then strain. Drink 1 cup in the morning and 1 at midday.

To increase urination
Dandelion (capsules, 300mg powder) Take 1 capsule with water, three times a day.
Java tea Put 5g into 1 litre of boiling water. Leave to infuse for 5 minutes. Drink 1-3 cups a day, the last several hours before bed.
Maize (tincture, 1:5 in 25% alcohol) Take 5-15ml three times a day.
Raspberry (tincture, 1:4 in 25% alcohol) Take 20 drops in water, three times a day, after meals.
Silver birch (tincture, 1:4 in 25% alcohol) Take 15 drops in a glass of water three times a day after meals.

To promote good circulation
Cinnamon Put 1g of Chinese cinnamon bark or 0.5-1g of Ceylon cinnamon bark into a cup of boiling water. Leave to infuse for 10 minutes. Drink 3 cups a day.
Ginkgo (tincture, 1:4 in 25% alcohol) Take 20 drops in water, three times a day, after meals.
Grape seed extract (capsules, 30-100mg) Take 1 capsule a day.

Other measures

- Restrict consumption of mineral waters with high sodium content, but especially most white wines. Drink plenty of fluids, preferable mineral waters with low sodium content.
- Do not cut out all salt from your diet, as this will only increase uraemia.
- Eat fruits, especially melon, watermelon and grapes.

DID YOU KNOW?
Kidney problems

Plant-power may help kidney problems. Researchers at the University of Metz, France have studied the effects of four plants used by medical herbalists to encourage the excretion of water and sodium chloride in urine. While common elder, Java tea, uva-ursi/bearberry and mouse-ear hawkweed all increase the volume of urine excreted, only an aqueous extract of common elder and a tincture of Java tea speed up the elimination of sodium.

Kidney stones

When urates, calcium or phosphates (substances present in urine) become concentrated in the kidneys, stones can form, which migrate towards the bladder or the ureter, producing severe pain.

Symptoms

- Sharp, recurring pain, in the kidney area, from the low back and side of the abdomen, into the pelvis
- Possibly, blood in the urine
- Fever, in cases of secondary infection

Causes

Kidney stones may be caused by metabolic disorders allied to a diet too rich in proteins and calcium. But an excess of calcium in the blood can be caused by osteoporosis, hyperthyroidism, excessive levels of vitamin D, or uric acid in those suffering from gout. Stones can also form following an infection or the slowdown of kidney function.

Consult your doctor or a medical herbalist

- If you suffer any of the symptoms above, it is important to consult a doctor, and possibly a urologist.
- A medical herbalist can also advise you on helpful plants.

WHICH PLANTS?

WARNING Use only one of the following at any given time

Internal usage

Alfalfa (tincture, 1:4 in 25% alcohol) Take 20 drops in a glass of water, three times a day, after meals.
Ash (capsules, 300mg powder) Take 2 capsules with a large glass of water, three times a day.
Bitter fennel Add ¼-½ teaspoon of crushed seeds to a cup of boiling water. Leave to infuse for 10 minutes. Strain. Drink 1 cup up to three times a day.
Dandelion (capsules, 300mg powder) Take 1 capsule with water, three times a day.
Goldenrod Put 1.5-3g of aerial parts into 1 cup of boiling water. Leave to infuse for 10-15 minutes and filter. Drink 3-5 cups a day.
Java tea Put 5g into 1 litre of boiling water. Leave to infuse for 5 minutes. Drink 1-3 cups a day, the last one several hours before bed.
Maize (tincture, 1:5 in 25% alcohol) Take 5-15ml three times a day.
Raspberry (tincture, 1:4 in 25% alcohol) Take 20 drops in water, three times a day, after meals.
Silver birch (tincture, 1:4 in 25% alcohol) Take 15 drops in a glass of water, three times a day, after meals.

Other measures

- Eat fruits such as melon and grapefruit, and especially watermelon and citrus fruits.
- Drink lots of water: tap or mineral, but preferably low in calcium.
- Take a course of trace elements: manganese or copper-manganese for infection or exhaustion.

Prostate disorders

At least 50 per cent of men over 40 will experience some of the disorders and diseases that can affect the prostate gland.

Benign prostatic hyperplasia (BPH) causes an enlargement of the prostate gland. This restricts the urethra (urinary canal) that passes through the prostate and causes urinary obstruction and retention. Because enlargement of the prostate gland is also a symptom of prostate cancer, a medical examination is essential.

Prostatitis, an infection or inflammation of the prostate gland, may be chronic or acute.

Symptoms

Prostatic enlargement

- Frequent feelings of wanting to urinate when there is no real need, especially at night
- A feeling of not being able to empty the bladder; (an ultrasound scan usually confirms the presence of a residue)
- Reduction in the flow of urine to a trickle or even droplets
- Tightness and burning in the bladder

Prostatitis

- A feeling of heaviness and pain in the groin and above the base of the penis
- Pain when urinating, with urgency and frequency. Also painful ejaculation
- Fever in cases of serious infection

Consult your doctor

- Only a medical examination can make the distinction between BPH, a prostate or urinary infection, and prostate cancer.
- Some forms of BPH require surgical intervention. Prostatitis is also potentially serious – it can lead to sterility and requires medical treatment.

Causes

Prostatic enlargement may be caused by a hormonal imbalance. This is a common development in men between middle and old age. Prostatitis is usually the result of an infection of the urinary tract caused by ureteritis, cystitis or sexually transmitted diseases.

WHICH PLANTS?

WARNING Use only one of the following at any given time

Internal usage

Prostatic enlargement
Horse chestnut (tablets, 300mg powder) Take 1 tablet a day.
Pumpkin (capsules, 430mg seed oil) Take 3 capsules a day.
Red clover (liquid extract, 1:1 in 25% alcohol) Take 1.5-3ml a day.
Saw palmetto (tincture, 1:5 in 75% alcohol) Take 10-20 drops in water, two to three times a day, after meals.
Stinging nettle (tincture, 1:4 in 25% alcohol) Take 20 drops in water, three times a day, after meals.

Prostatitis
See Cystitis.

Other measures

- Do not take decongestants or any other over-the-counter cold remedies: they could aggravate the symptoms.
- If you are having trouble urinating, do not strain; consult your doctor.

Pyelonephritis

Pyelonephritis is an acute inflammation of the urinary tracts and kidney that tends to affect pregnant women. However, it can also be chronic and start in childhood.

Symptoms

- Fever that escalates rapidly and is preceded by shivering
- Violent pains and a sense of heaviness in the lower back
- Infrequent urination and dark-coloured urine

Consult your doctor

- Acute pyelonephritis should be treated immediately. The diagnosis can be determined by tests carried out on the urine, which will reveal the nature of the bacteria involved.
- In the event of repeated urinary problems, medicinal plants can have a preventative effect.

Causes

Acute pyelonephritis can be a complication of cystitis or of a benign urinary infection. It can also be the result of a massive bacterial invasion of the urinary system, particularly in a hospital environment.

It also occurs when there is a previous history of urinary disorders (infections, acid reflux, gallstones). Chronic pyelonephritis may be caused by a malformation of the valve that prevents the backflow of urine into the ureter.

WHICH PLANTS?

WARNING Use only one of the following at any given time

Internal usage

To promote healthy kidneys
Globe artichoke (capsules, 300mg dried leaf extract) Take 1 capsule a day.

For inflammation and pain
Buchu (capsules, 350mg powder) Take 1 capsule with a large glass of water, twice a day, with meals.
Maize (tincture, 1:5 in 25% alcohol) Take 5-15ml three times a day.
Meadowsweet (tincture, 1:4 in 25% alcohol) Take 20 drops in water, three times a day, after or between meals.

To increase urination
Dandelion (capsules, 300mg powder) Take 1 capsule with water, three times a day.
Java tea Put 5g into 1 litre of boiling water. Leave to infuse for 5 minutes. Drink 1-3 cups a day, the last several hours before bed.

To treat infection
Garlic (capsules, 300mg powder) Take 1-3 capsules a day.
Goldenrod Put 1.5-3g of aerial parts into 1 cup of boiling water. Leave to infuse for 10-15 minutes and strain. Drink 3-5 cups a day.
Grapefruit seed extract (capsules, 125mg) Take 1 capsule twice a day for the first three days, then three times a day for days four to ten, and finally 2 capsules two to three times a day for days 11-28.
Silver birch (tincture, 1:4 in 25% alcohol) Take 15 drops in a glass of water, three times a day, after meals.
Uva ursi (tincture, 1:1 in 25% alcohol) Take 2-4ml a day.

As directed by a medical herbalist

- Barberry, Hemp agrimony

Other measures

- Increase your fluid intake to facilitate urination, bring down the fever and reduce inflammation.

Licensed herbal medicines

Thousands of herbal products are available in the UK over the counter, by mail order or via the internet. Among the safest and most effective of these are those that have been licensed by the Medicines and Healthcare products Regulatory Agency (MHRA). To obtain a licence for a herbal remedy, manufacturers have to submit bibliographic evidence for their product's efficacy, expert reports on its safety, and details of appropriate quality controls.

The products listed on the following pages are among those that the MHRA has licensed. They can be easily distinguished from other herbal remedies on the market by the Product Licence (PL) number on their labels.

Allergies

Boots Alternatives Hayfever Relief Tablets
To treat hayfever symptoms
Herbal constituents garlic, eyebright, sabadilla

Weleda Gencydo Ointment
To treat hayfever symptoms
Herbal constituents lemon juice, flowering quince

Blood, heart and circulatory problems

Aqualette
To treat water retention
Herbal constituents horsetail, dandelion

Bio-Health Lowater
To treat water retention, urinary tract inflammation
Herbal constituents buchu, uva ursi, dandelion root, parsley piert, cayenne

Boots Alternatives Haemorrhoid Relief Cream
To treat haemorrhoids
Herbal constituents horse chestnut, marigold, witch hazel, peony

Boots Alternatives Water Relief Tablets
To treat water retention
Herbal constituents uva ursi, clivers, burdock

Frank Roberts Anti-Irritant Ointment
To treat haemorrhoids
Herbal constituents pilewort

Frank Roberts Pilewort Compound Tablets (Green Label)
To treat haemorrhoids, constipation
Herbal constituents senna, pilewort, cascara, agrimony

Frank Roberts Pilewort Compound Tablets (Orange Label)
To treat haemorrhoids
Herbal constituents senna, pilewort, agrimony, cranesbill root

Gerard House Water Relief
To treat water retention
Herbal constituents bladderwrack, clivers, ivy, burdock

HRI Water Balance Tablets
To treat water retention
Herbal constituents dandelion, buchu, parsley piert, uva ursi

Lanes Water Retention Tablets (Modern Herbals)
To treat water retention
Herbal constituents burdock, clivers, uva ursi

Nelsons Chilblain Cream
To treat chilblains
Herbal constituents black bryony

Nelsons Haemorrhoid Cream
To treat haemorrhoids
Herbal constituents horse chestnut, marigold, witch hazel, peony

Potter's Diuretabs Tablets
To treat water retention
Herbal constituents buchu, juniper berry, parsley piert, uva ursi

Potter's Piletabs
To treat haemorrhoids
Herbal constituents pilewort, agrimony, cascara, collinsonia

Potter's Watershed Tablets
To treat water retention
Herbal constituents buchu, juniper berry, parsley piert, uva ursi

Weleda Fragaria/Urtica Drops
To treat anaemia
Herbal constituents wild strawberry, stinging nettle

Children's health

Boots Alternatives Nappy Rash Relief Cream
To treat nappy rash, chapped skin, cuts, minor burns
Herbal constituents witch hazel, eucalyptus, camphor

Boots Alternatives Teething Pain Relief
To treat teething pains
Herbal constituents chamomile

Weleda Chamomilla 3X Drops
To treat colic, teething pains
Herbal constituents: chamomile

Dental and gum problems

Weleda Medicinal Gargle
To treat mouth ulcers, sore gums
Herbal constituents rhatany, myrrh, clove oil, eucalyptus oil, geranium oil, lavender oil, peppermint oil, sage oil

Digestion

Bio-Health Digestive Tablets
To treat flatulence, indigestion.
Herbal constituents ginger, myrrh, golden seal, rhubarb, valerian

Bio-Health Natural Herb Laxative
To treat constipation
Herbal constituents senna, aloes, cascara, dandelion, valerian, holy thistle

Boots Alternatives Laxative Tablets
To treat constipation
Herbal constituents senna, cascara, aloin

Dual-Lax Extra Strong
To treat constipation
Herbal constituents senna, cascara, aloin

Equilon Herbal
To treat irritable bowel syndrome, bloating, flatulence, constipation,
Herbal constituents peppermint

Frank Roberts Althaea Compound Tablets
To treat acid indigestion, irritable bowel syndrome
Herbal constituents marshmallow, meadowsweet, slippery elm, liquorice

Frank Roberts B.&L. Tablets
To treat sluggish digestion, constipation
Herbal constituents aloin, black root, rhubarb, cascara, capsicum, ginger

Frank Roberts Black Root Compound Tablets
To treat indigestion, nausea (associated with fatty foods)
Herbal constituents black root, capsicum, fringetree bark, ginger

Frank Roberts Constipation Tablets
To treat constipation
Herbal constituents aloin, cascara, senna, valerian

Frank Roberts Cranesbill Compound Tablets
To treat digestive problems
Herbal constituents cranesbill root, slippery elm, marshmallow, echinacea

Frank Roberts Nervous Dyspepsia Tablets
To treat acid indigestion, heartburn, flatulence, nausea
Herbal constituents ginger, golden seal, myrrh, valerian, spearmint oil, dandelion, rhubarb

Fybogel
To treat constipation, irritable bowel syndrome
Herbal constituents ispaghula husk

Gerard House Herbulax
To treat constipation
Herbal constituents alder buckthorn, dandelion root

HRI Golden Seal Digestive Tablets
To treat indigestion, flatulence
Herbal constituents ginger, myrrh, golden seal, rhubarb, valerian

Lanes Laxative Tablets (Modern Herbals)
To treat constipation
Herbal constituents senna, aloin, cascara

Potter's Acidosis Tablets
To treat indigestion, stomach ache, acid stomach
Herbal constituents meadowsweet, rhubarb

Potter's Appetiser Mixture
To treat poor appetite, flatulence.
Herbal constituents chamomile, calumba, gentian

Potter's Cleansing Herb Tablets
To treat constipation
Herbal constituents senna, aloes, cascara, dandelion, fennel seed

Potter's GB Tablets
To treat indigestion (following meals)
Herbal constituents black root, wahoo bark, kava kava, burdock

Potter's Indian Brandee
To treat indigestion, stomach upsets
Herbal constituents capsicum, ginger, rhubarb

Potter's Indigestion Mixture
To treat indigestion
Herbal constituents meadowsweet, gentian, euonymus

Potter's Out of Sorts Tablets
To treat constipation
Herbal constituents senna, aloes, cascara, dandelion, fennel seed

Potter's Pegina Mixture
To treat indigestion, flatulence, stomach upsets
Herbal constituents capsicum, ginger, rhubarb, cassia oil, clove oil, fennel oil, lemon oil, orange oil, peppermint oil

Potter's Slippery Elm Tablets
To treat indigestion, heartburn, flatulence
Herbal constituents slippery elm bark, cinnamon oil, clove oil, peppermint oil

Potter's Spanish Tummy Mixture
To treat diarrhoea
Herbal constituents blackberry root, catechu

Licensed herbal medicines

Potter's Stomach Mixture
To treat stomach upsets
Herbal constituents dandelion, yellow gentian, rhubarb

Senokot Granules, Tablets and Syrup
To treat constipation
Herbal constituents senna

Sure-Lax Herbal
To treat constipation
Herbal constituents aloin, bitter fennel, valerian, milk thistle

Sure-Lax Senna
To treat constipation
Herbal constituents senna

Weleda Carminative Tea
To treat flatulence
Herbal constituents aniseed, fennel, caraway, yarrow, chamomile

Weleda Choleodoron Drops
To treat gall bladder problems
Herbal constituents celandine, turmeric

Weleda Clairo Tea
To treat occasional constipation
Herbal constituents aniseed, clove, peppermint, senna

Weleda Digestodoron Tablets and Drops
To treat indigestion, heartburn, flatulence, constipation
Herbal constituents fern leaf, willow leaf

Weleda Fragaria/Vitis Tablets
To treat nervous indigestion, nausea
Herbal constituents wild strawberry leaf, red vine leaf

Weleda Laxadoron Tablets
To treat occasional constipation
Herbal constituents aniseed, caraway, centaury, clove, wax plant nectar, peppermint, senna, yarrow

Weleda Melissa Comp Drops
To treat stomach ache, nausea, occasional diarrhoea
Herbal constituents Angelica, cinnamon, melissa, nutmeg

Ear, nose and throat problems

Benylin Active Response
To treat colds, influenza, nose and throat infections
Herbal constituents echinacea

Bio-Health Echinacea Tablets
To treat cold and flu symptoms, viral and bacterial infections
Herbal constituents echinacea

Bio-Health Garlic Tablets
To treat colds and flu symptoms, catarrh, sinusitis
Herbal constituents garlic

Bio-Health Lobelia Compound
To treat blocked sinuses, cold and flu symptoms
Herbal constituents lobelia, gum ammoniacum, squill, cayenne

Boots Alternatives Catarrh Relief Tablets
To treat catarrh, blocked sinuses
Herbal constituents echinacea, marshmallow, elderflower

Boots Alternatives Cold Relief Tablets
To treat cold and flu symptoms, nose and throat infections
Herbal constituents echinacea

Earex
To treat ear blockages due to wax build-up
Herbal constituents almond oil, arachis oil, camphor oil

Frank Roberts Catarrh Tablets
To treat catarrh, blocked sinuses
Herbal constituents lobelia, poke root, echinacea

Frank Roberts Cold Tablets
To treat cold and flu symptoms
Herbal constituents elderflower, ipecacuanha, poplar bark, yarrow, capsicum

Frank Roberts 'Drops of Life' Tablets
To treat cold and flu symptoms
Herbal constituents elderflower, peppermint oil, capsicum, yarrow

Frank Roberts Echinacea Tablets
To treat cold and flu symptoms
Herbal constituents echinacea

Frank Roberts Garlic Oil Capsules
To treat catarrh, blocked sinuses
Herbal constituents echinacea

Frank Roberts Rob-Bron Tablets
To treat nose, throat and bronchial infections
Herbal constituents ipecacuanha, lobelia, white horehound, liquorice

Frank Roberts Sinus and Hay Fever Tablets
To treat catarrh, blocked sinuses
Herbal constituents echinacea, elderflower, garlic

Gerard House Catarrh-Eeze
To treat catarrh
Herbal constituents white horehound, yarrow, elecampane

Gerard House Echinacea & Garlic
To treat cold and flu symptoms
Herbal constituents echinacea, garlic

Höfels Garlic Pearles
To treat cold and flu symptoms, catarrh
Herbal constituents garlic oil

Licensed herbal medicines

Höfels Garlic with Parsley Tablets
To treat cold and flu symptoms, catarrh
Herbal constituents garlic oil

Lanes Cold & Catarrh Tablets (Modern Herbals)
To treat cold and flu symptoms,
Herbal constituents lobelia, balsam of tolu

Olbas Oil
To treat catarrh, blocked sinuses
Herbal constituents cajuput oil, clove oil, eucalyptus oil, peppermint oil, juniper berry oil, wintergreen oil

Olbas Pastilles
To treat cold and flu symptoms, coughs, catarrh, blocked sinuses
Herbal constituents eucalyptus oil, peppermint oil, juniper berry oil, wintergreen oil

Phytocold (Arkocaps)
To treat cold and flu symptoms
Herbal constituents echinacea

Potter's Antibron Tablets
To treat coughs
Herbal constituents lobelia, wild lettuce, coltsfoot, euphorbia, pleurisy root, senega

Potter's Antifect Tablets
To treat catarrh, blocked sinuses
Herbal constituents garlic, echinacea

Potter's Balm of Gilead Cough Mixture
To treat coughs
Herbal constituents balsam of gilead, squill, lobelia, lungwort

Potter's Catarrh Mixture
To treat catarrh
Herbal constituents boneset, blue flag, burdock, hyssop

Potter's Chest Mixture
To treat chesty coughs, catarrh
Herbal constituents horehound, pleurisy root, senega, lobelia, squill

Potter's Elderflowers with Peppermint and Composition Essence
To treat cold and flu symptoms,
Herbal constituents bayberry, hemlock spruce, elderflower, peppermint oil

Potter's Elixir of Echinacea
To treat cold and flu symptoms,
Herbal constituents echinacea, fumitory, wild indigo

Potter's Garlic Tablets
To treat colds, catarrh, nose and throat infections
Herbal constituents garlic

Potter's Horehound and Aniseed Cough Mixture
To treat coughs
Herbal constituents pleurisy root, elecampane, white horehound, skunk cabbage, lobelia

Potter's Life Drops
To treat cold and flu symptoms, nose and throat infections.
Herbal constituents capsicum, elderflower, peppermint oil

Potter's Lightning Cough Remedy
To treat coughs
Herbal constituents liquorice, anise

Potter's Peerless Composition Essence
To treat cold and flu symptoms
Herbal constituents oak bark, pine bark, poplar bark, prickly ash bark, bayberry bark

Potter's Vegetable Cough Remover
To treat coughs
Herbal constituents black cohosh, ipecacuanha, lobelia, pleurisy root, elecampane, horehound, hyssop

Revitonil
To treat cold and flu symptoms, nose and throat infections
Herbal constituents marshmallow, echinacea, elderflower

Sinotar
To treat catarrh, blocked sinuses
Herbal constituents barberry, blackthorn, bryony, camphor, echinacea, eucalyptus oil, peppermint oil

Weleda Catarrh Cream
To treat catarrh, blocked sinuses
Herbal constituents echinacea

Weleda Cough Drops
To treat dry stubborn coughs
Herbal constituents angelica, cinnamon, clove, coriander, lemon oil, melissa oil, nutmeg

Weleda Cough Elixir
To treat coughs, catarrh
Herbal constituents aniseed, horehound, thyme, marshmallow

Weleda Herb and Honey Cough Elixir
To treat dry coughs
Herbal constituents aniseed, elderflower, horehound, Iceland moss, marshmallow, thyme

Weleda Oleum Rhinale Nasal Drops
To treat blocked sinuses
Herbal constituents marigold, eucalyptus oil, peppermint oil

Eye problems

Weleda Larch Resin Comp. Ointment and Lotion
To treat tired or strained eyes
Herbal constituents larch resin, lavender oil, pineapple

Hair and nail problems

Potter's Adiatine
To treat scalp problems (including dandruff)
Herbal constituents southernwood, witch hazel, bay oil, rosemary oil

Licensed herbal medicines

Potter's Medicated Extract of Rosemary
To treat poor hair condition
Herbal constituents rose geranium oil, rosemary oil, bay oil

Mental health

Bach Rescue Remedy
To treat stress, anxiety, shock
Herbal constituents rock rose, impatiens, clematis, cherry plum, star of Bethlehem

Bio-Health Good Night
To treat sleeping disorders, insomnia, anxiety, night sweats
Herbal constituents hops, valerian, vervain, wild lettuce, passionflower

Bio-Health Motherwort Compound Tablets
To treat nervous tension, menopausal stress
Herbal constituents motherwort, skullcap

Bio-Health Neurotone
To treat nervous tension, stress, irritability
Herbal constituents hops, valerian, skullcap, gentian

Bio-Health Passiflora Tablets
To treat insomnia, sleep problems
Herbal constituents passionflower

Bio-Health Reston Tablets
To treat nervousness, insomnia
Herbal constituents hops, vervain, skullcap, valerian

Boots Alternatives Sleep Well Tablets
To treat insomnia, nervous tension
Herbal constituents valerian, hops

Boots Alternatives Stress Relief Tablets
To treat stress, irritability
Herbal constituents valerian, lemon balm

Frank Roberts Avexan Tablets
To treat stress, nervous tension, irritability
Herbal constituents oats, prickly ash bark

Frank Roberts Calmanite Tablets
To treat insomnia
Herbal constituents hops, passionflower, pulsatilla, wild lettuce, valerian

Frank Roberts Nerfood Tablets
To treat stress, nervous tension, irritability
Herbal constituents asafetida, valerian, oats, passionflower

Frank Roberts Pulsatilla Compound Tablets
To treat stress, nervous tension, irritability
Herbal constituents asafetida, hops, valerian, pulsatilla

Frank Roberts Valerian Compound Tablets
To treat stress, nervous tension, irritability
Herbal constituents valerian, lime flowers, Jamaica dogwood, pulsatilla

Gerard House Serenity
To treat stress, irritability
Herbal constituents hops, passionflower, valerian

Gerard House Somnus
To treat insomnia, restlessness
Herbal constituents hops, valerian, wild lettuce

HRI Calm Life Tablets
To treat restlessness, irritability
Herbal constituents Jamaica dogwood, hops, chamomile, valerian, skullcap

HRI Night Tablets
To treat insomnia
Herbal constituents valerian, passionflower, wild lettuce, vervain, hops

Kalms
To treat stress, insomnia
Herbal constituents hops, valerian, gentian

Lanes Sleep Aid (Modern Herbals)
To treat insomnia
Herbal constituents passionflower

Lanes Stress Tablets (Modern Herbals)
To treat stress, nervous tension, irritability
Herbal constituents motherwort, vervain, valerian, passionflower

Natracalm
To treat stress, irritability
Herbal constituents passionflower

Natrasleep
To treat insomnia
Herbal constituents hops, valerian

Nytol Herbal Tablets
To treat insomnia
Herbal constituents hops, Jamaica dogwood, wild lettuce, passionflower, pulsatilla

Phytocalm (Arkocaps)
To treat stress, nervous tension, insomnia
Herbal constituents passionflower

Phytorelax (Arkocaps)
To treat insomnia, anxiety
Herbal constituents valerian

Potter's Ana-Sed Tablets
To treat tension headaches, stress, irritability
Herbal constituents hops, Jamaica dogwood, wild lettuce, passionflower, pulsatilla

Potter's Newrelax Tablets
To treat nervous tension, stress, irritability
Herbal constituents hops, skullcap, valerian

Potter's Nodoff Tablets
To treat insomnia
Herbal constituents passionflower

Potter's Valerian Tablets
To treat stress, irritability, insomnia
Herbal constituents hops, skullcap, valerian, vervain

Quiet Life
To treat stress, irritability, insomnia
Herbal constituents motherwort, hops, passionflower, wild lettuce, valerian

Seven Seas Slumber Tablets
To treat insomnia
Herbal constituents hops, wild lettuce, passionflower, Jamaica dogwood

Stressless
To treat stress, irritability
Herbal constituents hops, skullcap, valerian, vervain

Sunerven Tablets
To treat stress, nervous exhaustion
Herbal constituents motherwort, vervain, valerian, passionflower

Valerina Day-Time
To treat stress, irritability, nervous tension
Herbal constituents valerian, lemon balm

Valerina Night-Time
To treat insomnia
Herbal constituents valerian, lemon balm, hops

Weleda Avena Sativa Comp. Drops
To treat stress, irritability
Herbal constituents oats, hops, passionflower, valerian, coffee

Metabolism and immune-system disorders

Bio-Health Boldo Aid to Slimming
To treat excess weight
Herbal constituents dandelion, boldo, bladderwrack

Bio-Health Strength
To treat lack of vitality, exhaustion
Herbal constituents kola nuts, damiana, saw palmetto

Boots Alternatives Diet Aid
To treat overeating, obesity
Herbal constituents bladderwrack, boldo, dandelion

Frank Roberts Kelp & Nettle Compound Tablets
To treat overeating, obesity
Herbal constituents bladderwrack, blue flag, nettle

Frank Roberts Reducing Tablets
To treat overeating, obesity
Herbal constituents boldo, bladderwrack, dandelion

Frank Roberts Strength Tablets
To treat lack of vitality, exhaustion
Herbal constituents kola nut, damiana, saw palmetto

Frank Roberts Supa-Tonic Tablets
To treat lack of vitality, exhaustion
Herbal constituents saw palmetto, kola nut, damiana, rosemary

Gerard House Slimmers Aid
To treat obesity, overeating
Herbal constituents bladderwrack

Pharmaton Capsules and Pharmaton Vit-al Plus
To treat lack of vitality, exhaustion
Herbal constituents ginseng

Phytoslim (Arkocaps)
To treat overeating, obesity
Herbal constituents bladderwrack

Potter's Boldex Tablets
To treat overeating, obesity
Herbal constituents boldo, butternut bark, dandelion, bladderwrack

Potter's Chlorophyll Tablets
To treat lack of vitality, exhaustion
Herbal constituents kola nut

Potter's St John's Wort Compound
To treat exhaustion, listlessness
Herbal constituents juniper berry, St John's wort, white willow, black cohosh, skullcap

Potter's Strength Tablets
To treat lack of vitality, exhaustion
Herbal constituents kola nut, damiana, saw palmetto

Weleda Blackthorn Elixir
To treat lack of vitality, exhaustion
Herbal constituents blackthorn

Yariba
To treat lack of vitality, exhaustion
Herbal constituents kola nut

Muscles, bones and joints

Bio-Health Runo
To treat rheumatic pain
Herbal constituents guaiacum, poke root, burdock, sarsaparilla, black cohosh, prickly ash, capsicum

Boots Alternatives Rheumatic Pain Relief Tablets
To treat rheumatic pain, backache
Herbal constituents celery, bogbean, black cohosh

Cuxson Gerrard Belladonna Plaster
To treat muscular tension and strain, rheumatic pain, sciatica, backache, neuralgia
Herbal constituents belladonna

Licensed herbal medicines

Frank Roberts Buchu Backache Compound Tablets
To treat backache
Herbal constituents buchu, uva ursi, parsley piert

Frank Roberts Prickly Ash Compound Tablets
To treat muscular and rheumatic pain, stiffness
Herbal constituents capsicum, celery oil, guaiacum, prickly ash, poplar bark, uva ursi

Frank Roberts Rheumatic Pain Tablets
To treat rheumatic pain
Herbal constituents bogbean, guaiacum, capsicum, celery oil

Frank Roberts Sciatica Tablets
To treat sciatica
Herbal constituents bogbean, guaiacum, uva ursi, celery oil

Gerard House Reumalex
To treat rheumatic pain, backache, stiffness
Herbal constituents poplar bark, sarsaparilla, black cohosh, guaiacum, willow bark

Nelsons Rhus Tox Cream
To treat rheumatic pain
Herbal constituents poison ivy

Nelsons Strains Cream
To treat sprains
Herbal constituents rue

Potter's Backache Tablets
To treat backache
Herbal constituents gravel root, hydrangea, buchu, uva ursi

Potter's Comfrey Ointment
To treat sprains, bruises
Herbal constituents comfrey

Potter's Malted Kelp Tablets
To treat rheumatic pain
Herbal constituents kelp, malt

Potter's Nine Rubbing Oils
To treat muscular pain and stiffness, backache, sciatica, lumbago, fibrositis, rheumatic pain and strains
Herbal constituents amber oil, arachis oil, clove oil, eucalyptus oil, linseed oil, mustard oil, peppermint oil, thyme oil

Potter's Rheumatic Pain Tablets
To treat rheumatic pain, backache
Herbal constituents bogbean, burdock, yarrow, guaiacum resin

Potter's Sciargo Tablets
To treat sciatica, lumbago
Herbal constituents shepherd's purse, wild carrot, clivers, uva ursi, juniper berry

Potter's Tabritis Tablets
To treat rheumatic pain, stiffness
Herbal constituents elderflower, prickly ash bark, yarrow, burdock, clivers, poplar bark, uva ursi

Weleda Birch Elixir
To treat rheumatic pain
Herbal constituents birch leaf

Weleda Massage Balm with Arnica
To treat muscular pain, stiffness, backache
Herbal constituents arnica, birch leaf, lavender oil, rosemary oil

Weleda Massage Balm with Calendula
To treat muscular tension
Herbal constituents birch leaf, marigold, German chamomile, lavender oil

Weleda Rheumadoron Ointment and 102A Drops
To treat rheumatic pain
Herbal constituents aconite, arnica, birch leaf, mandrake

Weleda Rhus Tox. Ointment
To treat rheumatic pain
Herbal constituents poison ivy

Weleda Ruta Ointment
To treat sprains
Herbal constituents rue

Reproduction and sexuality

Bio-Health Damiana Tablets
To treat low libido and depression
Herbal constituents damiana

Frank Roberts Alchemilla Compound Tablets
To treat menstrual problems
Herbal constituents lady's mantle, motherwort, valerian, pulsatilla, vervain

Frank Roberts Motherwort Compound Tablets
To treat menopausal problems
Herbal constituents motherwort, lime flowers, valerian, pulsatilla

Potter's Elixir of Black Haw and Golden Seal
To treat menopausal problems
Herbal constituents black haw, golden seal

Potter's Elixir of Damiana and Saw Palmetto
To treat lack of libido in men
Herbal constituents cornsilk, damiana, saw palmetto

Potter's Prementaid Tablets
To treat premenstrual bloating
Herbal constituents vervain, motherwort, pulsatilla, uva ursi, valerian

Potter's Raspberry Leaf Tablets
To treat menstrual pain
Herbal constituents raspberry leaf

Potter's Wellwoman Tablets
To treat menopausal problems
Herbal constituents yarrow, motherwort, lime flowers, skullcap, valerian

Weleda Menodoron Drops
To treat menstrual problems
Herbal constituents shepherd's purse, yarrow, oak, stinging nettle, marjoram

Skin problems

Bio-Health Blue Flag Root Compound
To treat: skin irritations, psoriasis
Herbal constituents blue flag, burdock, yaw root, sarsaparilla

Boots Alternatives Bruise Relief Cream
To treat bruises
Herbal constituents arnica

Boots Alternatives Skin Care Tablets
To treat skin irritations, acne, eczema
Herbal constituents echinacea, burdock, stinging nettle

Boots Alternatives Sore Skin Relief
To treat skin irritations, sores
Herbal constituents marigold

Gerard House Skin Tablets
To treat acne, minor skin problems, eczema
Herbal constituents burdock, wild pansy

HRI Clear Complexion Tablets
To treat acne, minor skin problems
Herbal constituents sarsaparilla, blue flag, burdock

Kamillosan
To treat sores, cracked and chapped skin
Herbal constituents chamomile

Nelsons Arnica Cream
To treat bruises
Herbal constituents arnica

Nelsons Burns Cream
To treat burns
Herbal constituents marigold, nettle, echinacea, St John's wort

Nelsons Hypercal Cream
To treat cuts, sores
Herbal constituents marigold, St John's wort

Potter's Sarsaparilla Jamaica Mixture
To treat skin blemishes, rashes
Herbal constituents sarsaparilla, capsicum, liquorice, peppermint oil

Potter's Skin Clear Tablets
To treat skin blemishes
Herbal constituents echinacea

Potter's Skin Eruptions Mixture
To treat skin blemishes, eczema, psoriasis
Herbal constituents blue flag, burdock, yellow dock, sarsaparilla, buchu, cascara

Snowfire Healing Tablet Ointment
To treat chapped skin, chilblains
Herbal constituents benzoin, cade oil, citronella oil, clove oil, thyme oil, lemon thyme oil

Weleda Balsamicum Ointment
To treat minor wounds, abrasions, boils, nappy rash
Herbal constituents marigold, dog's mercury, balsam of Peru

Weleda Calendula Lotion and Ointment
To treat cuts, abrasions
Herbal constituents marigold

Weleda Combudoron Lotion, Ointment and Spray
To treat minor burns, insect bites
Herbal constituents arnica, nettle

Weleda Hypericum/Calendula Ointment
To treat painful cuts, minor wounds
Herbal constituents St John's wort, marigold

Witch Doctor Gel
To treat skin irritations, rashes, itching, insect bites and stings, sunburn, minor burns
Herbal constituents witch hazel

Urinary tract and kidney problems

Bio-Health Parsley Piert Compound
To treat urinary tract infections, kidney and bladder problems
Herbal constituents buchu, uva ursi, dandelion, parsley piert

Boots Alternatives Bladder Discomfort Relief Tablets
To treat female bladder discomfort and urinary infections
Herbal constituents bearberry, dandelion

Potter's Antiglan Tablets
To treat male urinary discomfort
Herbal constituents kava kava, saw palmetto, horsetail, hydrangea

Potter's Antitis Tablets
To treat urinary tract and bladder infections, including cystitis
Herbal constituents buchu, clivers, couchgrass, horsetail, shepherd's purse, uva ursi

Potter's Kas-Bah Herb Remedy
To treat urinary and bladder problems
Herbal constituents buchu, clivers, couchgrass, horsetail, uva ursi, senna leaf

Sabalin
To treat male urinary discomfort
Herbal constituents saw palmetto

Uvacin
To treat female bladder discomfort, including cystitis
Herbal constituents bearberry, dandelion, peppermint

Glossary

Type in **bold** indicates entry in glossary

acid Having a pH value below 7, pH being a measure of the acidity or alkalinity of a substance (such as soil) or a solution.

acute Arising suddenly, and usually of short duration.

aerial parts The parts of a plant that grow above the ground.

aggregation of platelets Coagulation of blood **platelets** causing the formation of a blood clot, involved in the healing of wounds.

AHA Acronym for alpha-hydroxy-acid, a substance composed of fruit acids.

alcoholate An alcohol-based preparation of a plant.

alkaline Having a pH value of more than 7, pH being a measure of the acidity or alkalinity of a substance (such as soil) or solution.

alkaloids Organic compounds of plant origin, with a marked pharmacological action, whose molecules contain at least one nitrogen atom.

allergen A substance or molecule that can trigger an allergic reaction in those sensitive to that substance.

allergenic Provoking an allergic reaction.

analgesic Prevents or reduces the perception of pain.

anethole A compound found in volatile oils with an odour of anise. It is extracted from, for example, anise (*Pimpinella anisum*) and star anise (*Ilicium verum*) and used in flavourings.

annual A plant that lives for one year, during the course of which it grows from a seed, reproduces and dies.

anorexia Loss of appetite. Anorexia nervosa is a psychological condition related to the fear of becoming fat.

anthelmintic or vermifuge Acting to expel or destroy intestinal worms.

anthocyanins Vegetable pigments found mainly in plants that are blue, mauve or purple. They form part of the **polyphenol** group.

anthraquinones Quinones (molecules with a cyclical structure) deriving from anthracene that have laxative properties.

antibiotic Kills bacteria or prevents their proliferation.

antifungal Kills microsopic fungi or prevents their proliferation.

anti-inflammatories Class of drug designed to relieve inflammation in the body. Common examples are ibuprofen, aspirin and paracetamol.

antioxidant Combats the actions of free radicals, which are produced naturally by the body during cell metabolism but when produced to excess can have a harmful degenerative effect.

antipruritic Acts against itchiness.

antipyretic Reduces fever.

antiseptic Destroys or weakens micro-organisms, such as bacteria, microscopic fungi, parasites.

anxiolytics, tranquillisers, sedatives Drugs or herbal medicines reducing anxiety or nervousness.

aphrodisiac Substance that stimulates or intensifies sexual desire.

aqueous extract Preparation obtained after treating a plant with water, at which point the solution obtained is concentrated.

arrhythmia Irregularities of the heartbeat.

asthenia General fatigue, weakening of the body.

astringent Tightens tissue, in particular the skin, such as tannin.

auricles The two small chambers of the heart that receive blood back from the rest of the body, before pumping it into the ventricles. Also known as atria.

autoimmune disease The body's allergic reaction to part of itself, mistaking it for a foreign agent or chemical. Rheumatoid arthritis is an example, where the body attacks the synovial tissue of its own joints.

Ayurvedic medicine Ancient system of holistic medicine originating in India.

bacterium (plural bacteria) Infectious agents usually comprising a single cell, living and reproducing on living or dead organic matter, sometimes capable of causing disease in humans. Staphylococcus and streptococcus are examples of bacteria.

benign Not very serious. Not cancerous.

berberine A bitter-tasting yellow alkaloid, obtained from barberry and other plants, and used in medicine as a tonic.

betacarotene Orange-coloured pigment from the **carotenoid** group, used by the body to produce vitamin D.

biennial Plant whose lifecycle is two years. The first year the plant forms leaves and builds up reserves and in the second produces an upright stem that carries flowers.

bile duct Canal that links the gall bladder to the small intestine and through which bile flows during digestion.

bitter principles A range of organic compounds, characterised by their bitter taste, that stimulate the secretion of saliva and digestive juices.

blood platelets See platelets.

blood serum Clear liquid that separates from a blood clot after coagulation.

bract A leaf-like structure situated at the base of a flower or a group of flowers (inflorescence). Often smaller than the other leaves, it can, however, be well developed and brightly coloured in certain species.

bronchodilator Increases the diameter of the bronchi (airways in the lungs).

calcareous Containing calcium – alkaline, chalky.

calculus Hard stone-like mass that can form in the kidneys, the salivary gland or the gall bladder.

capillaries Tiny vessels with very thin walls that ensure the body's cells are supplied with fluids and nutrients. Blood capillaries carry blood, and lymphatic capillaries transport lymph.

capsule Dry fruit that opens when ripe to disperse its seeds via a cap of small holes (pores) or a transversal slit, such as the fruit of the poppy.

Glossary

carbohydrate Sugars and starches. Foods such as flour, potatoes, rice and bread consist mostly of carbohydrates. Used to produce energy in the body.

carcinogenic Potentially causing cancer.

cardiovascular system The parts of the body relating to the flow of blood. This includes the heart, arteries, capillaries and veins.

carminative Facilitates the expulsion or absorption of intestinal gas.

carotenoids Group of orange, red or yellow-coloured pigments, very common in vegetables and present in the animals that consume them.

catecholamines Group of organic molecules that are the body's neurotransmitters (messengers from the nervous system) or hormones and which include adrenaline.

catkin In botany, a collection of very small flowers (inflorescence) in a simple spike, generally drooping, eg the inflorescence of the poplar.

cholesterol In the body, blood cholesterol – a fat-like waxy material that is a component of all cells – is manufactured by the liver. It is also involved in the creation of some hormones and helps to make vitamin D and bile acids to aid digestion. High levels of blood cholesterol (inherited, or associated with poor diet and obesity) are a major risk factor for heart disease. Dietary cholesterol is the cholesterol contained in food; it is now not generally considered to affect blood cholesterol levels to any significant degree in healthy people, though the debate continues.

chronic Persistent.

colic Pain which waxes and wanes in a rhythmic fashion.

collagen Fibrous protein that is an important constituent of skin in particular and which improves its elasticity.

connective tissue Tissue such as collagen that fills and supports body organs.

corm A swollen underground stem, similar to a bulb, having papery rather than fleshy scale leaves. It is used by the plant for storage and propagation.

cornea The clear convex part of the front of the eye which allows the passage of light.

corticosteroids Hormones produced by the adrenocortex (outer region of the adrenal gland) from cholesterol, and their synthetic equivalents. Cortisone is a corticosteroid.

cortisone Corticosteroid hormone that plays an important role in the regulation of the metabolism, including the processing of fats, sugars and proteins.

coumaric (derivative) Vegetable compounds derived from coumarins.

coumarins Aromatic compounds with various properties. Often acting as an anticoagulant in the blood, they are commonly used as a venous tonic.

decoction Water-based preparations, used for the tough parts of herbs, such as seeds, barks and roots, that release their active constituents only if cut or broken into small pieces and simmered.

demulcent Soothing, usually mucilaginous or oily substance, used especially to relieve pain in inflamed or irritated mucous surfaces.

depurative Encouraging elimination of waste products from the body.

dermatitis Inflammation of the skin. Also known as eczema.

dermis Lower layer of skin covered by the epidermis (outer layer) consisting of tissue composed of blood vessels, nerves, the base of hair follicles and sweat glands.

DEXA-scan An X-ray used to measure bone density.

diuretic Increases the production of urine.

division Type of propagation in which a plant is split into parts, one or more of which can be replanted.

dopamine Molecule acting as a neurotransmitter (transmits messages between nerves). Found largely in the brain.

double blind study or trial Experiment in which neither the patient nor the doctor knows whether the patient is taking the real substance under evaluation (for example, a new drug or herbal medicine), or a placebo (ineffective substance, often a sugar pill). Thought to be the most objective and reliable way to test the effectiveness of new medicines or treatments.

dried extract Formed when a plant is extracted with a solvent (Aqueous extract if extracted only with water). The resulting solution is filtered and the solvent removed to produce a solid or semi-solid dry extract.

dyspepsia Indigestion.

emollient Softens tissue, notably the skin.

encephalitis Inflammation or infection of the brain.

endocrine Relating to the organs and tissues that secrete hormones.

ENT Ear, nose and throat.

enzyme Protein that accelerates the biochemical reactions that occur in living organisms.

epidermis Outer layer of the skin.

erythema Redness of the skin.

Escherichia coli Parasitic bacterium that lives in the intestine, not virulent in its normal state, but which, in certain cases, can cause various ailments (infections of the urinary or biliary tracts, septicaemia, etc). Synonym: colibacillus or coliform.

essential oil Volatile, highly aromatic oil contained in certain plants that have medicinal properties. Obtained by steam distillation.

excitant Causing stimulation.

expectorant Aids evacuation of any secretions that have accumulated in the air passages, by encouraging coughing.

fatty acids Organic molecules that are the principal constituents of lipids (fats). Fatty acids are known as **saturated** when all the carbon-carbon links are single. They are known as **unsaturated** when at least two carbon atoms are linked by a double bond.

Glossary

fissure Split in the skin or membrane, for example, an anal fissure – split in the skin of the anus.

fistula Abnormal channel linking two hollow organs, or one of them and the skin, often caused by ulceration or congenital malformation (such as an anal fistula).

flavones Vegetable compounds belonging to the flavonoid group, present in vegetables, fruit, wine or tea.

flavonoids Vegetable pigments with diuretic, anti-inflammatory and anti-spasmodic properties.

flora (intestinal, buccal, skin) The types of microbes living in or on a particular part of the body – mostly bacteria. They are often harmless and can be protective, if they prevent other more pathological microbes from establishing themselves.

flowerheads A flower cluster (inflorescence) which, when gathered, includes petals, sepals, bracts, small leaves and flower stalks.

follicle Name given to various anatomical structures such as a cluster of cells (ovarian follicle) or a structure in the form of a small cavity (hair follicle) all generally having a secretory, excretory or protective function.

free radicals Atoms or group of atoms produced during cell **metabolism** and by the action of certain rays (especially light rays). They are highly reactive and unstable. When they occur in large numbers, they are liable to degrade cell membranes and are thought therefore to represent a potential risk of heart disease, cancer and other serious conditions. **Antioxidants** help to limit their harmful effects.

fungi Infectious agents that, unlike plants, have no green chlorophyll, stems, roots or leaves. They live in or off living or dead organic material, sometimes causing disease. Examples include yeasts, tinea, moulds, mushrooms, *Candida*. They reproduce through spores.

glomerulus Small knot of blood vessels in the kidneys whose role is to filter waste matter from the blood into the urine. Each kidney contains about a million glomeruli.

glucosides Vegetable substances consisting of compounds that have at least one glucose molecule attached.

glucosinolates Sulphurated vegetable compounds that are mainly only present in plants of the Brassica genus (including hedge mustard and horseradish) and which have expectorant properties.

glycerides Category of lipids composed of a fatty acid combined with one or more glycerine molecules.

glycogen A carbohydrate found in the liver and muscles, which is used by the body as an energy store.

gullet *See* oesophagus.

haematoma Accumulation of blood in tissue, often following a blow and commonly called a bruise.

haemoglobin Major oxygen-bearing protein in red blood cells which gives blood its red colour. It is made up of an iron-containing compound haem (approx 6 per cent) and the protein globin (approx 94 per cent). It carries oxygen in the blood and supplies it to the tissues.

haemorrhage Bleeding.

Helicobacter pylori Bacterium suspected of causing chronic gastritis and stomach ulcers.

hepatic Relating to the liver.

herb Term used to describe a plant used in medical herbalism, without its roots but with or without flowering tops.

herbaceous (plant) Plant characteristic of a herb and without a woody stem.

hermaphrodite In botany, a flower that has both male (stamen) and female (pistil) organs.

heteroside Complex sugar composed of a glucose molecule combined with a non-sugar molecule.

histamine Compound in plant and animal tissue, notably released during allergic reactions, causing characteristic inflammation and itching.

hormone Substance secreted by an endocrine gland which, after having been transported through the blood to a target organ, modifies that organ's activity.

hyperglycaemia Higher than normal level of sugar in the blood.

hyperparathyroidism Condition caused by overactive parathyroid gland (glands situated behind the thryroid).

hypersensitivity Condition of heightened sensitivity of the immune system when in contact with an allergen already experienced, which causes an allergic reaction.

hypertension High blood pressure.

hypotension Low blood pressure.

immune system The organs, tissues, cells and molecules that protect the body against invading pathogens or abnormal body cells.

immunodeficiency Weakness of the immune system.

immunosuppression Abnormally weak activity of the immune system following a disease such as HIV/AIDS or leukaemia; or chemotherapy for tumours or organ transplants, or removal of the spleen.

inflammation A protective reaction by the body to injury, infection, allergy or cancer: the affected tissue becomes hot, red, swollen and painful.

in vitro Designating biological processes or experiments conducted in an artificial environment outside the living organism.

in vivo Designating biological processes or experiments conducted or occurring within the living organism.

iridoids Vegetable compounds belonging to the terpene group with various medicinal properties, such as anti-inflammatory.

ischaemia Reduced blood supply to an area of the body resulting in inadequate oxygenation of the tissues.

isoflavones Vegetable compounds belonging to the flavonoid group that have an action similar to that of **oestrogen**.

keratin Fibrous protein that is the principal constituent of nails and hair.

ketones Substances produced in the body as a by-product of the burning of fats to produce energy – often found in people who can't use, or don't have, any glucose as an energy source, such as in diabetes or starvation.

latex The usually milky, viscous sap of certain trees and plants, containing substances such as alkaloids, mineral salts, starch and sugars.

laxative, purgative A substance that stimulates evacuation of the bowels.

leaflets Division of a compound leaf.

lesion Any visible abnormality, caused by disease. Most common on the skin.

linalool (or linalol) A colourless, fragrant compound found in many volatile oils and used in perfume manufacture.

liniment A fluid preparation used externally on the skin.

lipids Any of numerous fats and fatlike substances which, with carbohydrates and proteins, constitute the principal structural material of living cells.

lymphatic Concerning the lymph fluid. The lymphatic system includes lymph nodes and all the capillaries and vessels that transport the lymph fluid.

lymphocyte Type of white blood corpuscle, which plays a part in the working of the immune system.

malignant Of disease, a tumour or other disorder that tends to become progressively worse and result in death.

medicinal wine Preparation obtained by macerating medicinal plants in wine.

meningitis Inflammation or infection of the outer covering of the brain.

metabolism All the biochemical reactions that take place in the body and keep it supplied with energy.

monoterpenes Vegetable compounds containing 10 carbon atoms from the **terpene** group, whose molecules have one cycle (or none), with medicinal properties, present in most essential oils.

mucilage Sticky carbohydrate substance present in many plants, such as Aaron's rod.

mucous membrane Membrane lining the ducts or cavities of the digestive tube, the urogenital and respiratory systems and the interior of the eye socket that ensures they keep moist through the production of mucus.

myxoedema Thickening and roughening of the skin, a symptom of hypothyroidism (an underactive thyroid gland) when generalised, and of hyperthyroidism (an overactive thyroid gland) when limited to the shins.

narcotic A substance that dulls the senses, induces sleep and with prolonged use becomes addictive.

necrosis Death of tissue.

nervous system Body's control system. The central nervous system (brain and spinal column) works with the peripheral nerve system (consisting of billions of nerve cells) to relay sensory and motor impulses throughout the body.

neuropathy Generic term describing all illnesses of the central nervous system.

neurotoxic Toxic to the central nervous system.

neutral Having pH value of 7, so neither acid or alkaline, pH being a measure of the acidity or alkalinity of a substance (such as soil) or solution.

neurotransmitters Chemicals produced in the body to enable communication between one nerve cell and another, or between a nerve and a muscle.

node In botany, the point at which a leaf's stalk (petiole) joins a stem.

noradrenalin Substance that acts on the sympathetic nervous system (that stimulates the body's involuntary functions: digestive, respiratory, cardiac and urogenital) as a neurotransmitter (messenger from the nervous system).

oedema Abnormal accumulation of fluid in the body tissues causing swelling.

oesophagus Tube connecting the mouth to the stomach, also known as gullet.

oestrogen Female sex hormone secreted by the ovaries and playing a major role in the regulation of the menstrual cycle.

oestrogenic Having an action identical to that of oestrogen cells.

officinal Designating a plant used in medicine (from Latin *officinalis* 'used or kept in a [medical] workshop'), and apparent in many plant names such as dandelion (*Taraxacum officinale*) or sage (*Salvia officinalis*)

oilcake The solid residue that remains after the oil has been extracted from the fruits and seeds of oleaginous plants.

opiate Derived from opium.

opposite In botany, describing leaves, opposite each other on the same node (point at which the leaf joins the stem).

organic Relates to the constituents of living organisms, for example organic acids, organic compounds.

osteo-densitometry An X-ray used to measure bone density, sometimes also called a DEXA-scan.

palmate Describes a leaf divided into elongated leaflets arranged like the fingers of an open hand.

papule A skin lesion forming a small, firm elevation.

pathological Causing disease

pectin An organic substance, produced by plants and abundant in fruits such as plums. Its structure is similar to that of starch. Pectin is the substance that makes jams and jellies set.

perineum Area between the anus and the genitalia.

periodontal disease Any disease affecting tissues that surround and support the teeth, such as gums and bones.

peristalsis Involuntary, wavelike muscular contractions that propel undigested food and digestive wastes along the alimentary canal.

petiole The small stem (leafstalk) that forms the narrow part of a leaf and attaches it to the stem of the plant.

phenols A family of organic compounds in plants. They include salicylic acid (found in willow) and thymol (in thyme).

photosensitivity Sensitivity to sunlight caused by certain substances known as photosensitisers.

physiological Relating to the way the body functions.

Glossary

phytochemicals The chemical components of plants.

phyto-oestrogens Organic compounds with a similar structure and action to oestrogens.

phytoprogesterone An organic compound with a similar structure and action to progesterone.

phytosterols **Sterols** produced by plants.

pituitary gland Small gland situated at the base of the brain (beneath the hypothalamus) which secretes several hormones that are very important for the functioning of the body.

platelets The smallest of the three types of blood cell, responsible for clotting the blood when there is an injury or inflammation in the blood vessel.

pod In botany, dry fruit characteristic of the genus Leguminosae (peas, beans, broad beans…) that opens into two halves on maturity, seeds being born in each of the two halves.

polyp The medical term for a benign tumour that develops on a mucous membrane.

polyphenols Compounds that contain phenol groups, often with antibacterial and antioxidant properties..

polysaccharide A class of complex carbohydrates, whose molecules contain several monosaccharide molecules. Examples include starch and cellulose.

polyunsaturated fats The oils largely found in plants (such as sunflower, safflower) consisting of long chains of carbon connected with multiple bonds. They are less likely to be made into cholesterol in the body, so less likely to cause atherosclerosis. Olive oil is monounsaturated, so contains only one multiple bond.

proanthocyanins, proanthocyanidins Polymeric, phenolic ompounds often referred to as condensed tannins or **polyphenols**.

probiotics In alternative medicine, beneficial bacteria used as food additives to replace or promote the development of normal intestinal flora.

progesterone Female sex hormone secreted during the second phase of the ovarian cycle and during pregnancy.

prolactin Hormone secreted by the pituitary gland after giving birth, and while the new baby continues to suckle at the breast. It stimulates the production of progesterone from the ovary, so preventing menstruation, and maintains the milk flow.

prolapse The displacement of an organ (womb, rectum, bladder) due to a weakness in the structures that hold it in place within the body.

prostaglandins Any of various substances composed of fatty acids that have a hormone-like activity and are found especially in mammals.

protein Molecule used by the body as building blocks (for example, in muscle, skin, hormones or enzymes) and made up of various amino acids.

proteolytic Describes an enzyme that hydrolyses proteins.

provitamin A substance such as carotene from which vitamins are made within the body.

prurigo An inflammatory disease of the skin characterised by the formation of **papules** and intense itching.

pruritis Intense itching.

psychomotor skills Muscular activity related to mental processes, such as driving a car.

psychosomatic Describes physical symptoms that result from emotional states, either repressed or excessive.

purgative (*See* laxative, purgative)

pyrrolizidine alkaloids A group of plant alkaloids that are found in herbs such as borage (*Borago officinalis*), some of which can cause liver damage if taken in excess.

red cells The cells in the blood responsible for carrying oxygen, through its constituent haemoglobin.

remission Marked improvement or temporary absence of symptoms in a disorder (such as cancer or multiple sclerosis), sometimes ending in relapse.

renal Related to the kidneys.

respiratory system The parts of the body related to breathing, which allow the exchange of oxygen and carbon dioxide with the inhaled air. This includes the diaphragm, lungs, bronchi and the trachea.

retina The lining of the back of the eye which perceives light and images.

rhizome A bulbous underground stem, which usually grows horizontally, and bears roots and aerial stems.

saponins Organic compounds (found in the roots, rhizomes and bulbs of plants) that foam like soap when shaken with water. The term derives from the Latin *saponis* meaning 'soap'.

saturated fats Animal fats, containing single bonds between the atoms. Excess saturated fats in the diet can lead to atherosclerosis. Dairy products, eggs and meat therefore contain saturated fats.

sebaceous gland A small gland at the base of the hair follicle that produces the oily secretion known as sebum.

seborrhoea Greasiness of the skin due to the over-production of sebum by the sebaceous glands of the skin and hair follicles.

secoiridoids Plant substances based on the **iridoid** group of compounds.

sedative A drug or treatment that has a calming effect.

senescence The ageing of body tissue.

serotonin A compound that occurs in the brain and acts as a neurotransmitter.

sesquiterpenes Organic compounds that have medicinal – especially anti-inflammatory – properties and are found in certain essential oils.

spasm A muscular contraction which is both involuntary and painful.

sphincter (muscle) Ring of muscle under the control of the autonomic nervous system, which opens or closes to regulate the passage of material in the body (for example, the anal sphincter opens to allow the passage of stools).

spike Cluster of flowers (inflorescence) that are attached without petioles (stalks) along a central axis called a raceme.

Glossary

spore A cell ensuring the dispersal and reproduction of fungi and ferns.

stamen The male organ of a flower that produces pollen.

staphylococcus A bacterium found commonly on the skin, often benign, but sometimes pathological, causing boils and abscesses. *S. aureus* (Latin for 'gold') is responsible for impetigo, an infection of the skin with yellow crusts.

sternum The breastbone.

steroids Organic compounds belonging to the larger **sterol** group and including corticosteroid hormones, cholesterol and certain sex hormones (oestradiol, testosterone).

sterols Alcohols of the steroid group, such as cholesterol and ergosterol, found in animals and plants and that have various physiological effects.

stigma The upper part of the pistil (the female organs of a flower) that receives the pollen.

succulent A plant, usually native to arid areas, that has fleshy leaves or stems that can store water.

syndrome A group of symptoms which, considered as a whole, are characteristic of a particular disease or condition.

synovial Relating to synovia or synovial fluid, the viscous liquid that lubricates the joints. It is secreted by the synovial tissue, which forms the membrane that surrounds the joints.

tannins Phenolic, organic compounds that can combine with proteins and are used in herbal remedies for their medicinal (especially astringent) actions. The name derives from the fact that they were originally used to tan hides.

terpenes Organic compounds whose molecules are usually characterised by a ring system. They are generally aromatic and found in essential oils.

testosterone A male sex hormone secreted by the testicles (and in smaller quantities by the ovaries in women).

thiamine Another name for vitamin B_1.

thujone A volatile oil found in plants including sage (*Salvia officinalis*), that has carminative and antiseptic effects in therapeutic doses. Higher amounts can cause convulsions in people susceptible to epilepsy.

tic The regular or recurrent twitching or spasm of a muscle or group of muscles.

toxin Poisonous substance, secreted by certain organisms, that can cause adverse effects in the body.

trace elements Chemicals that are vital for the healthy functioning of the body, but are only needed in very small quantities, such as selenium and zinc.

triglycerides Basic building blocks of fats, linked to glycerol and constituting a storage medium for lipids (fats) in the body's adipose tissues.

triterpenes Organic compounds belonging to the larger group of **terpenes** whose molecules comprise 30 carbon atoms and one or more ring systems. They have medicinal properties such as anti-inflammatory and are found in certain essential oils.

tryptophan One of the 20 amino acids involved in the composition of proteins.

tuber A large, usually underground stem that stores food reserves for the growth of the plant, such as the potato, and is involved in its propagation.

uraemia The accumulation in the blood of urea, usually excreted in the urine, due to kidney failure.

urea A toxic ammoniac compound produced by protein **metabolism** and excreted in non-toxic form in urine.

ureter The canal that conveys urine from the kidney, where it is produced, to the bladder, where it is stored.

urethra The canal that conveys urine from the bladder out of the body.

urethritis Inflammation of the urethra.

vascular system The network of blood vessels in the body.

vasodilator An agent, drug or nerve that causes the walls of a blood vessel to dilate.

veinotonic A substance that strengthens the walls of blood vessels.

venous Related to the veins and venous system.

ventricles (heart) The two major chambers of the heart that pump blood around the body.

virus Infectious agent comprising a genetic core (DNA or RNA) and outer coat made of protein, only able to live and reproduce within the cells of another living organism, sometimes causing disease in humans. The common cold, warts, flu, glandular fever, and HIV are all examples of viral infections.

volatile oils Fragrant oils extracted or distilled from plants, and thought to be produced by the plant to attract pollinating insects and to deter animals and predatory insects. They are commonly known as essential oils.

white cells The blood cells produced by the immune system, to help protect the body against infection and cancer. The main types are neutrophils and lymphocytes. Some of them produce antibodies, molecules that also help to ward off infection and cancer.

xanthone A bright yellow substance with fungicidal properties found in plants including St John's wort and centaury.

Addresses & web sites

Addresses

National Institute of Medical Herbalists
56 Longbrook Street
Exeter, Devon EX4 6AH
Tel: 01392 426022
www.nimh.org.uk

Association of Master Herbalists
The Bield, Lewes Road, Forest Row
East Sussex RH18 5AF
Tel: 01342 826899
www.associationofmaster-herbalists.co.uk

International Register of Consultant Herbalists & Homeopaths
32 King Edward Road
Swansea, South Wales SA1 4LL
Tel: 01792 655 886
www.irch.org

College of Phytotherapy
Rutherford Park, Marley Lane
Battle, East Sussex TN33 0TY
Tel: 01424 776780
www.collegeofphytotherapy.com

British Complementary Medicine Association
PO Box 5122
Bournemouth BH8 0WG
Tel: 0845 345 5977
www.bcma.co.uk

British Herbal Medicine Association
1 Wickham Road, Boscombe
Bournemouth, Dorset BH7 6JX
Tel: 01202 433691
www.bhma.info

British Holistic Medical Association
59 Lansdowne Place
Hove, East Sussex BN3 1FL
Tel: 01273 725951
www.bhma.org

European Herbal Practitioners Association (EHPA)
45A Corsica Street
London N5 1JT
Tel: 020 7354 5067
www.users.globalnet.co.uk/~ehpa/

Institute for Complementary Medicine (ICM)
PO Box 194
London SE16 7QZ
Tel: 020 7237 5165
www.icmedicine.co.uk

Web sites

The internet is a valuable resource for anyone interested in alternative or complementary therapies. Many sites are devoted to herbs and their uses, and most sell herbal remedies online.

http://www.botanical.com
Online version of the definitive reference work, *A Modern Herbal* by Mrs. M. Grieve, first published in 1931. Fascinating folklore and history of herbs, as well as their medicinal and culinary uses. Many of the entries contain advice on cultivation.

http://www.holisticonline.com
This US site has a huge database of herbs (go into the site and click 'herbs' in the 'most popular destinations' box), listed both by their scientific names and their common names. A typical entry will give the plant's other names, its application in herbal medicine – European, Chinese or Indian uses may be listed – and safety advice. Some entries give a short history of the herb and list its active components.

http://www.rain-tree.com
Raintree is a well-designed site specifically about tropical plants found in the Amazon rain forest. Plants are listed by their scientific and their common names. The site is run by Raintree Nutrition Inc, a US company that markets medicinal plants, and aims to prevent further destruction of the rain forests.

http://www.nimh.org.uk/
The National Institute of Medical Herbalists is a British association of practitioners of herbal medicine. You can use the site to find a qualified medical herbalist, to read the latest research, and to keep up to date on the politics of herbal medicine.

http://www.herbmed.org
HerbMed is an electronic herbal database with useful links to other relevant sites. The US based site is clearly laid out and easy to use. It describes itself as 'an evidence-based information resource for professionals, researchers, and general public'.

http://naturalhealthweb.com
An Internet directory of articles related to natural health and complementary medicine.

http://www.mhra.gov.uk
The Medicines and Healthcare products Regulatory Agency is part of the UK Department of Health. The web site has good sections for consumers on the new Directive, buying and using herbal medicines, and safety.

http://www.bbc.co.uk/health/complementary/therapies_herbal.shtml
The BBC's Healthy Living web site offers articles on various alternative therapies including herbal medicine. The site is regularly updated and has links to other sites of interest.

http://www.naturalark.com/herbenc.html
The Herbal Encyclopedia is a US site written by a naturopath trained in the use of herbs. Its clear layout makes it easy to use. Each herbal entry has three sections covering the plant's medicinal use, its religious significance and how it is grown.

http://www.nhsdirect.nhs.uk
Symptoms, diagnosis, causes and conventional treatment of disease can all be found on this excellent site.

http://holisticmed.com/www/herbalism.html
Herbal Medicine Internet Resources is a US site compiled by the Holistic Medicine Resource Center. It has numerous links to herbal medicine web sites, organisations, practitioner databases, training, publications and discussion groups.

http://www.herbsociety.co.uk
This is the web site of The Herb Society, which aims to increase the understanding, use and appreciation of herbs. There are articles on herbs and botanic gardens open to the public.

http://www.choicesforhealth.com
Health WWWeb is a US site that provides resources on traditional herbal medicine and how this can be combined with modern science.

http://www.ipni.org
The International Plant Names Index (IPNI) is a database of the names and associated basic bibliographical details of all known seed plants. It has been compiled by The Royal Botanic Gardens, Kew, The Harvard University Herbaria and the Australian National Herbarium.

Index

Bold indicates main entries. Italics indicate remedies with preparation instructions given.